The National Ski Patrol's
Outdoor Emergency Care Study Book

Third Edition

National Ski Patrol System, Inc.
133 South Van Gordon Street, Suite 100
Lakewood, Colorado 80228
303-988-1111
FAX 1-800-222-4754
or 303-988-3005
Email: nsp@nsp.org

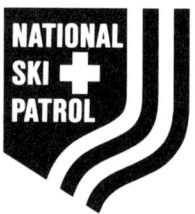

National Ski Patrol System, Inc. is a federally chartered educational association serving the ski and outdoor recreation community by providing exceptional education programs.

Credits

Education Director: Judy Over
Education Assistant: Elizabeth Mason
Communications Director: Rebecca Ayers
Graphic Design: Ken Grasman
Cover Illustration: Heather Haworth
Cover Design: 601 Design, Inc.

Copyright ©1998 by the National Ski Patrol System, Inc.

All rights reserved. No part of The *Outdoor Emergency Care Study Book* may be reproduced, stored in a retrieval system, or transmitted, in any form or by any means—electronic, mechanical, photocopying, recording, or otherwise—without the prior written permission of the National Ski Patrol System, Inc.

ISBN: 0-929752-09-0

Printed in the United States of America

The National Ski Patrol System, Inc. is a federally chartered educational association serving the ski and outdoor recreation community by providing exceptional education programs.

The *NSP Policies and Procedures* as amended constitutes the approved national policies of the National Ski Patrol System, Inc. All other publications are educational documents and may or may not reflect current NSP policies.

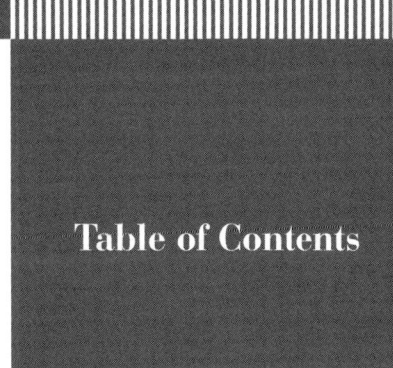

Table of Contents

Acknowledgements	iv
Introduction	1
Study Checklist for Content Objectives	2
Study Checklist for Routine OEC Skills	6
Chapter 1 Adapting to the Outdoor Environment	13
Chapter 2 Human Anatomy and Physiology	21
Chapter 3 Surface Anatomy and Vital Signs	41
Chapter 4 Introduction to Patient Assessment	55
Chapter 5 Patient Assessment and Life Support Interventions	63
Chapter 6 Oxygen and Other Types of Respiratory System Support	89
Chapter 7 Bleeding and Shock	103
Chapter 8 Skin and Soft Tissue Injuries, Burns, and Bandaging	111
Chapter 9 Emergency Care of Bone and Joint Injuries: General Principles	121
Chapter 10 Mechanisms and Patterns of Injury	135
Chapter 11 Specific Injuries to the Upper Extremity	141
Chapter 12 Specific Injuries to the Lower Extremity and Pelvis	155
Chapter 13 Injuries to the Head, Eye, Face, and Soft Tissues of the Neck	175
Chapter 14 Neck and Back Injuries	185
Chapter 15 Chest Injuries	203
Chapter 16 Injuries to the Abdomen, Pelvis, and Genitalia	209
Chapter 17 Common Medical Complaints	215
Chapter 18 Medical Emergencies	225
Chapter 19 Environmental Emergencies	237
Chapter 20 Emergency Care of Infants and Children	249
Chapter 21 Advanced Assessment	257
Chapter 22 Rescue Techniques	267
Chapter 23 Snowsport and Mountain Bike Injuries	281
Chapter 24 Triage	291
Chapter 25-28	297
Poisoning	
Hazardous Plants and Animals	
Water Emergencies	
Emergency Childbirth	
Answer Key	305
Found an Error?	393

Acknowledgments

Many thanks to the OEC supervisors, instructor trainers, instructors, and patrollers who participated in the development and review of materials for the *OEC Study Book, third edition.*

Study Book Task Committee
- Cathy LaMarre, Southern
- Pam Mead, Eastern
- John Keith, Intermountain

National OEC Committee 1998-1999
- Mary Murrett, National OEC Program Director
- Sue Gormley, Assistant National Program Director
- Paul Brooks, Alaska
- Kathleen Ferrigan, Central
- Janet Bell, Central
- Dagmar Prout, Central
- William Halsey, Eastern
- Ken LaPlante, Eastern
- Terry Randolph, Eastern
- James Miller, Eastern
- Karin Sandowski, European
- Guylene Tree, Far West
- Arnie Kay, Far West
- Jim Fillmore, Intermountain
- Russell Sigman, Northern
- Elizabeth Dodge, Pacific Northwest
- Jan Stanford, Pacific Northwest
- William Kyrioglou, Rocky Mountain
- Charles Lentz, Southern

National Staff
- John J. Clair, National Chairman
- Jeffrey Olsen, Assistant National Chairman
- Michael Baker, Assistant National Chairman
- Warren D. Bowman, M.D., National Medical Director

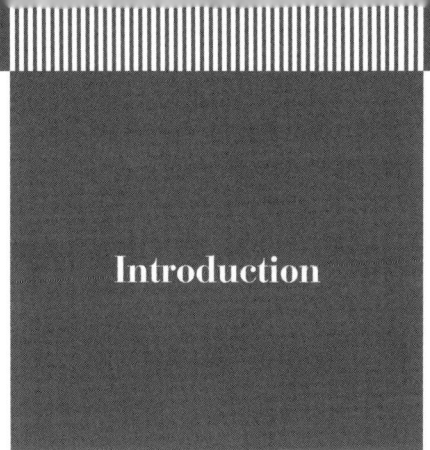

Introduction

This study book has been designed to accompany the National Ski Patrol's *Outdoor Emergency Care*, third edition textbook. It is intended to reinforce the most important concepts and skill performance guidelines for NSP's Outdoor Emergency Care course. Suggested uses for the *OEC Study Book* include interactive learning, home study, verification of knowledge and skills, reducing classroom sessions, and reviews for final practical and written evaluations.

The *OEC Study Book*, third edition, follows the *Outdoor Emergency Care,* third edition chapters. Each chapter is divided into three sections:

- **Content and Skill Objectives**
    An OEC trainee is expected to apply and demonstrate all concluding objectives at the end of each lesson.

- **Study Questions**
    After thoroughly studying each chapter in the *Outdoor Emergency Care* text, the study questions reinforce the most important content for each lesson following the concluding objectives. The **local protocol** section is designed to help the OEC trainee obtain and review knowledge on standards of care, techniques, and equipment based on the resort's patrol protocols. A checklist is included at the beginning of this book to help document comprehension of content.

- **Skill Performance Requirements**
    Reference is made to the scenarios described in *Outdoor Emergency Care* chapters. They are written in the form of a script, are quite detailed, and are intended to be realistic. The intent is to give a short summary of a situation and involve the OEC trainee in applying his or her knowledge to provide appropriate care for the patient.
    The skill performance objectives are restated and appropriate skill performance guidelines are illustrated for student-based practice. OEC trainees (basic course and challenge) are expected to demonstrate **routine skill** techniques before applying their skills to scenario exercises. Skill performance guidelines are referenced in each chapter and printed in the first appropriate *OEC Study Book* chapter. These guidelines can be used as a study tool and also may be used by your instructors during skill and scenario evaluations. A checklist is included at the beginning of this book to help document skill progress.
    Additional chapter scenarios are included to provide the OEC trainee with realistic situations to which they can apply the knowledge and skills learned in the chapter. These can be used for a mental exercise or actual hands-on practice.

An answer key, located at the end of the *OEC Study Book,* provides the OEC trainee and the OEC instructors with opportunities to check answers and assist in strengthening the learning process.

OUTDOOR EMERGENCY CARE
Study Checklist for Content Objectives

This checklist provides the opportunity for students and instructors to monitor the comprehension of content objectives during OEC course training.

OEC Trainee _____

Chapter	Content Objectives	Completed	Date
1	Identify the survival requirements of the human body		
	Explain how the outdoor environment effects the major systems of the body		
	Identify methods of adapting to functioning in the outdoor environment		
	Identify nutritional needs of the human bod		
	Explain the importance of physical conditioning in adapting to the outdoor environment		
2	Identify anatomical descriptive terms		
	Describe the functions of the primary and supportive organ systems of the human body and relate how they interact in the healthy body		
3	Recognize and locate important landmarks of the body		
	Recognize and locate vital signs and other important signs		
4	Explain the purpose of patient assessment		
	Explain the techniques that make up basic life support (BLS)		
	Explain the four major parts of patient assessment		
	Define key patient assessment terminology		
	Explain the methodology and psychology of dealing with patients and the potential reactions of rescuers		
	Explain the importance of body substance isolation (BSI) precautions when using equipment and techniques that allow contact with body fluids		
	Explain the importance of dealing with and disposing of hazardous materials		
	Explain the legal aspects of emergency care		
5	Explain the basic components of a first impression		
	Explain the components and differences of a rapid body survey and a whole body survey		

		Explain the basic components of an urgent survey for the unresponsive patient		
		Explain the basic components of an urgent survey for the responsive patient (both injured and ill)		
		Explain trauma/medical history and focused body survey		
		Explain the following mnemonics: AVPU, SAMPLE; DCAP-BTLS; OPQRST; and CMS		
		Explain the significance of interventions		
		Explain transport decisions and considerations		
		Explain the basic components of the nonurgent and ongoing surveys		
	6	Recognize the body's need for oxygen		
		Explain the use of oxygen systems and other mechanical aids to resuscitation		
	7	Describe the types and causes of bleeding		
		Describe the types of shock		
	8	List and describe closed soft-tissue injuries		
		List and describe open soft-tissue injuries		
		Describe the three degrees and three classifications of thermal burns, and their significance		
		Describe the characteristics of chemical and electrical burns		
		List and describe types of dressings and bandages		
		Describe special techniques for problem surfaces		
	9	Describe the general characteristics of fractures, dislocations, and sprains		
		Explain the general principles of emergency care for musculo-skeletal injuries		
		Name the types of splints and explain the general principles of their application		
	10	Describe how trauma is influenced by laws of physics		
		Distinguish between various types of trauma and their implications		
	11	Describe the general characteristics of sprains, dislocations, and fractures of the upper extremities		
		Describe the principles of emergency care for upper extremity injuries		

12	Describe the features of sprains, dislocations, and fractures of the lower extremities			
	Describe the principles of emergency care for lower extremity injuries			
13	List possible causes of unresponsiveness and appropriate emergency care			
	Describe and provide appropriate emergency care for a responsive patient with injuries to the head, eye, face, and soft tissues of the neck			
14	Describe characteristics of spine and spinal cord injuries			
15	List the causes and mechanisms of common types of chest injuries			
	Describe signs and symptoms of common types of chest injuries			
16	List the types and causes of injuries to the abdomen, pelvis, and genitalia			
	Describe signs and symptoms of injuries to the abdomen, pelvis, and genitalia			
17	Describe the characteristics of common medical complaints			
	Describe the general principles of emergency care for patients with common medical complaints			
18	Describe the characteristics of common medical emergencies			
	Describe the general principles of emergency care for patients with common medical emergencies			
19	Describe injuries and illnesses caused by exposure to certain environmental conditions			
	Describe the emergency care measures as necessary for cases of environmental emergencies			
20	Describe the causes of and emergency care for illnesses and injuries to infants and children			
	Identify anatomical differences between pediatric and adult patients			
	Describe special aspects of pediatric emergency care			
21	Further develop assessment techniques as initially learned in Chapter 4 and 5			
22	Describe techniques for obtaining access to, extricating, transferring, packaging, and transporting patients who may be found in remote areas, unstable positions, and/or awkward positions			
23	Describe basic types of skiing (alpine, nordic) and snowboarding accidents and common injuries resulting from each accident type			

	Describe the safety aspects of modern alpine and nordic ski equipment, and of snowboards		
	Describe ways of preventing accidents		
	Describe the correct approach to an accident scene with a rescue toboggan		
	Describe positioning of patients in the toboggan		
	Describe common off-road bicycling injuries		
24	Explain the purpose and use of the triage process		
25	Describe the causes of and the general emergency care for illness and injuries from poisoning through ingestion, inhalation, injection, or absorption		
26	Describe the causes of and general emergency care for illness and injury from contact with hazardous plants and animals		
27	Describe the dangers of and typical injuries associated with water sport recreation activities and the emergency care for submersion injuries		
28	Describe the handling and treatment for newborn and mother prior to, during, and following a normal out-of-hospital childbirth delivery		

I certify that this OEC trainee has satisfactorily demonstrated his or her comprehension of OEC content objectives.

OEC Instructor_____Date_____

COMMENTS

OUTDOOR EMERGENCY CARE
Study Checklist for Routine OEC Skills

This checklist provides the opportunity for students and instructors to monitor the satisfactory completion of routine skills during OEC course training and before completing a professional challenge or course evaluation. These skills are to be demonstrated as rote skills using local patrol equipment and protocols. Complete problem solving, i.e., identification of specific incident problem(s), patient assessment, and emergency care are to be demonstrated in scenarios at the end of each lesson and during the final evaluation, *not* with rote skill performance.

OEC Trainee _____

Chapter	Skill Performance Objectives	Demo	Demo	Final Check	Date
1	Demonstrate layering principles using typical ski clothing				
2	Demonstrate comprehension of anatomical positions				
3	Demonstrate the techniques for taking and recording vital signs				
4	Demonstrate BSI precautions with the use and disposal of personal protective equipment and hazardous materials				
5	Demonstrate single-rescuer turning techniques				
	Demonstrate the techniques for a rapid body survey and a whole body survey				
	Demonstrate the technique for removing contact lenses				
	Demonstrate the basic assessment techniques as they pertain to the urgent survey for the unresponsive patient				
	Demonstrate the basic assessment techniques as they pertain to the urgent survey for the responsive patient which includes the trauma history and focused body survey				
	Demonstrate the basic assessment techniques as they pertain to the urgent survey for the responsive patient which includes the medical history and focused body survey				
	Demonstrate the basic assessment techniques as they pertain to the nonurgent and ongoing surveys				
	Demonstrate a complete patient assessment for an unresponsive patient				

	Demonstrate a complete patient assessment for a responsive injured (trauma) patient				
	Demonstrate a complete patient assessment for a responsive ill (medical) patient				
6	Demonstrate the basic techniques used for oxygen administration				
	Demonstrate the use of airway adjuncts: non-rebreather masks, pocket masks, mouth shields, nasal cannulas, bag-valve-masks, oral airways, and suction devices				
7	Demonstrate the emergency care techniques for controlling external bleeding				
	Demonstrate the emergency care techniques for managing internal bleeding				
	Demonstrate the appropriate care for shock				
8	Demonstrate basic emergency care techniques for open soft-tissue injuries				
	Demonstrate basic emergency care techniques for closed soft-tissue injuries				
	Demonstrate basic emergency care techniques for burns				
	Demonstrate basic techniques of applying dressings and bandages				
	Demonstrate basic techniques of applying special types and improvised dressings and bandages				
9	Demonstrate techniques for long spineboard immobilization				
	Demonstrate techniques for traction splint immobilization				
10	Inspect an accident scene and reconstruct the probable sequence of events				
11	Demonstrate the appropriate technique(s) for assessment and emergency care for sprains of the upper extremity • Shoulder • AC separations • Elbow • Wrist, hand, and finger				

	Demonstrate the appropriate technique(s) for assessment and emergency care for fractures of the upper extremity • Clavicle • Scapula • Upper arm • Forearm • Wrist • Hand					
	Demonstrate the appropriate technique(s) for assessment and emergency care for dislocations of the upper extremity • Shoulder • Elbow • Wrist • Finger					
12	Demonstrate the appropriate assessment and emergency care for technique for splinting pelvic and hip fractures and hip dislocations					
	Demonstrate the appropriate technique for splinting a femoral shaft fracture					
	Demonstrate the appropriate technique for splinting an above-knee femur fracture, and a knee or patella dislocation					
	Demonstrate the appropriate technique for splinting lower leg, ankle, and foot fractures; knee and ankle sprains; and ankle dislocations					
13	Demonstrate assessment techniques for a patient with a head injury					
	Demonstrate basic techniques of emergency care for an unresponsive patient					
	Demonstrate basic techniques of emergency care for injuries to the • Head • Eye • Face • Soft tissues of the neck					
14	Demonstrate the appropriate care of a patient with suspected spine or spinal cord injuries					
	Demonstrate the procedures for logrolling					
	Demonstrate the procedures for helmet removal					

	Demonstrate the procedures for the long-axis drag					
	Demonstrate the procedure for multi-person direct ground lift					
	Demonstrate the procedures for bridge lift					
	Demonstrate the procedures for immobilizing a patient on a long spineboard					
	Demonstrate the procedure for immobilizing a patient on a standing spineboard					
15	Demonstrate basic techniques for emergency care of a patient with injuries to the chest					
16	Demonstrate basic techniques of emergency care for a patient with specific injuries to abdominal and pelvic areas					
17	Demonstrate assessment and management of common medical complaints • Respiratory • Gastrointestinal • Genitourinary • Miscellaneous complaints					
18	Demonstrate assessment and management of common medical emergencies • Angina pectoris • Heart attack • Stroke • Diabetes • Seizures • Carbon monoxide poisoning • Substance abuse					
19	Demonstrate assessment and management of environmental emergencies • Frostbite • Hypothermia • Heat illness • Acute mountain sickness • Sunburn • Windburn • Snowbliindness • Lightning and electrical injury • Avalanche injury					
20	Demonstrate assessment of the pediatric patient					

	Demonstrate the emergency care for illnesses and injuries of infants and children				
21	Fully assess a situation, name and describe probable injuries or illnesses, and report emergency care				
	Obtain a relevant medical history from a responsive patient				
	Properly prioritize treatment of multiple injuries and/or multiple patient situations				
22	Align an injured person into a supine neutral position				

	Perform emergency and non-emergency patient moves, lifts, and carries
	• Emergency, One-Rescuer Techniques—Spine Injury Unlikely
	    Fireman's Drag
	    Fireman's Carry
	    Human Crutch
	    Front Cradle
	    Back Carries				

	Perform emergency and non-emergency patient moves, lifts, and carries • Emergency One-Rescuer Moves—Possible Spine Injury Long Axis Drag				

	Perform emergency and non-emergency patient moves, lifts, and carries
	• Emergency Two-Rescuer Moves—No Spine Injury
	    Seated Carries
	    Fore-and-Aft Carry				

	Perform emergency and non-emergency patient moves, lifts, and carries
	• Nonemergency Moves—One or Multiple Rescuers
	    Direct Ground Lift and Carry—No Spine Injury
	    Direct Ground Lift and Carry—Possible Spine Injury
	    Extremity Lift, Fractures Splinted—Two or More Rescuers
	    Canvas Stretcher or Blanket Lift and Carry—No Spine Injury
	    Bridge Lift—Possible Spine Injury				

	Demonstrate extricating or moving an injured person from a difficult or confining location				

23	Demonstrate loading an injured skier into a toboggan and securing the patient				
	Demonstrate the principles of boot removal				
24	Apply the four color-coded categories to a multiple-casualty incident				
	Apply proper sequence of emergency care for a single patient with multiple injuries				
25-28	Explain and demonstrate (where appropriate) the local procedures for handling illness and injuries that are not typical in the winter environment • Poisoning • Hazardous plants and animals • Submersion injuries • Out-of-hospital childbirth delivery				

I certify that this OEC trainee has satisfactorily demonstrated his or her ability to perform these routine skills in accordance with Outdoor Emergency Care procedures.

OEC Instructor_____Date_____
(signature)

COMMENTS

CHAPTER 1

Adapting to the Outdoor Environment

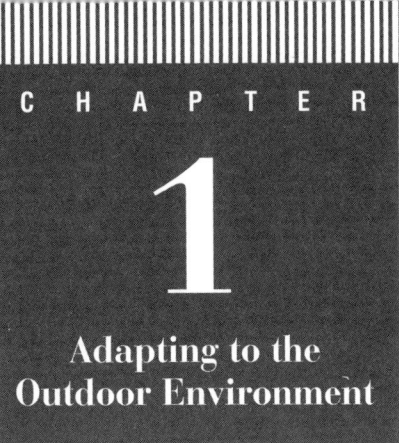

CONCLUDING OBJECTIVES

The learner will:

Content

- Identify the survival requirements of the human body

- Explain how the outdoor environment effects the major systems of the body

- Identify methods of adapting to functioning in the outdoor environment

- Identify nutritional needs of the human body

- Explain the importance of physical conditioning in adapting to the outdoor environment

Skill Performance

- Demonstrate layering principles using typical ski clothing

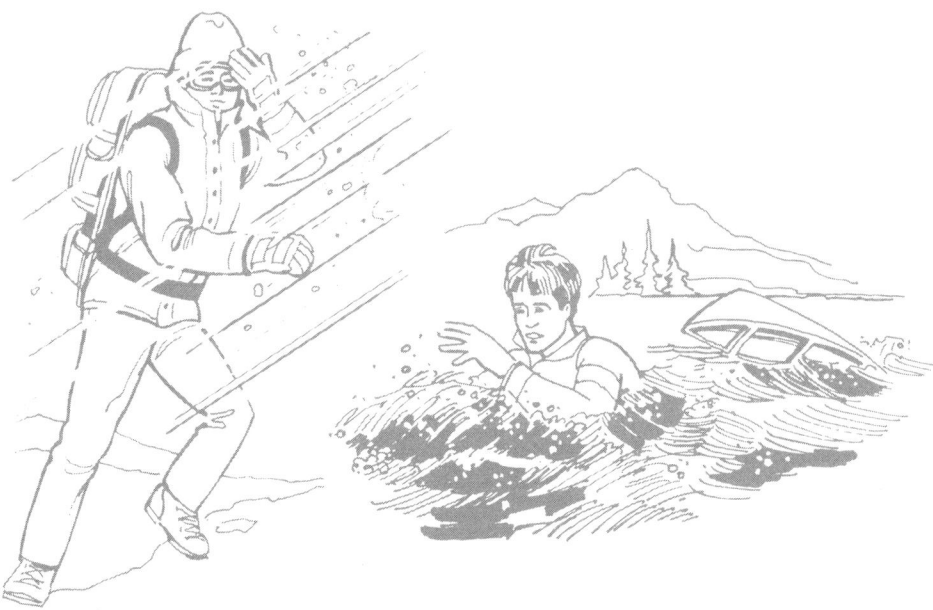

OEC Study Book 13

CHAPTER 1 STUDY QUESTIONS

1. List six survival requirements.

   _____
   _____
   _____
   _____
   _____
   _____

2. Where does the exchange of oxygen and carbon dioxide occur?

   _____

3. Identify ways in which the oxygen supply can be interrupted.

Insufficient oxygen in the outside air	
Obstruction of the upper airway	
Obstruction of the lower airway	

Interference with lung function
        Acute
 	
        Chronic	

Interference with chest integrity or function	
Interference with the brain's control of breathing	

Abnormal function of the circulatory system
        Illness
         Injury	

Interference with the blood's oxygen-carrying capacity	

4. How does the body adjust to high altitude?

   _____
   _____
   _____

5. The condition that denotes a lack of oxygen is called
   A. hypoxia
   B. hyperventilation
   C. hypoventilation
   D. apnea

6. Identify involuntary and voluntary methods of increasing heat gain.

Increasing Heat Gain
Involuntary
Voluntary

7. Define mechanisms of heat loss.

Physical Mechanisms of Heat Loss
Conduction
Convection
Evaporation
Radiation
Respiration

8. Identify involuntary and voluntary methods of decreasing heat loss.

Decreasing Heat Loss
Involuntary
Voluntary

9. Explain wind chill effects.

   _____
   _____

10. What are some ways to prevent problems from excessive heat?

    _____
    _____
    _____

11. Wool garments are effective as cold weather clothing because they
    A. dry quickly
    B. are warm even if wet
    C. are well constructed
    D. are windproof

12. Detail methods of decreasing body heat loss using the layering principle.

    _____
    _____
    _____
    _____

13. Describe the layering principle.

    _____
    _____

14. Describe the adage "if your feet are cold, put on your hat."

    _____
    _____

15. Water makes up about _____ of the body weight of the average young adult male.

16. Emergency food taken on rescues should have what four characteristics?

    _____
    _____
    _____
    _____

17. List the food sources for the six groups of nutrients.

Nutrients	Food Sources
Carbohydrates	
Proteins	
Fat	
Minerals	
Vitamins	
Water (amount required daily)	

18. A good physical training program should start off moderately but eventually aim for a minimum workout of 45 to 60 minutes how many times a week?
    _____

19. The best way to develop effective pulmonary function is to incorporate aerobic activity that uses the _____ and _____ _____ at the same time.

20. The physical training program should include four phases. What are they?
    _____
    _____
    _____
    _____

21. What are the two significant types of physical fitness? Explain each type.
    _____
    _____
    _____
    _____

Chapter 1 Local Protocol

1. List personal clothing and equipment available to you for patrolling activities in the more extreme weather conditions in your area.
    _____
    _____
    _____
    _____
    _____

2. List equipment maintained at your area for use in cold-weather search and rescue assignments.
    _____
    _____
    _____
    _____
    _____

CHAPTER 1 SKILL PERFORMANCE REQUIREMENTS

- Demonstrate layering principles using typical ski clothing

Skill Performance Guidelines

- No skill performance guidelines (SPG) in this chapter

Chapter 1 Scenario

1. You and a friend are planning a two-day winter camping/ski-touring trip for the weekend. Your local weather forecast says there is a 20 percent chance of precipitation and strong winds, with temperatures ranging from 30 to 40 degrees. What preparations do you make, including equipment and clothing? Why?

STUDY NOTES

CHAPTER 2

Human Anatomy and Physiology

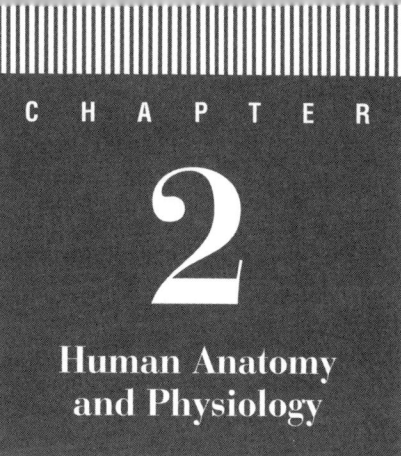

CONCLUDING OBJECTIVES

The learner will:

Content

- Identify anatomical descriptive terms

- Describe the functions of the primary and supportive organ systems of the human body and relate how they interact in the healthy body

Skill Performance

- Demonstrate comprehension of anatomical terms

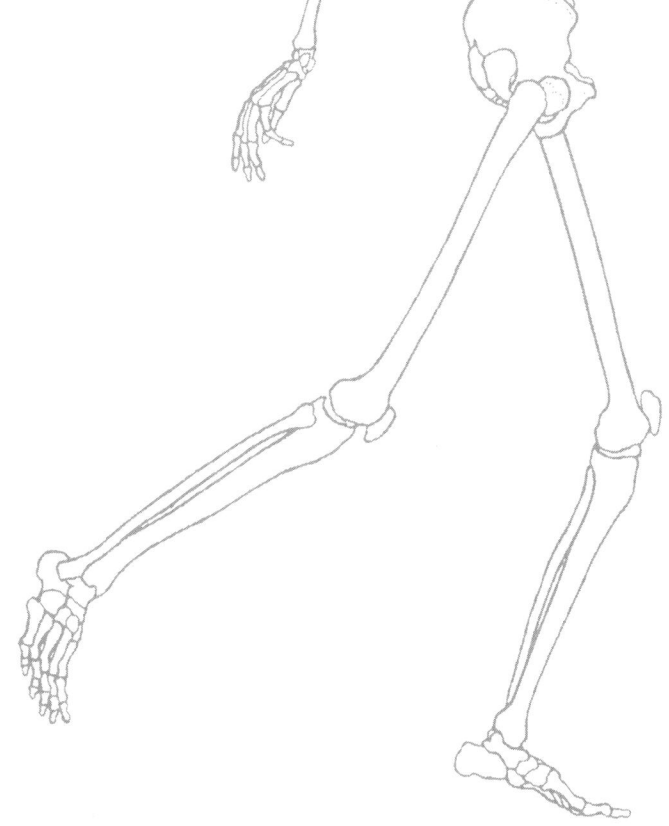

CHAPTER 2 STUDY QUESTIONS

1. Label the anatomical terms for the human body.

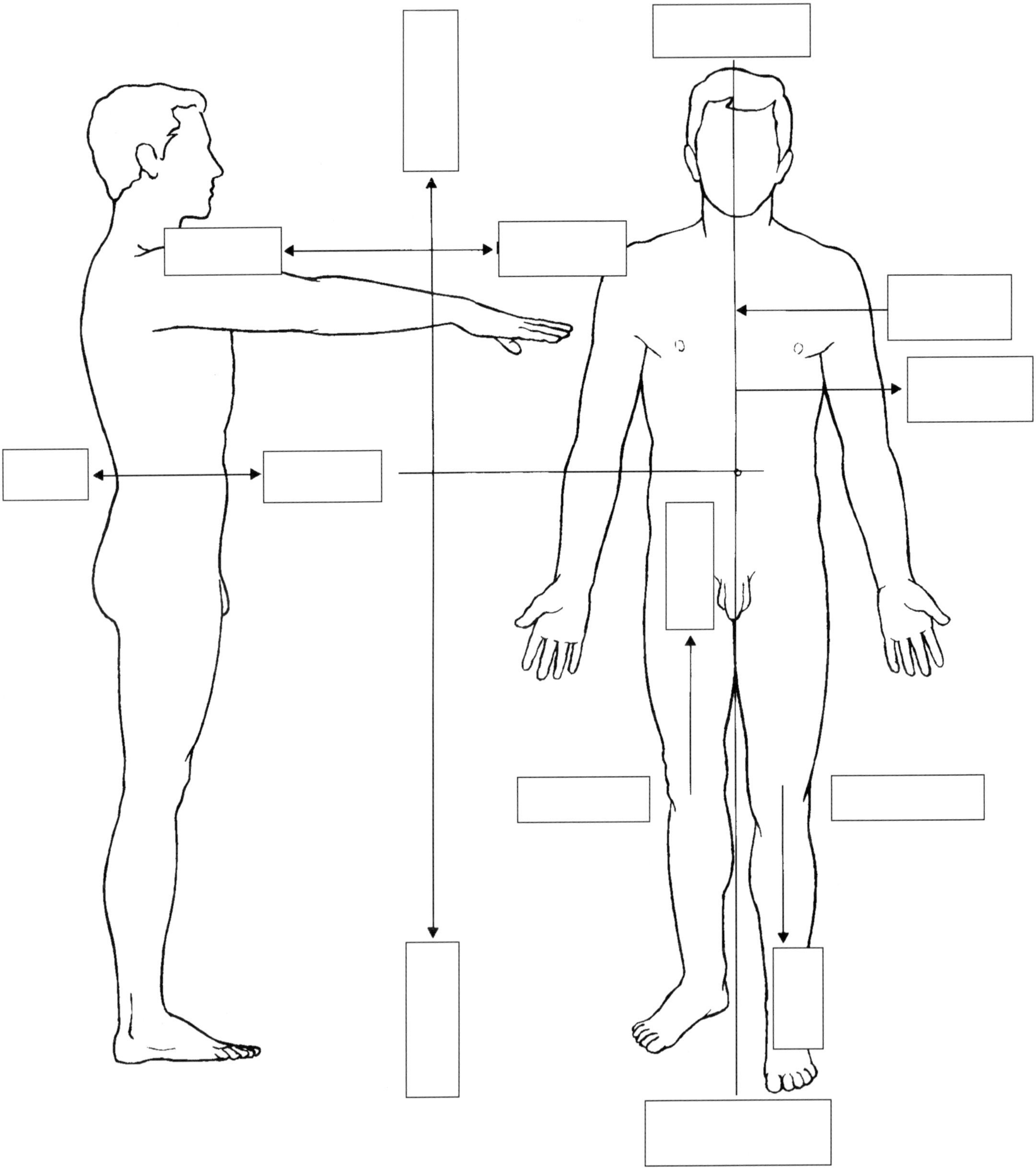

2. Match the organ system to a function that it performs.

    ___ Pumps oxygenated blood to the organs and gets rid of carbon dioxide
    ___ Brings oxygen into the body and expels carbon dioxide
    ___ Ingests, digests, and absorbs food and fluid, and eliminates wastes
    ___ Cleans blood and expels waste
    ___ Gives protection, form, and support to the body
    ___ Permits movement
    ___ Aids in keeping the body from drying out and protects from invasion by bacteria and other infectious organisms
    ___ Somatic (voluntary) and autonomic (involuntary systems)
    ___ Glands that produce the chemical substances that regulate body cells or organs
    ___ Means of procreating

    A. Cutaneous
    B. Nervous
    C. Respiratory
    D. Digestive
    E. Muscular
    F. Skeletal
    G. Circulatory
    H. Urinary
    I. Endocrine
    J. Reproductive

3. Match the anatomical term to its location on the body.

    ___ Nearer to the front of the body
    ___ Nearer to the back of the body
    ___ Nearer to the midline of the body
    ___ Farther from the midline of the body
    ___ Nearer to the top of the head
    ___ Nearer to the soles of the feet
    ___ Closer to the trunk of the body
    ___ Closer to the tips of the extremities

    A. Posterior
    B. Superior
    C. Proximal
    D. Anterior
    E. Lateral
    F. Medial
    G. Inferior
    H. Distal

4. What is oxygen debt?

    _____
    _____
    _____
    _____

5. Describe the circulatory system by tracing the flow of blood from the capillaries through the heart and back to the capillaries.

_____
_____
_____
_____
_____
_____
_____
_____
_____
_____
_____
_____

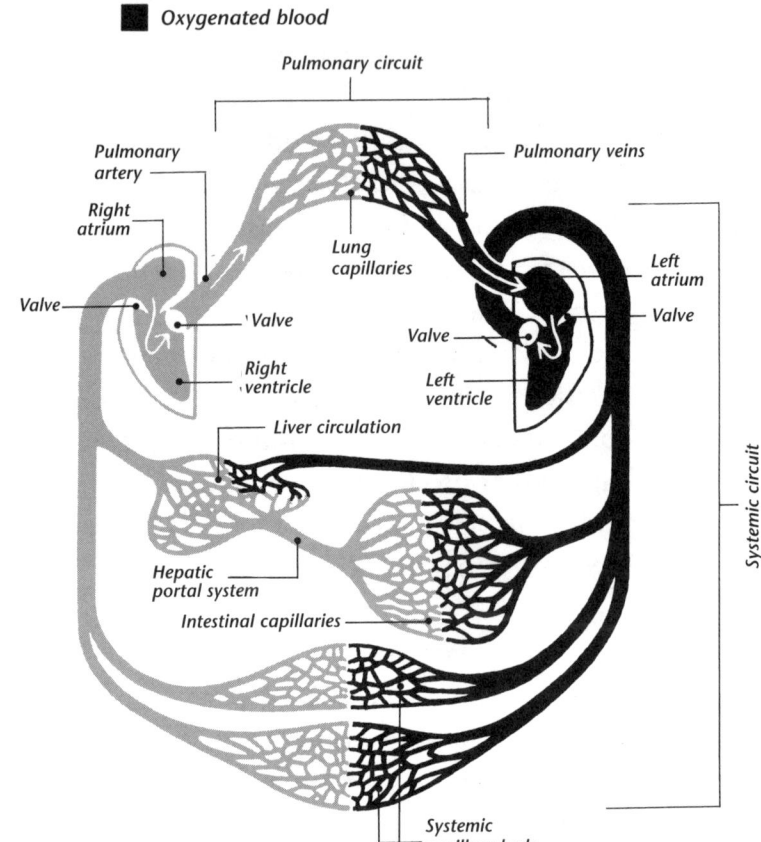

For clarity, the two sides of the heart are shown separated

6. The major artery of the body is called the
   A. brachial artery
   B. femoral artery
   C. aorta
   D. carotid artery

7. Label the major parts of the heart.

_____
_____
_____
_____
_____
_____

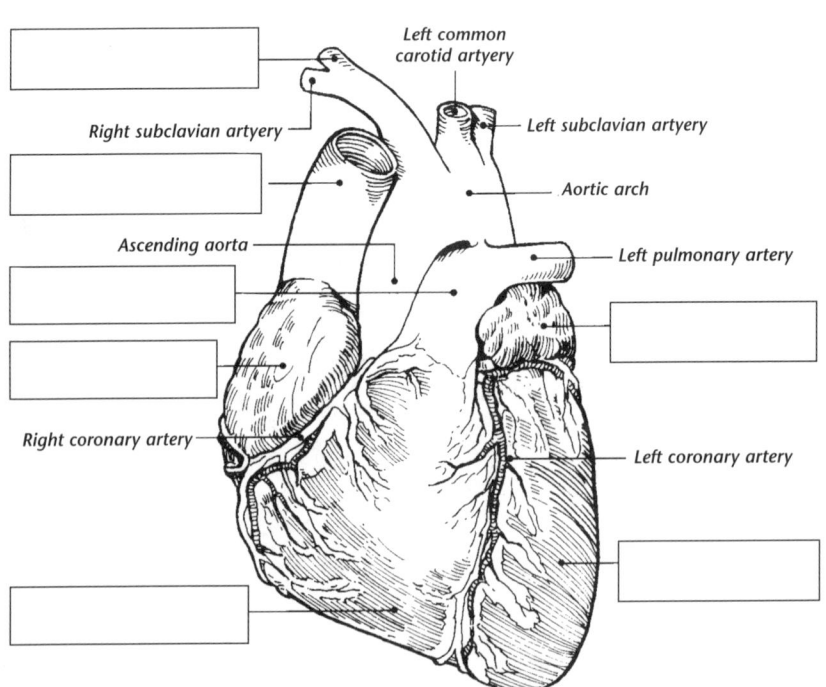

8. Label the major arteries.

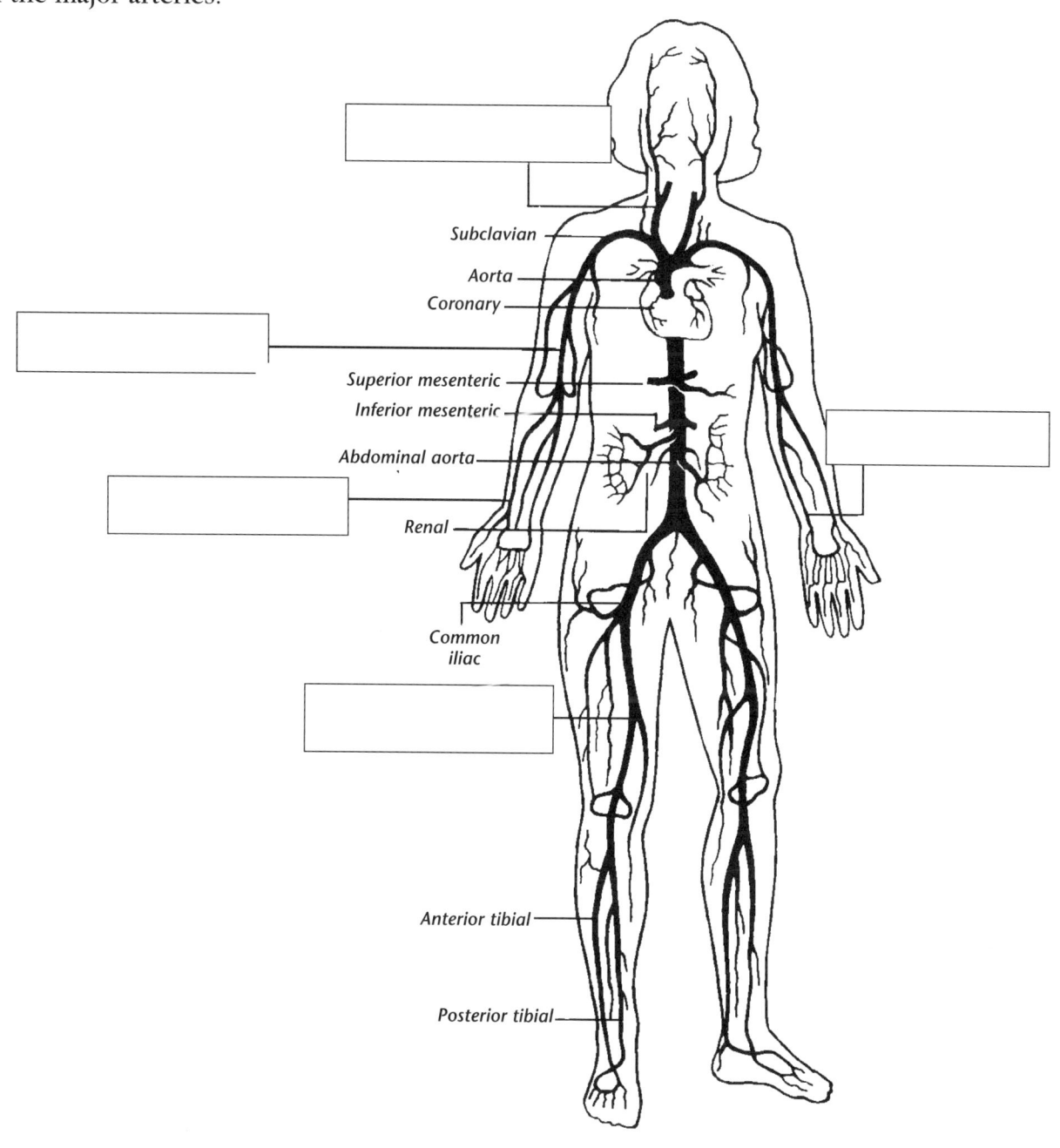

9. Define the purpose of the three types of blood cells.

Platelets _____

White _____

Red _____

OEC Study Book 25

10. Identify the major components of the respiratory system.

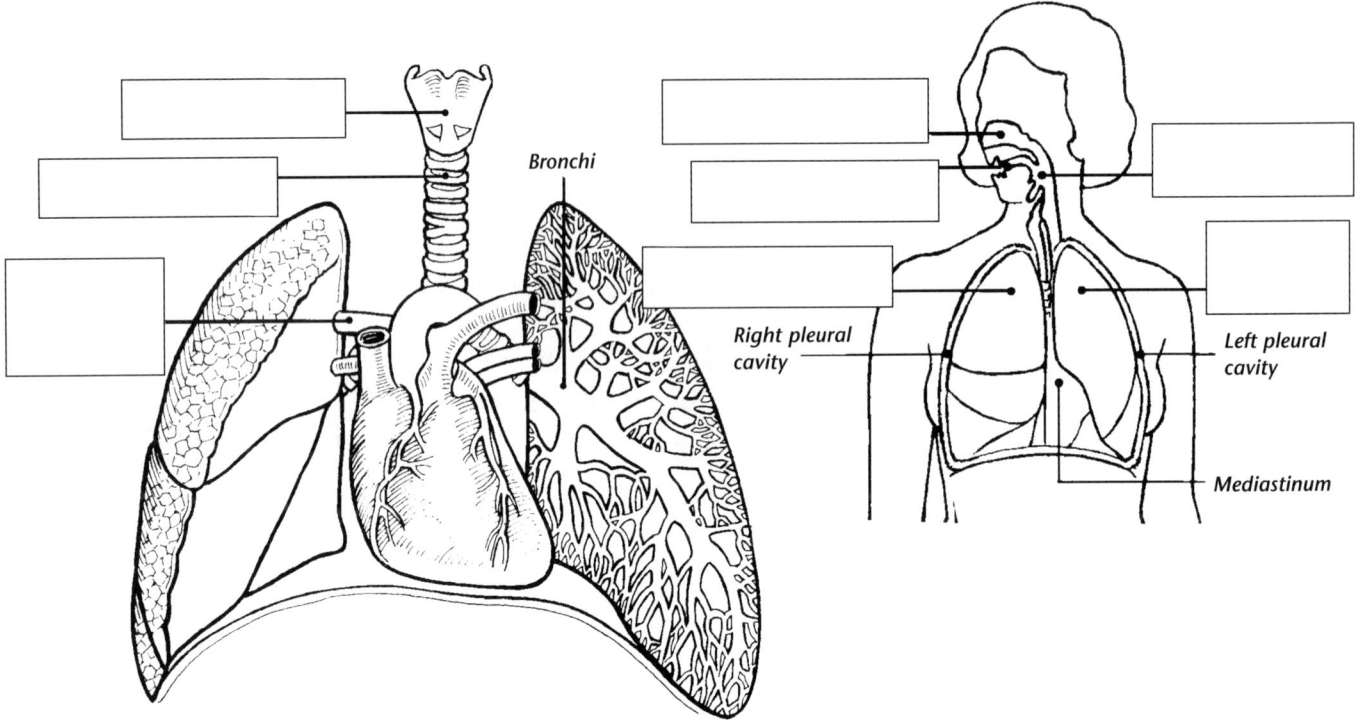

11. The upper airway includes all except the
    A. nasal cavity
    B. mouth
    C. larynx
    D. pharynx

12. Describe the role air pressure plays in the breathing process.

_____
_____
_____
_____

13. During the inhalation phase of breathing:
    A. The diaphragm rises into the chest.
    B. The thoracic cage enlarges.
    C. The lungs expand when pushed out from within.
    D. B and C.
    E. All of the above.

14. On the diagrams below, identify the breathing processes and their effects on the chest.

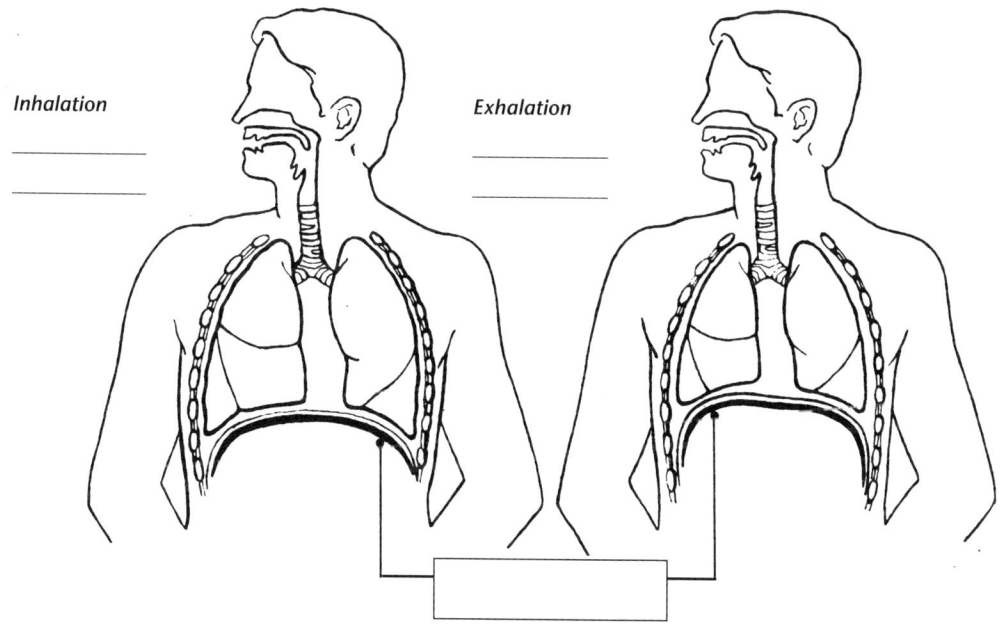

Inhalation   Exhalation
_____   _____

15. The nervous system is divided into two parts. What are they?
_____
_____

16. The brain and spinal cord are part of the _____.

17. Describe what each nervous system controls.

Somatic Nervous System	Autonomic Nervous System

18. Match the following terms with their definitions.
    ___ Neuron   A. One of several short processes of a neuron
    ___ Axon   B. Insulation that covers nerve tissue
    ___ Synapse   C. Special cells of the nervous system
    ___ Dendrite   D. Allows nerve impulses to be transmitted
    ___ Myelin   E. The long process of a neuron

19. Match the following terms with their definitions.
    ___ Meninges   A. Inner layers of the meninges
    ___ Cerebrospinal fluid B. Outermost layer of meninges
    ___ Pia mater   C. Triple-layered covering and arachnoid of brain and spinal cord
    ___ Dura mater   D. Circulates between spaces in brain and spinal cord

20. Which nervous system controls the heart, digestion, sweating, and shivering?
    _____

21. Where is the brain stem located?
    _____

22. To what part of the body do cranial nerves supply sensory and motor fibers?
    _____

23. Where do motor fibers carry information?
    _____

24. Where do sensory fibers carry information?
    _____

25. "Wrist drop" indicates damage to a certain nerve. Which nerve is it?
    _____

26. If a person has suffered damage to the median and/or ulnar nerve, he or she may not be able to _____ his or her fingers.

27. Label the major components of the digestive system.

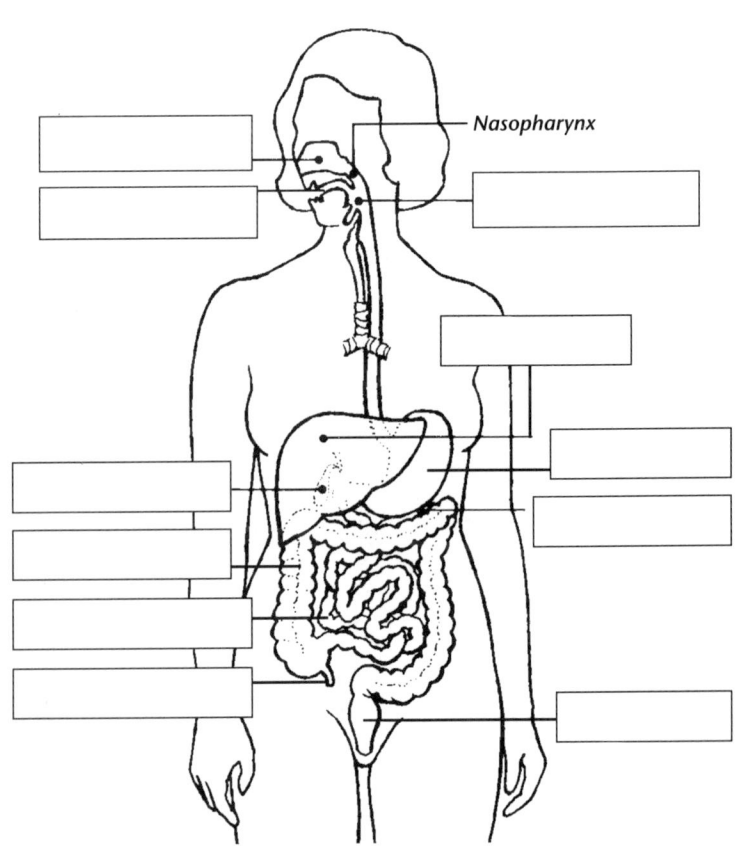

28 OEC Study Book

28. Describe and trace how food proceeds through the digestive tract.

_____
_____
_____
_____
_____
_____
_____
_____

29. The urinary system consists of two _____; the two _____, which drain urine from the kidneys; the _____, which stores urine; and the _____, which drains urine to the outside.

30. Kidneys filter:
    A. Oxygen
    B. Urine
    C. Blood

31. Identify the major components of the urinary system.

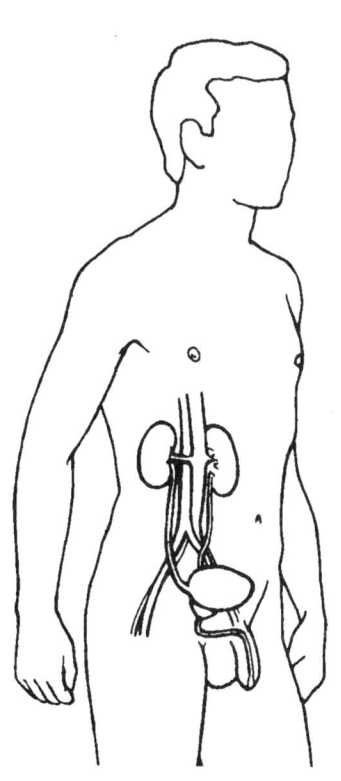
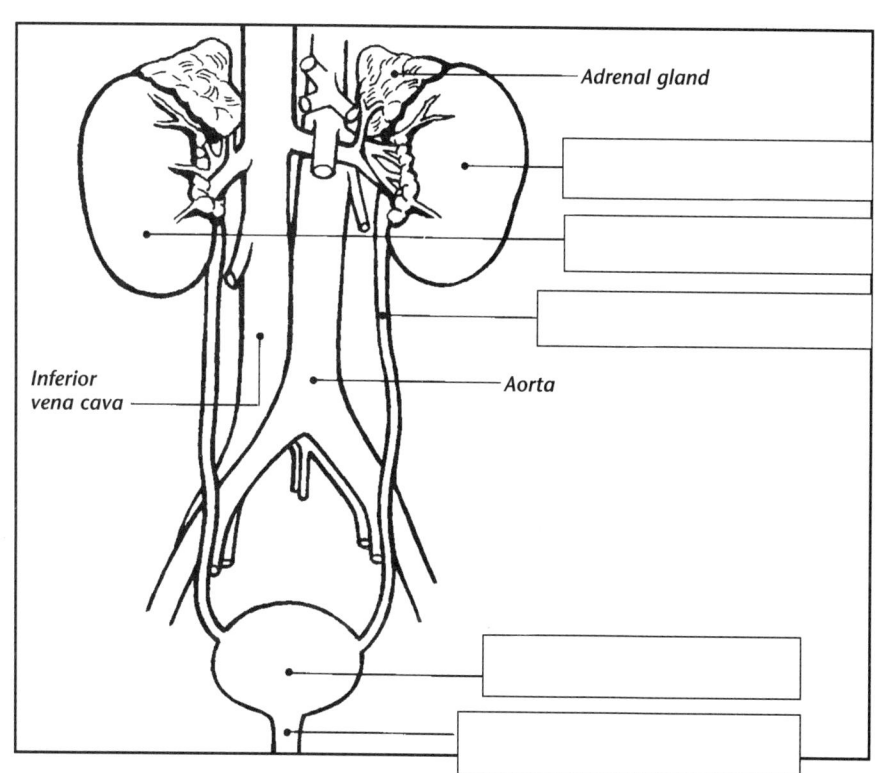

32. Identify the major bones of the human skeleton.

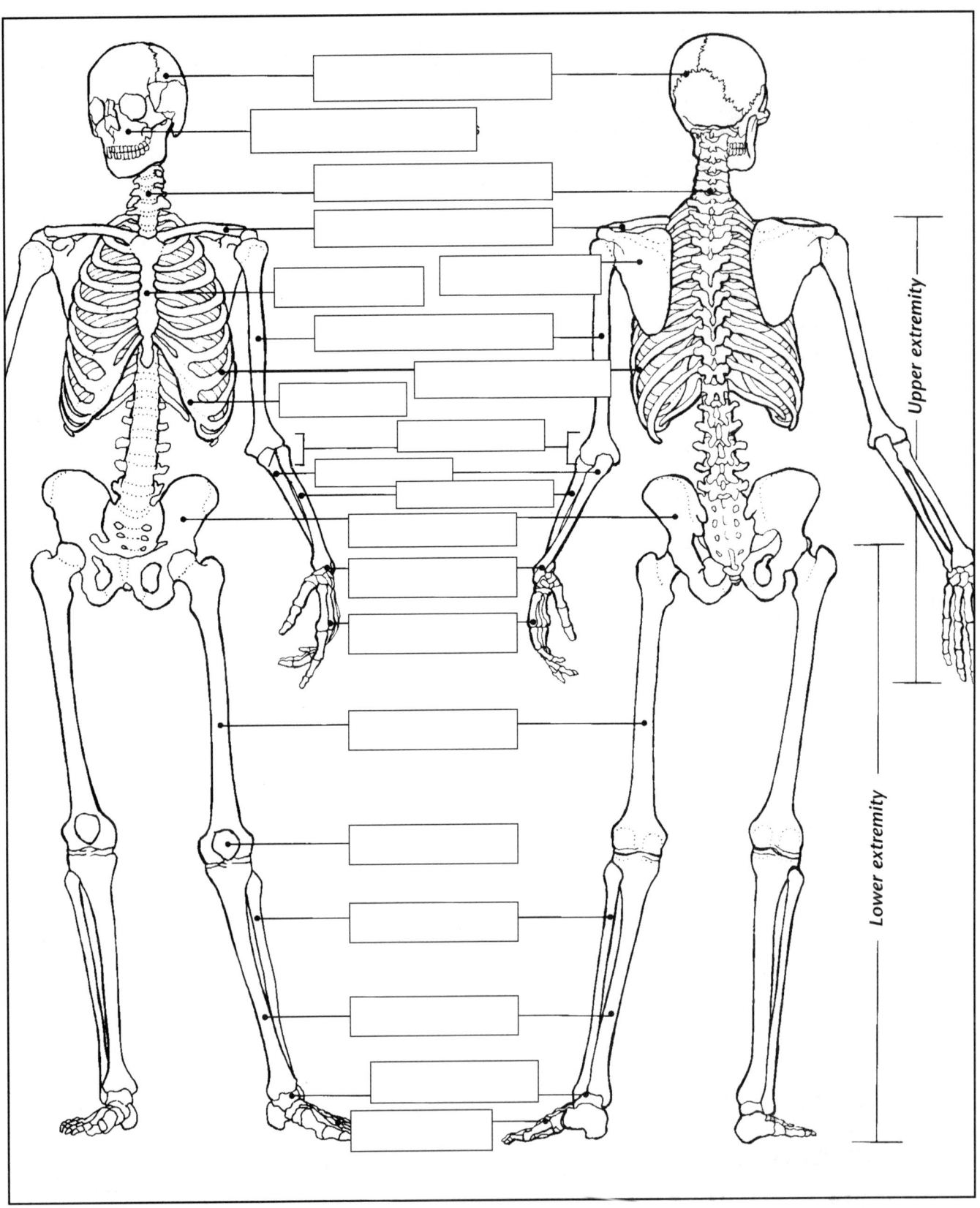

33. Identify and describe the major types of joints.

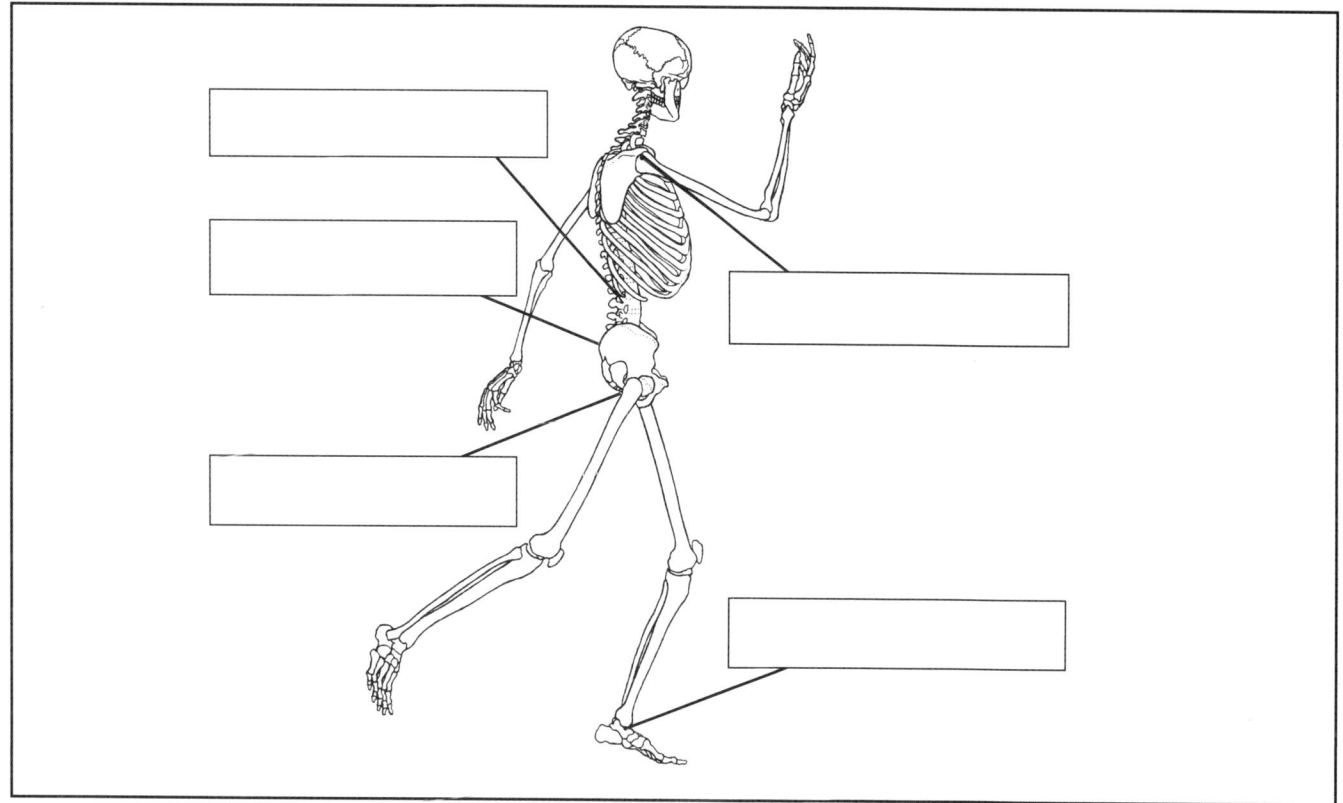

34. Identify the bones of the skull.

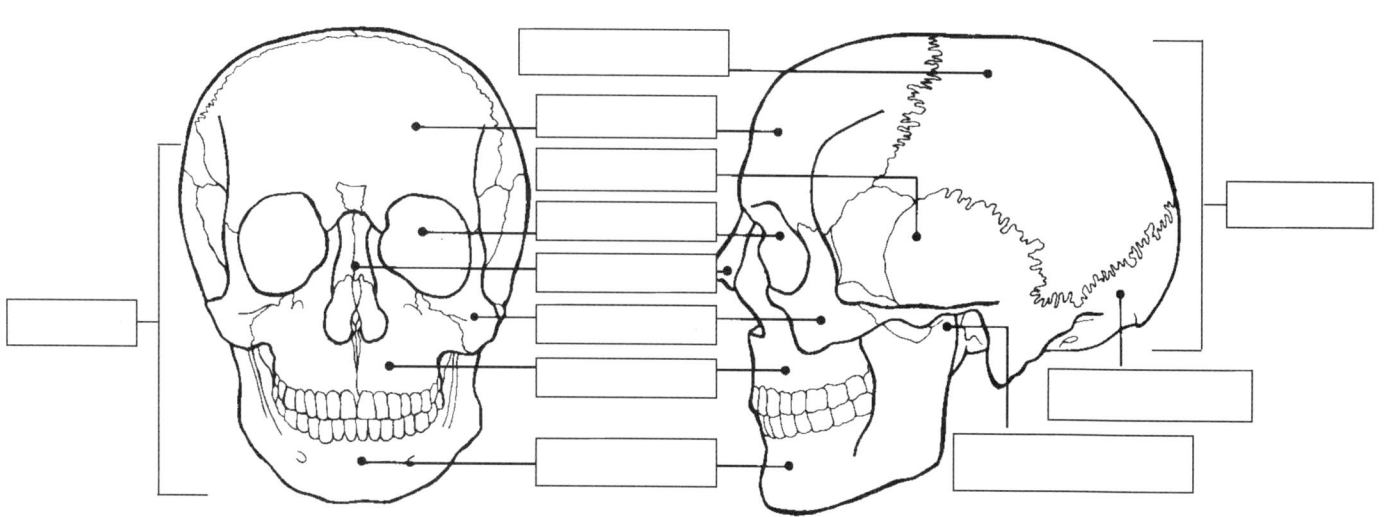

35. Identify the five regions of the spine and the number of vertebrae with each region

Five Regions of the Spine

36. Label the parts of the vertebrae.

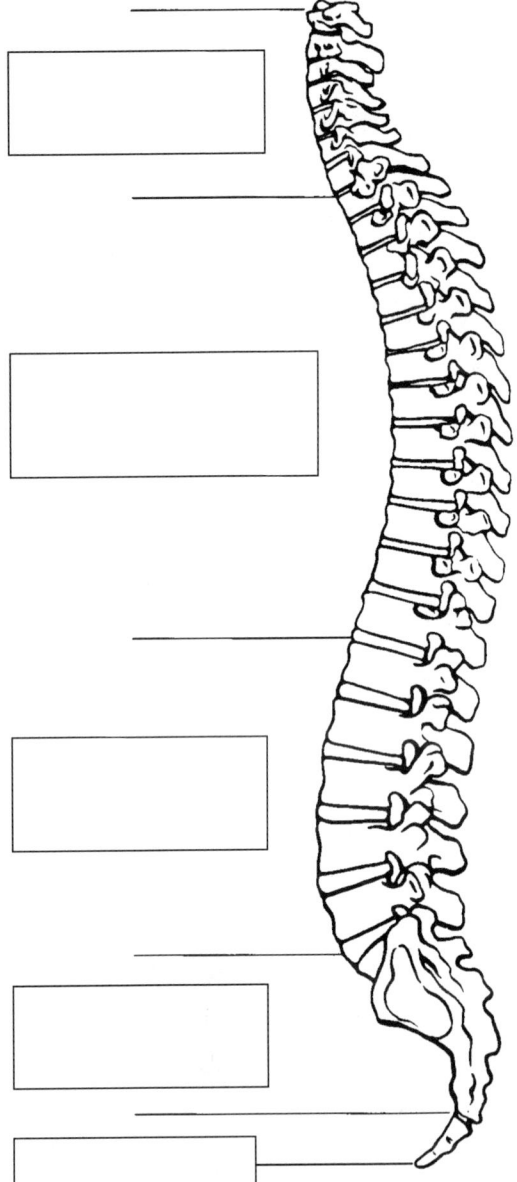
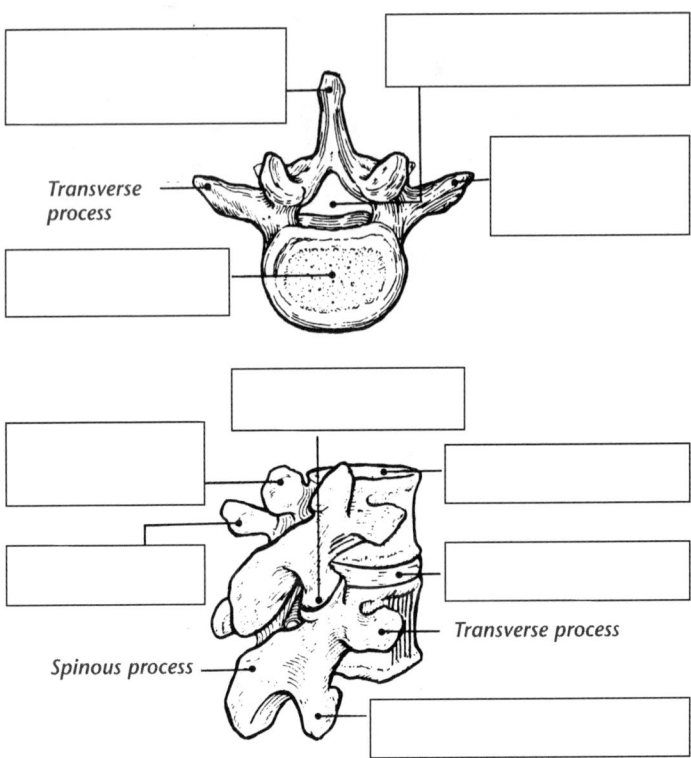

Transverse process

Spinous process

Transverse process

37. Label the upper extremity bones.

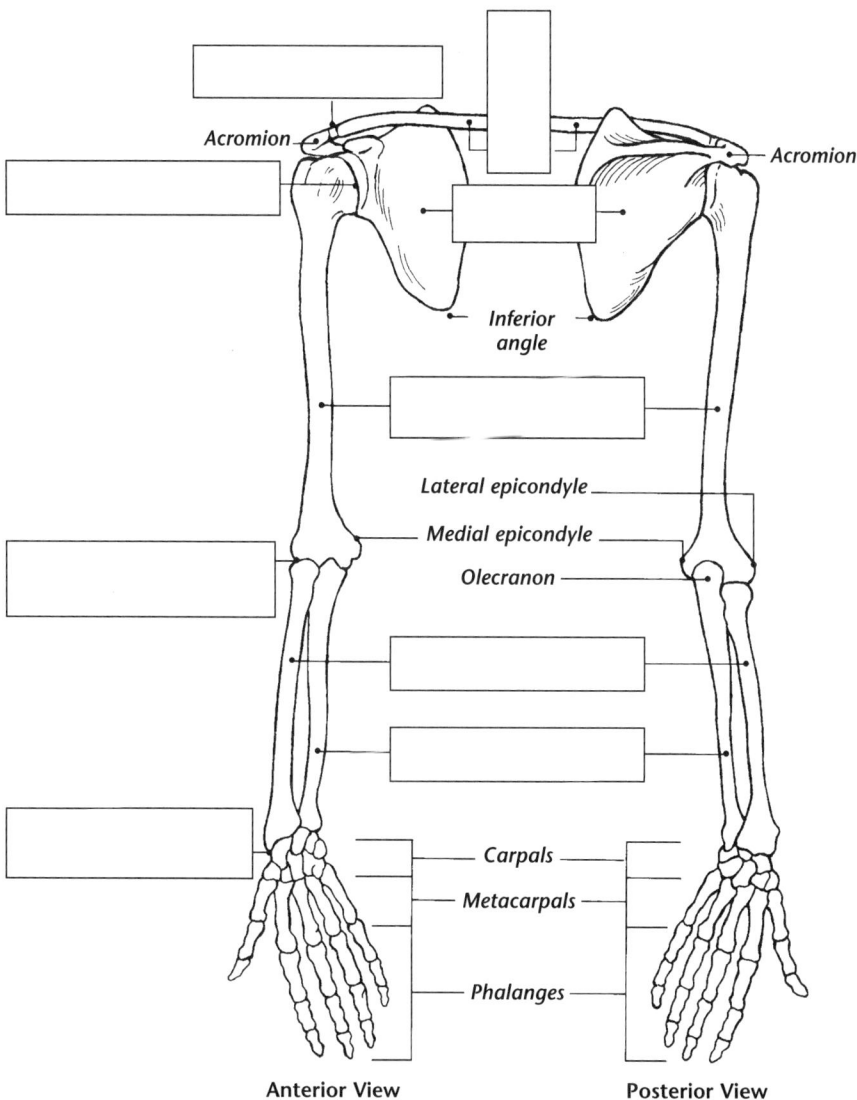

Anterior View   Posterior View

38. Match the name of the upper extremity bone(s) with the location or common name.

  ___ Shoulder blade   A. Clavicle
  ___ Carpals   B. Hand
  ___ Metacarpal   C. Scapula
  ___ Condyle   D. Elbow
  ___ Radius and ulna   E. Humerus
  ___ Collarbone   F. Wrist
  ___ Upper arm   G. Forearm
  ___ Fingers   H. Phalanges

39. Label the lower extremity bones.

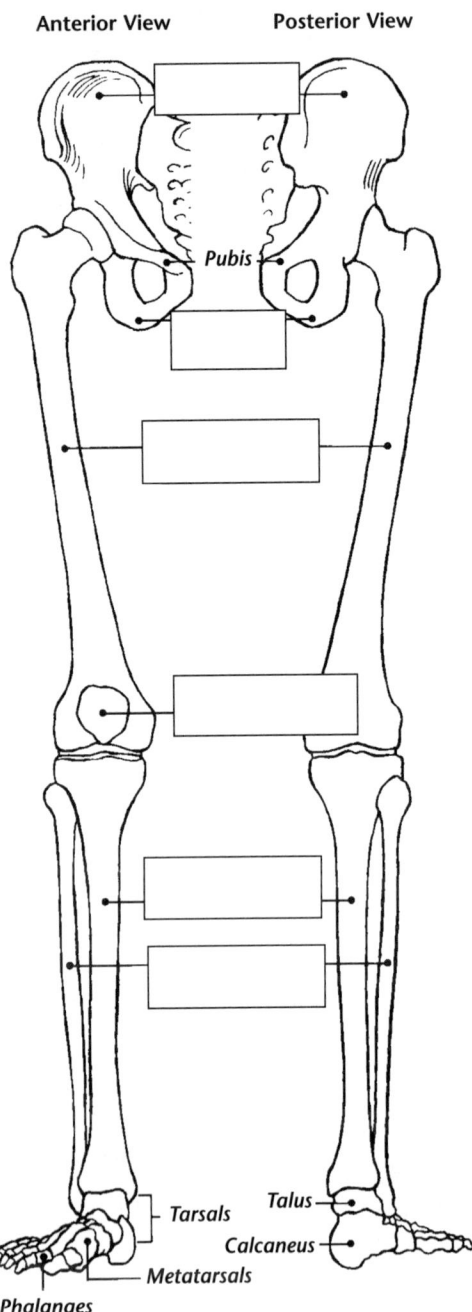

40. The part of the spine between the lowest ribs and the top of the pelvis is the:
    A. Thorax
    B. Lumbar
    C. Sacrum
    D. Coccyx

34 OEC Study Book

41. Identify the three major body cavities

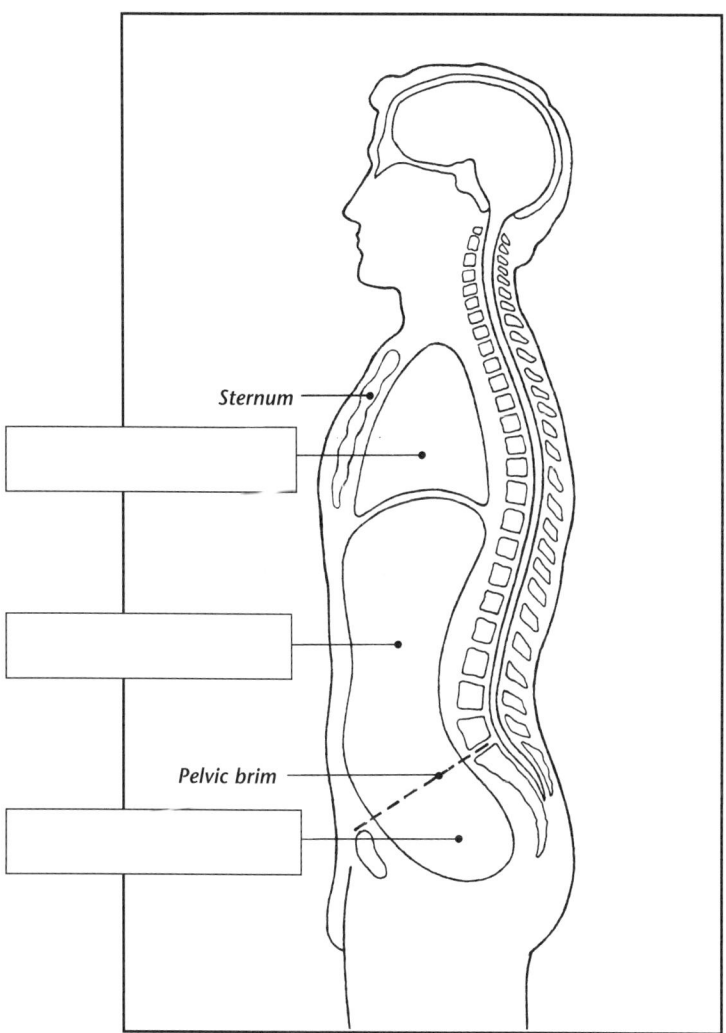

42. Identify the organs of the pelvic cavity.

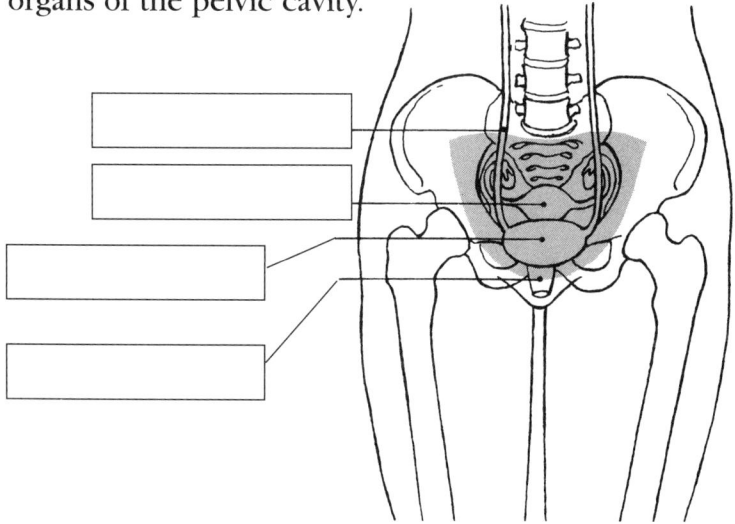

43. Label the organs of the abdominal cavity.

Organs of the Abdominal Cavity — Gallbladder, Transverse colon, Ascending colon, Descending colon

Organs Behind the Abdominal Cavity — Adrenal gland, Diaphragm, Inferior vena cava, Ureter, Urethra

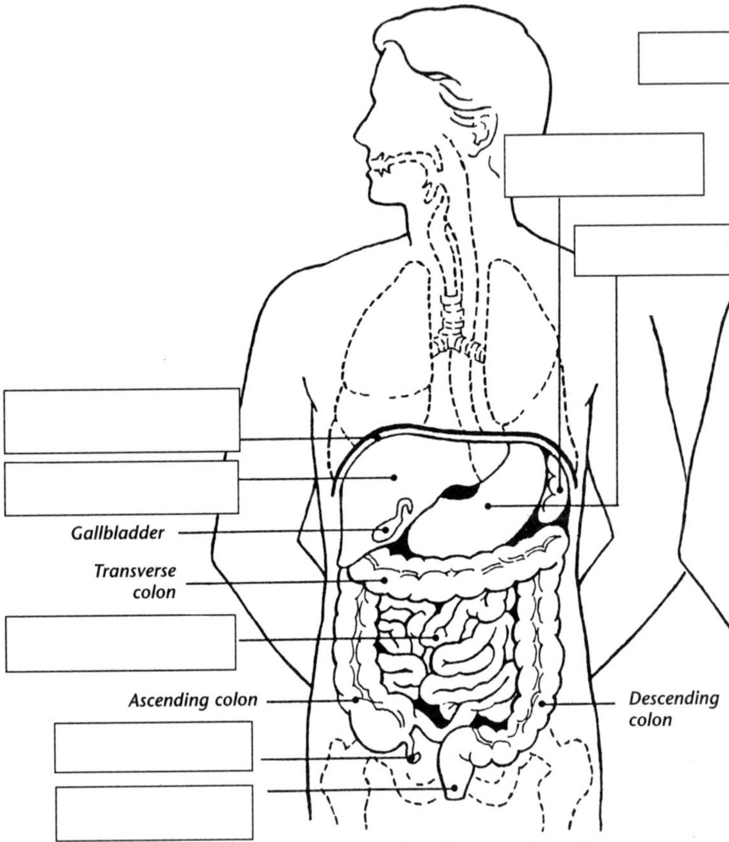

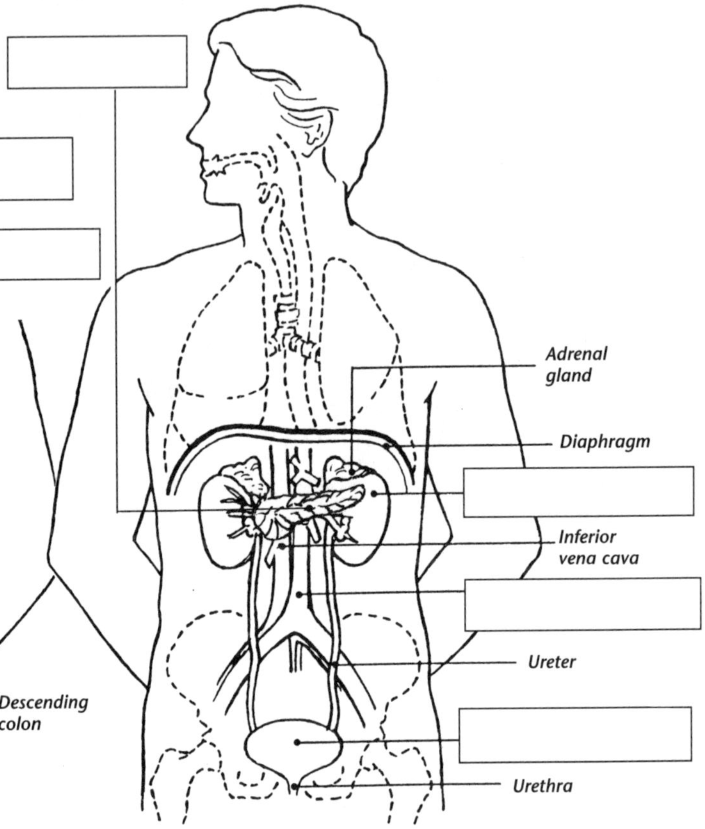

44. List the different kinds of muscle tissue and their characteristics in the table below.

Muscle Types	Characteristics
A.	
B.	
C.	

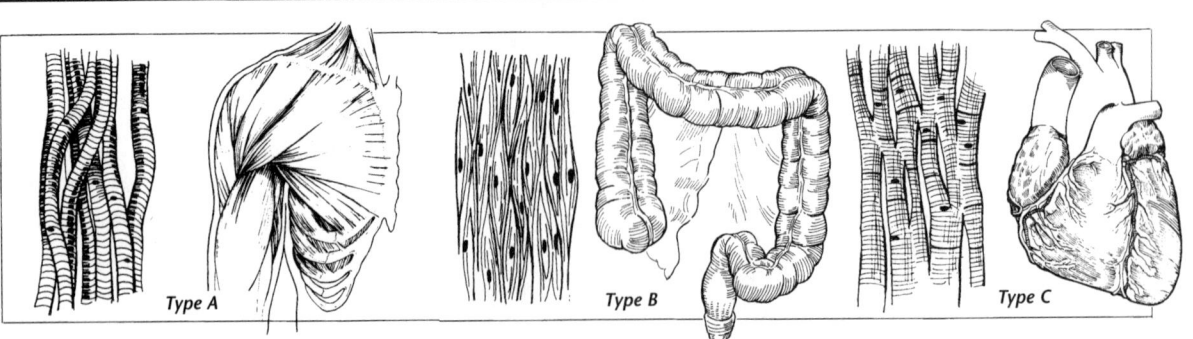

Type A   Type B   Type C

45. Match the following muscles to their description.

___ bicep
___ deltoid
___ hamstring
___ intercostal
___ latissimus dorsi
___ pectoralis
___ quadraceps
___ sternomastoid
___ trapezius
___ tricep

A. found attached to shoulders and spine
B. found on either side of the anterior portion of the neck and act to turn and flex the neck
C. found attached to the lumbar portion of the spine and act to adduct the upper extremities
D. found on the anterior chest and act to adduct the upper extremities
E. found in between the ribs and aid in the breathing process
F. found on the anterior thigh and act to extend the knee
G. found on the posterior thigh and act to extend the knee
H. found on the top of the shoulder and act to abduct the upper extremities
I. found on the anterior aspect of the upper arm and act to flex the elbow
J. found on the posterior aspect of the upper arm and act to extend the elbow

46. The skin is made up of two layers; the outer layer is called the _____, and the inner layer is called the _____.

47. The layer of the cutaneous system that contains hair follicles, sweat glands, nerves, and blood vessels is:
   A. Sub-cutaneous
   B. Dermis
   C. Epidermis
   D. Sub-epidermis

48. Identify the female genitourinary system.

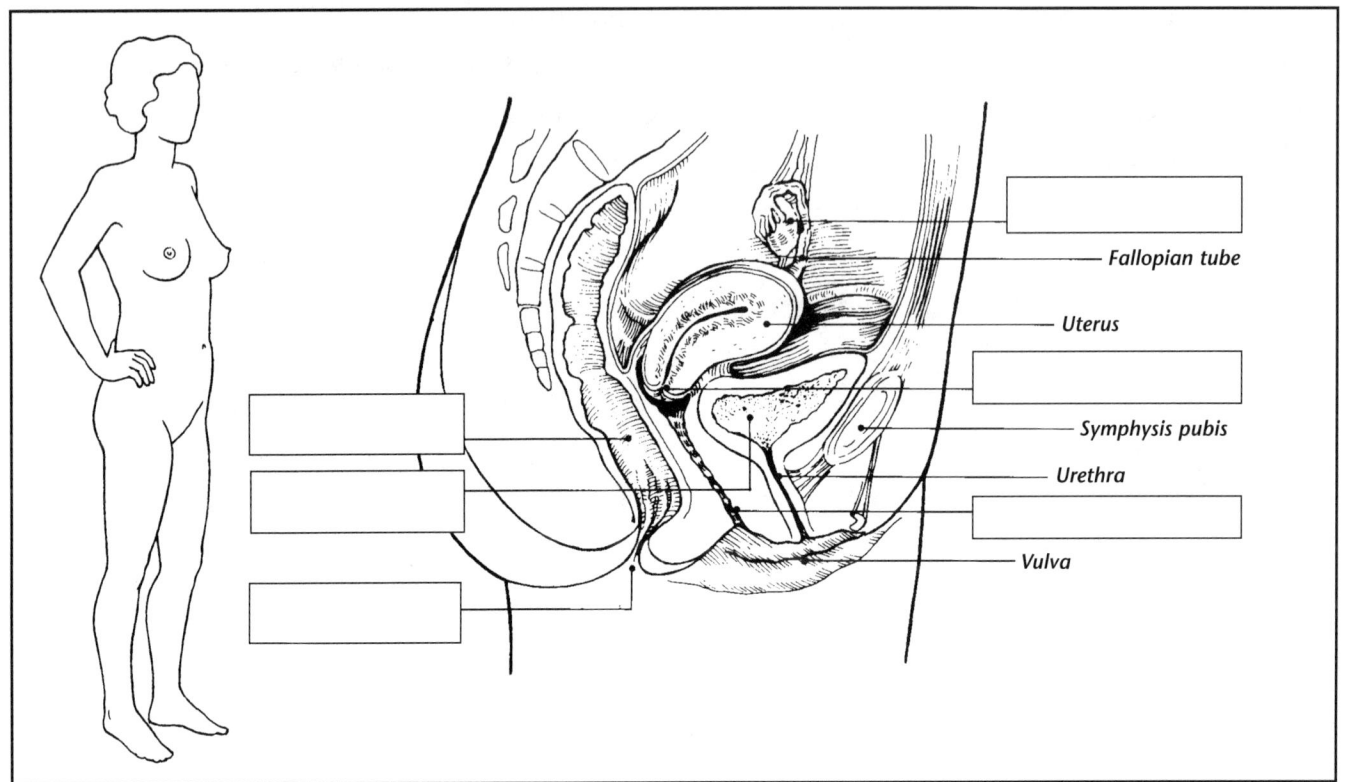

49. Identify the male genitourinary system.

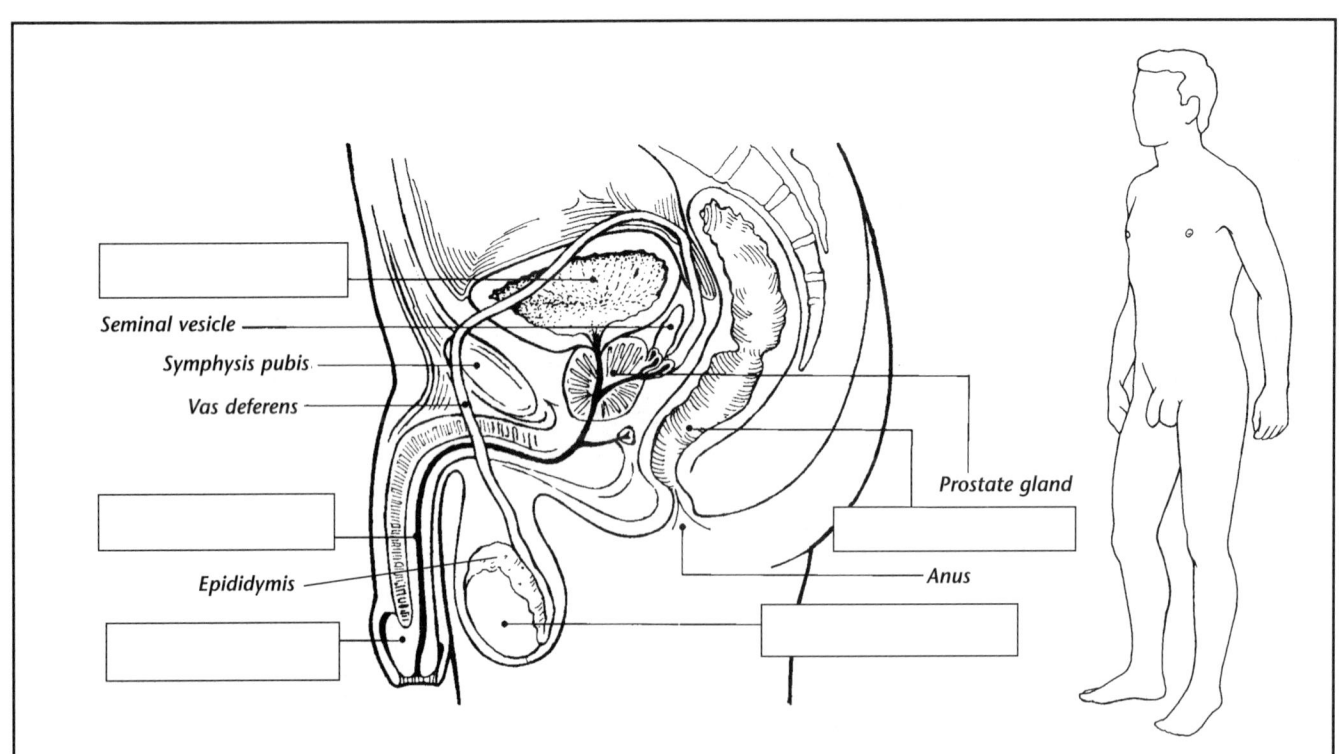

38 OEC Study Book

50. What controls both male and female reproductive systems?

   _____

51. Fill in the endocrine gland that performs the described function.

   A. _____ secretes epinephrine that regulates heart action and blood vessel tone

   B. _____ secretes many hormones including growth hormone and it controls many other glands

   C. _____ secretes hormones that control metabolism and the calcium in bones

   D. _____ secretes insulin to control carbohydrate metabolism and glucagon to control the release of glucose from the liver

   E. _____ produces estrogen that controls the development of secondary female sex characteristics

   F. _____ produces testosterone that controls the development of secondary male sex characteristics

CHAPTER 2 SKILL PERFORMANCE REQUIREMENTS

- Demonstrate comprehension of anatomical terms

Skill Performance Guidelines

- No skill performance guidelines (SPG) in this chapter

STUDY NOTES

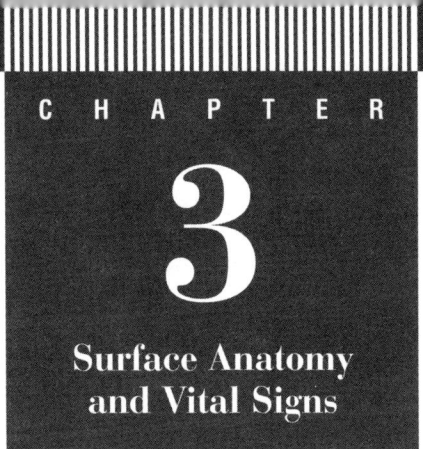

CHAPTER 3
Surface Anatomy and Vital Signs

CONCLUDING OBJECTIVES

The learner will:

Content

- Recognize and locate important landmarks of the body

- Recognize and locate vital signs and other important signs

Skill Performance

- Demonstrate the techniques for taking and recording vital signs

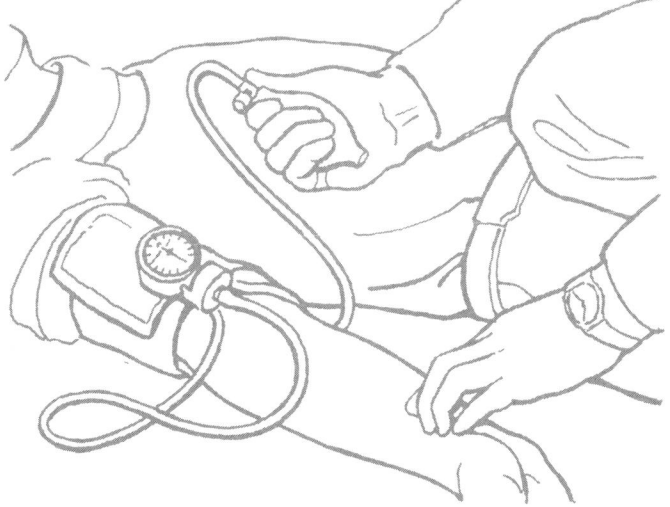

CHAPTER 3 STUDY QUESTIONS

1. Label the surface anatomy of the head.

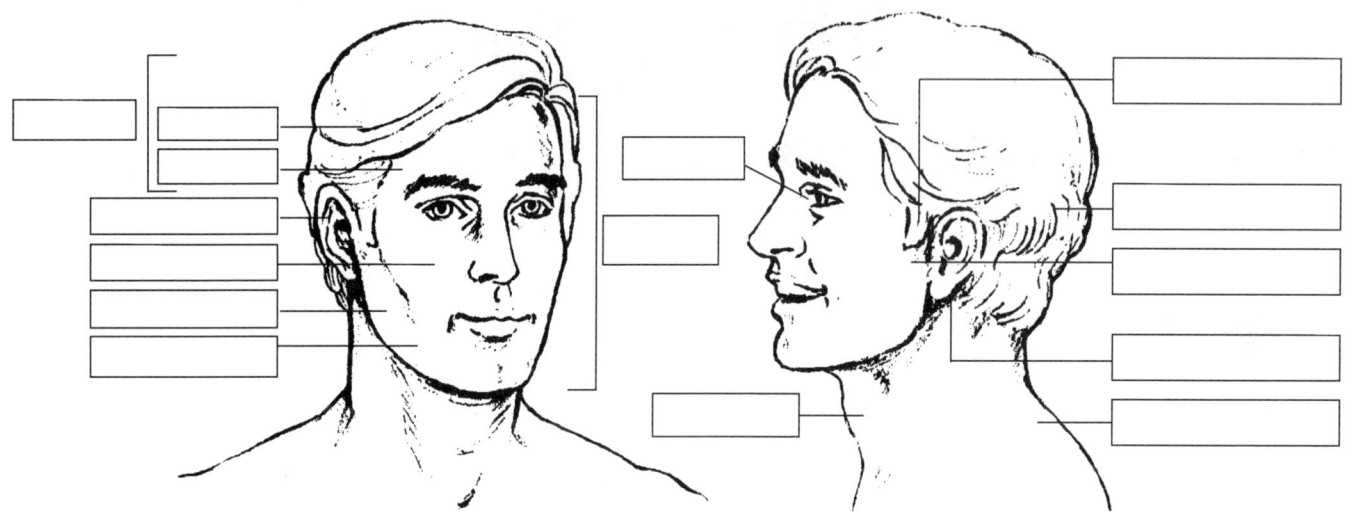

2. Match the name of the surface anatomy with the location or common name.

   ___ Cheekbone
   ___ Bony sockets that contain and protect the eyes
   ___ Head
   ___ External ear
   ___ Jawbone
   ___ Adams's apple

   A. Cranium and the face
   B. Bony ridge of the maxilla
   C. Pinna
   D. Orbits
   E. Mandible
   F. Thyroid cartilage

3. Label the surface anatomy of the mouth.

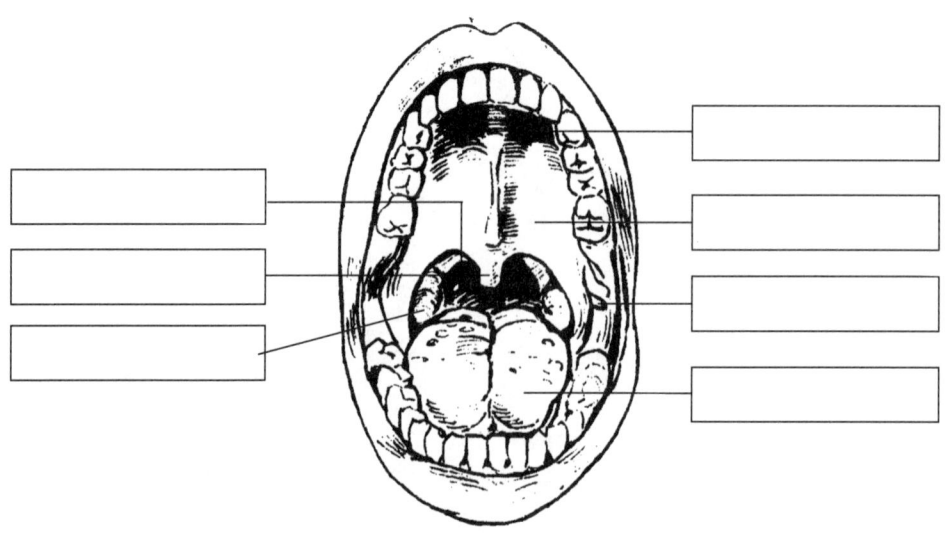

4. Label the surface anatomy of the neck.

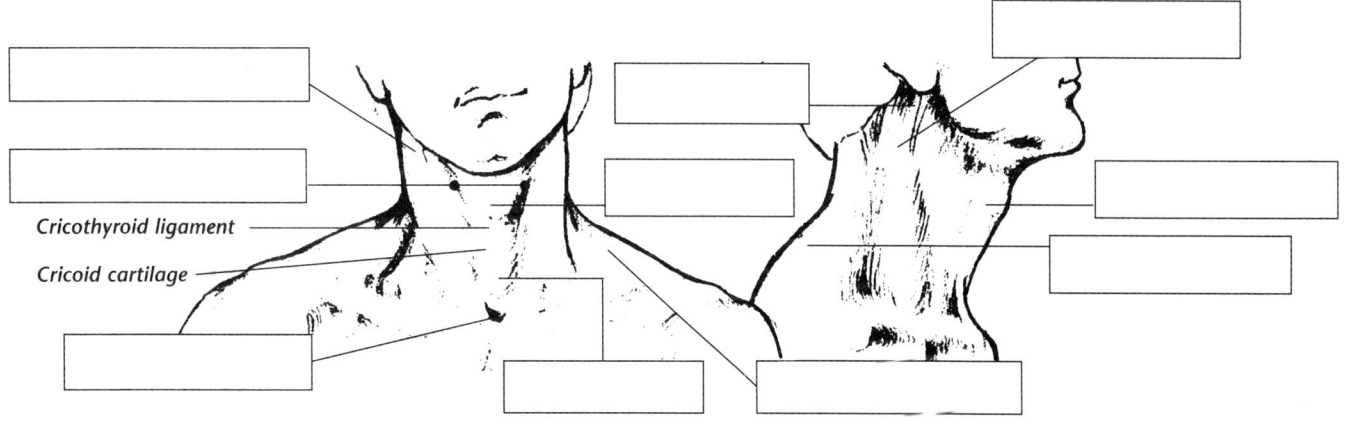

5. The neck contains _____ cervical vertebrae.

6. Label the areas of the chest.

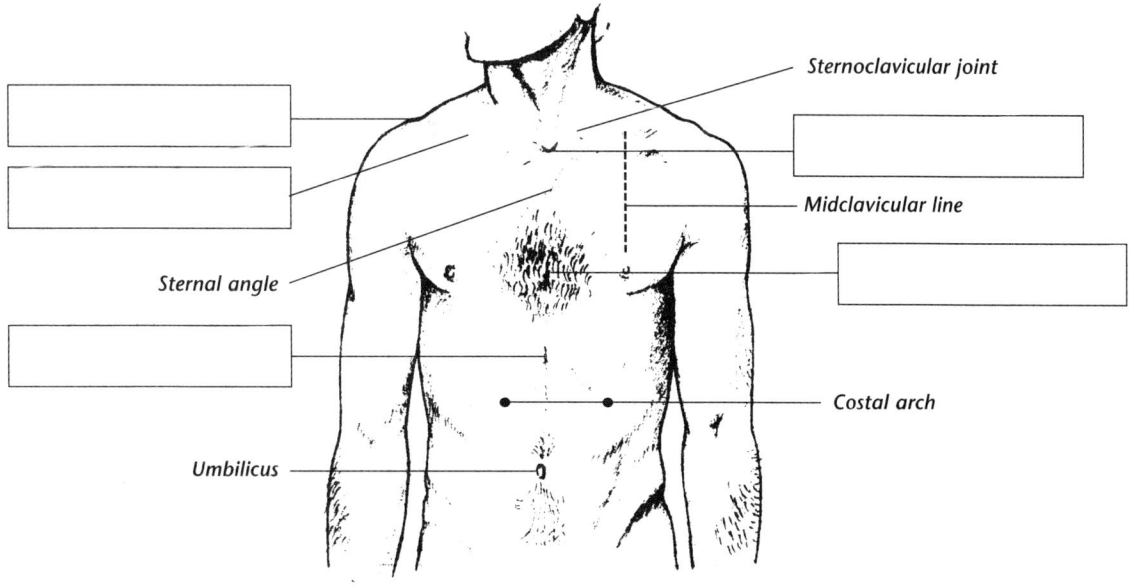

7. Label the chest, abdomen, and pelvic areas.

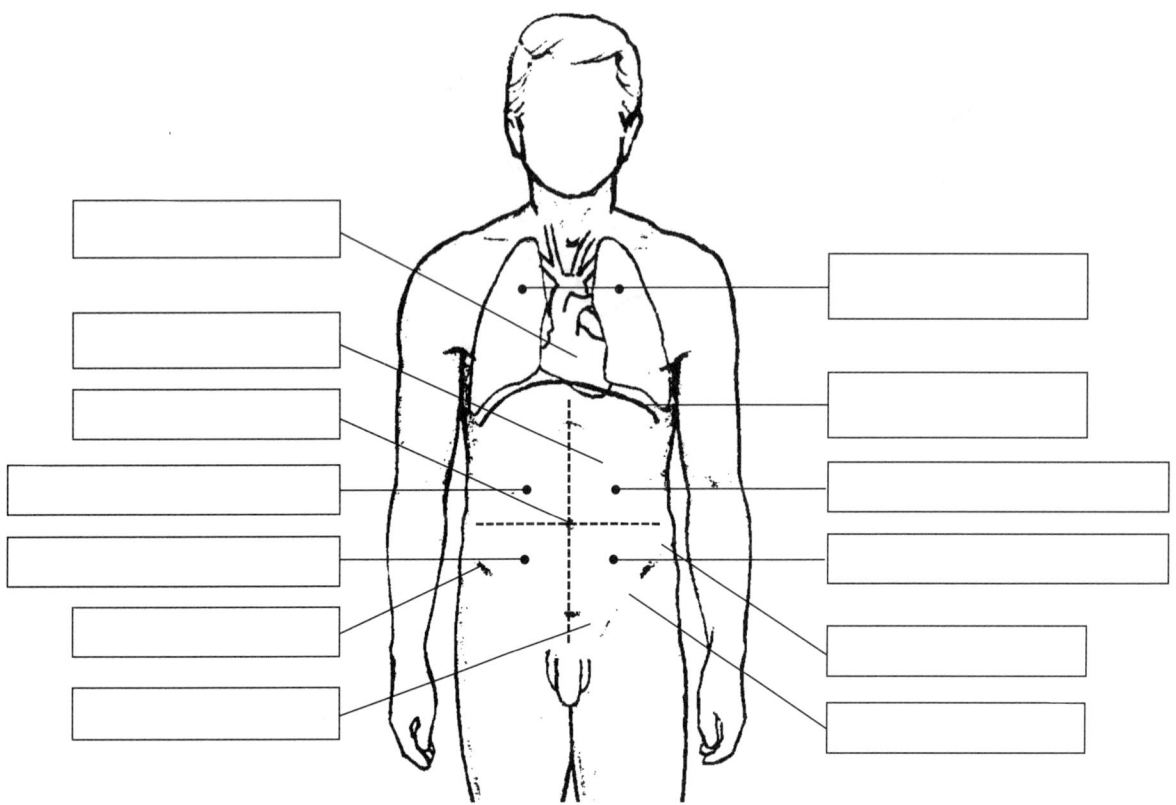

8. Label the anterior and posterior organs of the human body.

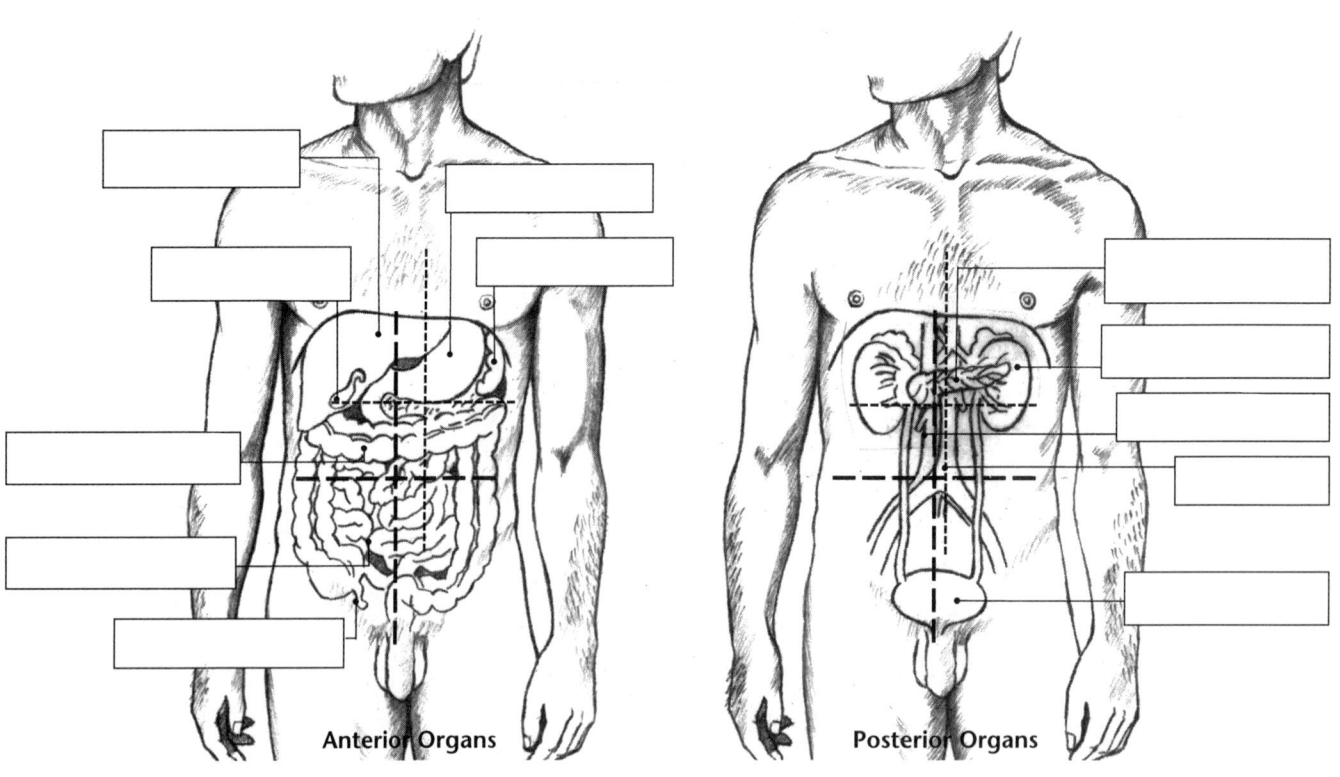

Anterior Organs   Posterior Organs

9. Label the surface anatomy of the leg.

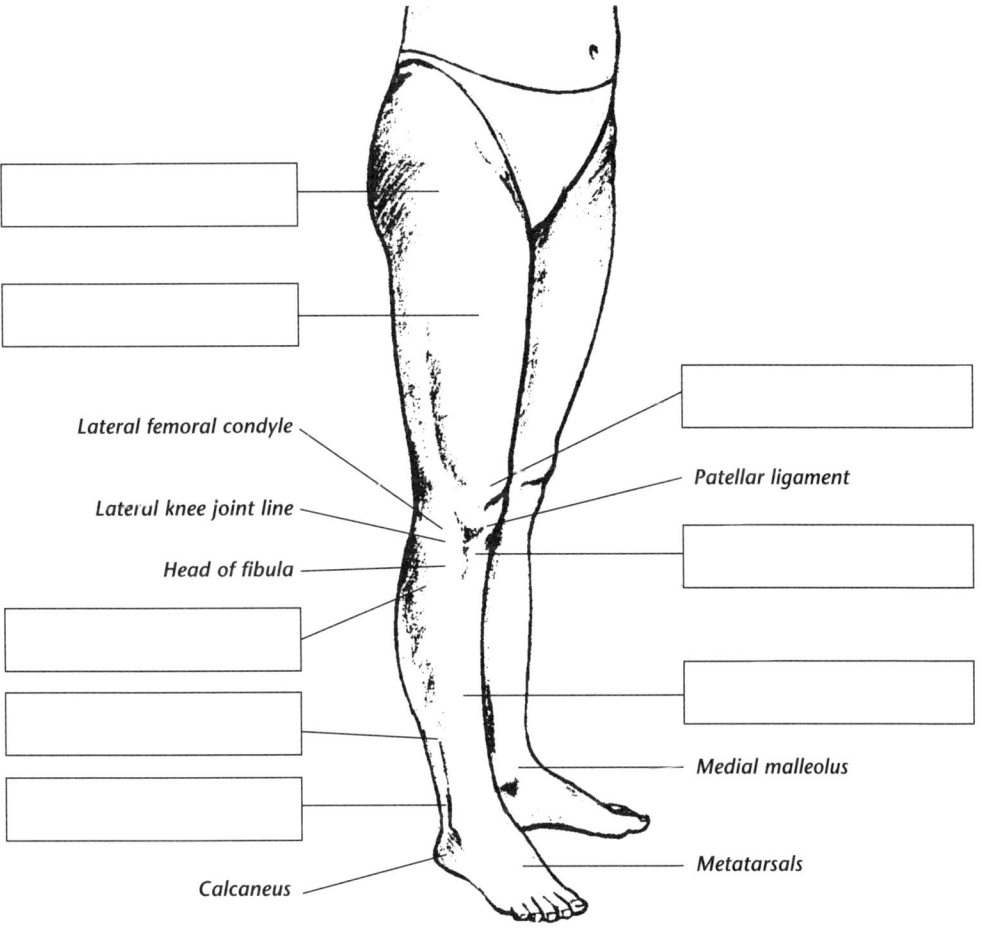

10. Label the surface anatomy of the foot.

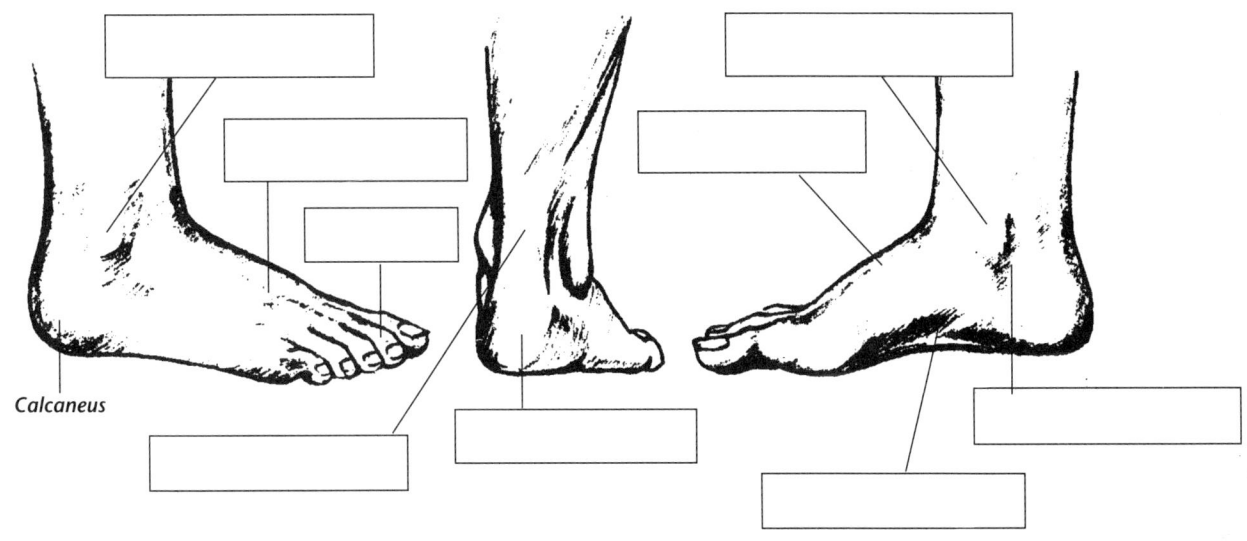

11. Label the surface anatomy of the arms and hands.

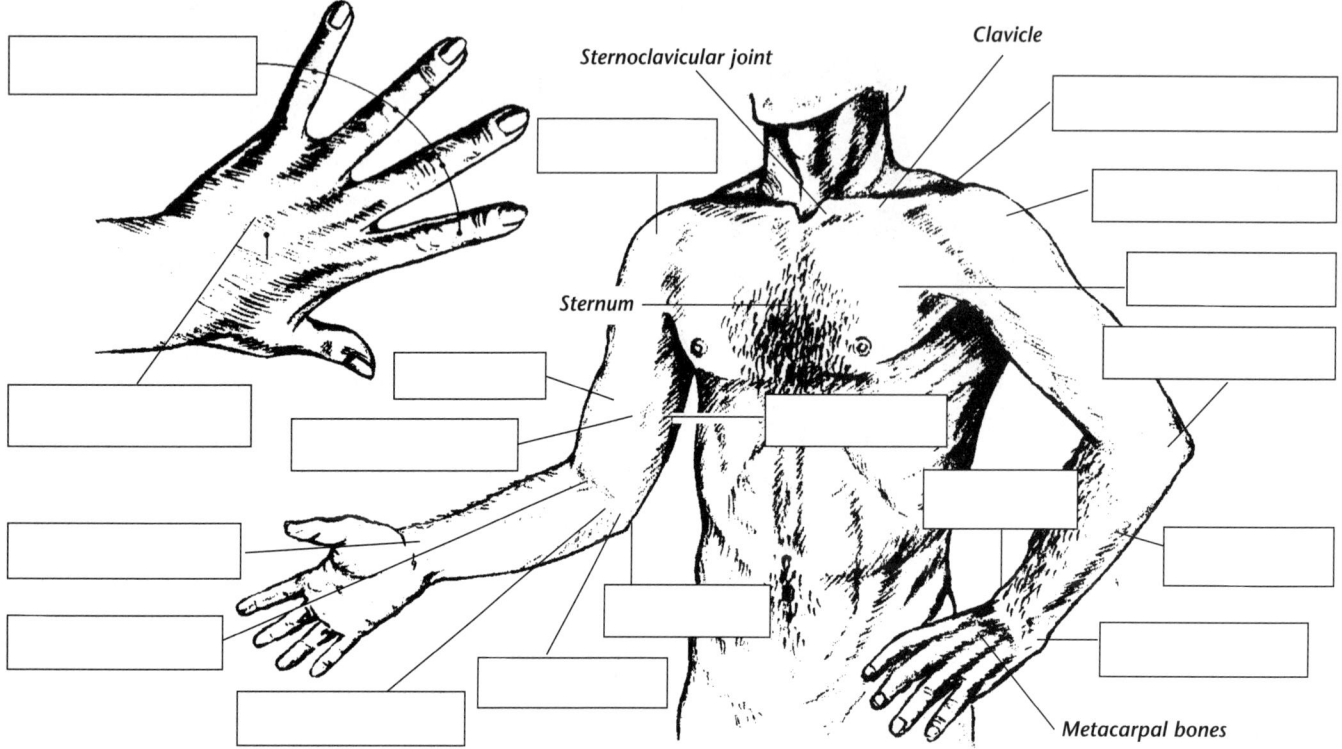

12. Label the surface anatomy of the back.

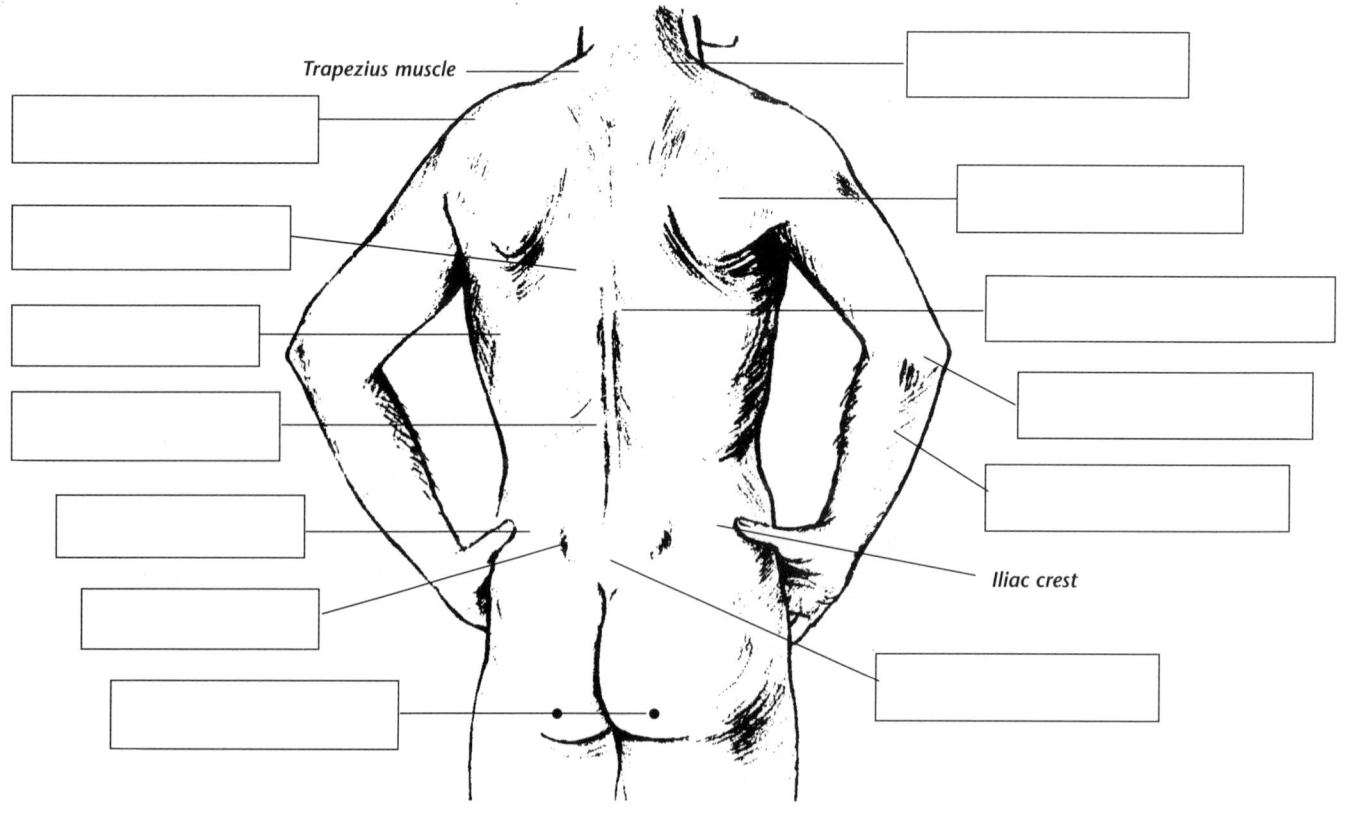

13. List the five vital signs.

   _____
   _____
   _____
   _____
   _____

14. Define a sign and a symptom.

Sign	
Symptom	

15. Define a normal level of responsiveness and any state of responsiveness other than the completely responsive state.

   _____
   _____
   _____

16. Define the AVPU Scale.

A	Alert	
V		
P		
U		The patient does not respond to verbal stimuli or to pain.

17. What does the pulse represent?

   _____
   _____

18. What does the presence of a pulse indicate to the examiner?

   _____

19. What does the absence of a pulse indicate to the examiner?

   _____
   _____

20. What are the three features of the pulse that should be checked during a survey?
    _____
    _____
    _____

21. Normal blood circulation is a continuous process, with the heart normally beating _____ to _____ times a minute in an adult.

22. A person's pulse may indicate shock if it is _____ and _____.

23. What are the two best anatomical sites to locate a patient's pulse?
    _____
    _____

24. Why should an OEC technician never use his or her thumb to feel for a patient's pulse?
    _____
    _____

25. Locate the important pulses.

26. The normal resting breathing rate for adults is between _____ and _____ respirations per minute.

27. Breathing that is abnormal and associated with obvious distress is called _____ _____.

28. Cyanosis is defined as a bluish discoloration of the skin, fingernails, and mucous membranes that occurs
    A. because of pre-existing asthma
    B. only when a patient has carbon monoxide poisoning
    C. because the blood is not properly oxygenated
    D. due to chemical dependence

29. Name three ways to measure body temperature and their normal degrees.

30. Name three possible body temperatures and how they are caused.

31. Blood pressure varies depending on what four components?

32. When taking someone's blood pressure, the highest point of the curve corresponds to the _____ and the lowest point to the _____.

33. In addition to the vital signs, list five important diagnostic signs.

34. To successfully complete a thorough patient assessment, the rescuer must have an understanding of the important elements of the assessment process. Summarize the normal functions of the characteristics below for an adult.

Elements	Normal Function
Level of Responsiveness	
Pulse	
Respiration	
Temperature	
Blood Pressure	
Skin Temperature, Moisture, and Color	
Capillary Refill Time	
Reaction of the Pupils	
Reaction to Pain	
Ability to Move	

Chapter 3 Local Protocol

1. Describe your local technique(s) for obtaining and recording vital signs.

   _____

   _____

   _____

   _____

2. Identify local storage area(s) for equipment and documentation papers used in taking and recording vital signs.

   _____

   _____

   _____

   _____

CHAPTER 3 SKILL PERFORMANCE REQUIREMENTS

- Demonstrate the techniques for taking and recording vital signs

Skill Performance Guidelines
- Vital Signs Determination

Vital Signs Determination

Pulse
- Palpates the radial pulse and determines the rate.

- Verbally describes the rhythm and strength.

- Palpates the carotid pulse and determines the rate.

- Demonstrates palpation of the dorsalis pedis pulse.

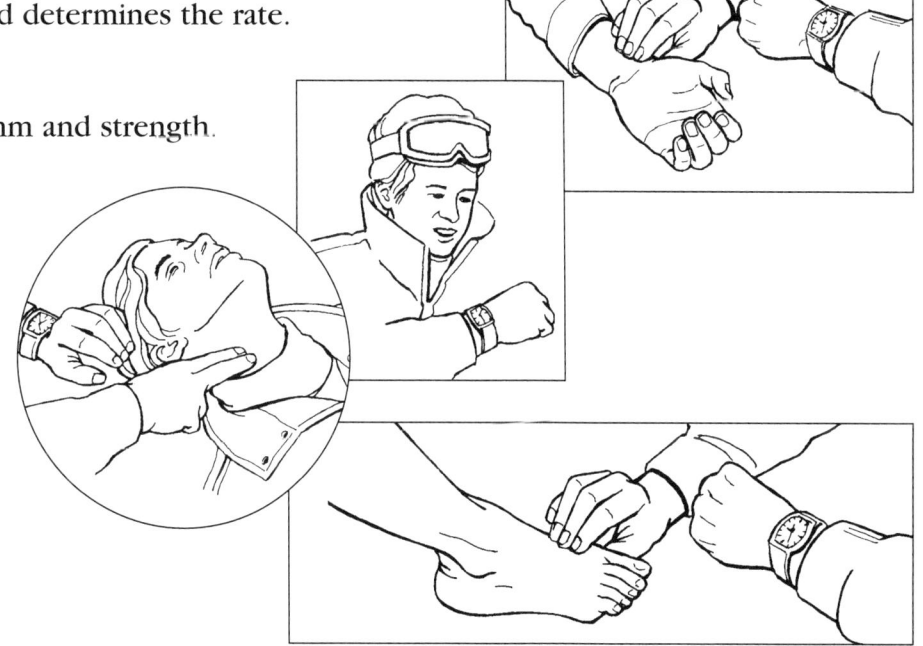

Respirations
- Observes the rise and fall of the chest wall over a 15-second period to determine the rate.

- Observes chest action for unequal rise, diaphragmatic breathing, flail segments, etc.

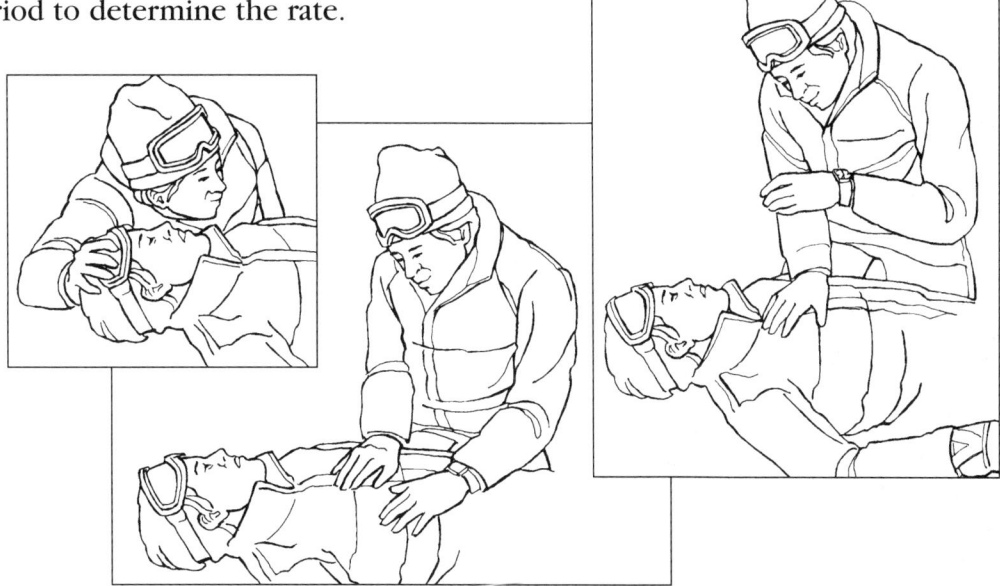

Blood Pressure by Auscultation

- Applies the blood pressure cuff to the arm above the elbow and centered over the brachial artery.

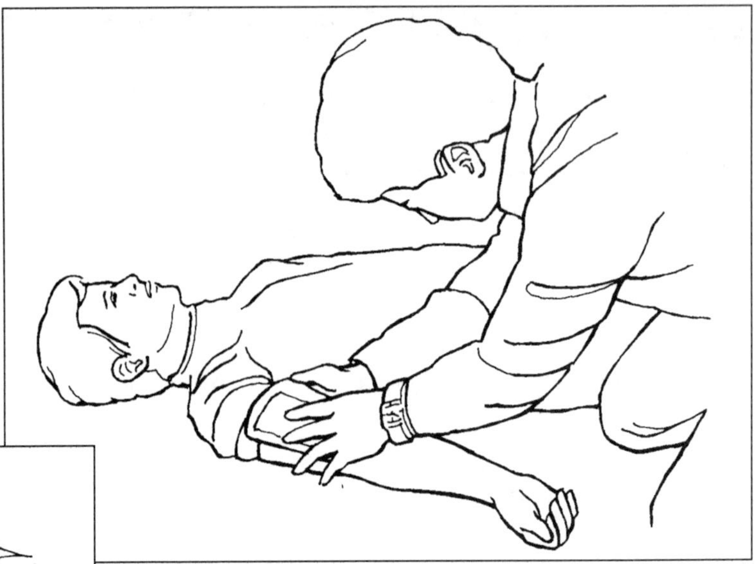

- Inflates the cuff while palpating the radial pulse.

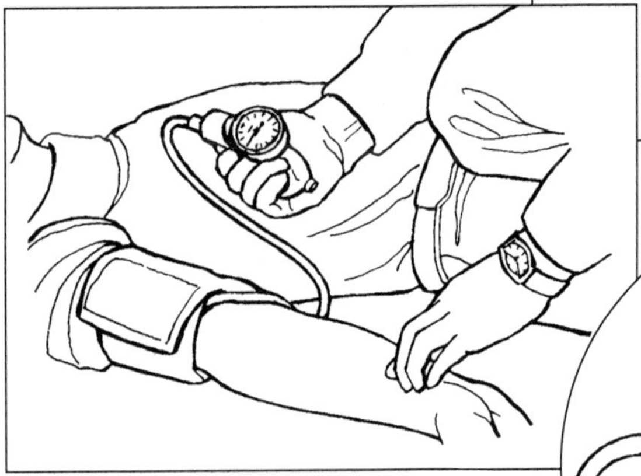

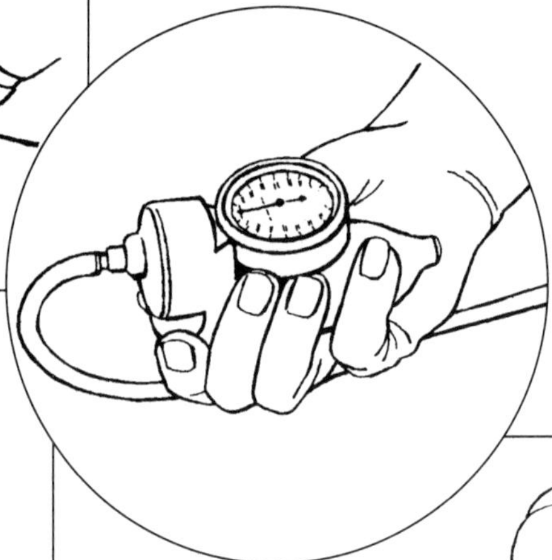

- Inflates the cuff to 30-mm Hg *above the approximate systolic*.

- Replaces stethoscope over the artery and slowly releases the pressure, noting when sound is first heard (systolic) and again when absent (diastolic). Report the values.

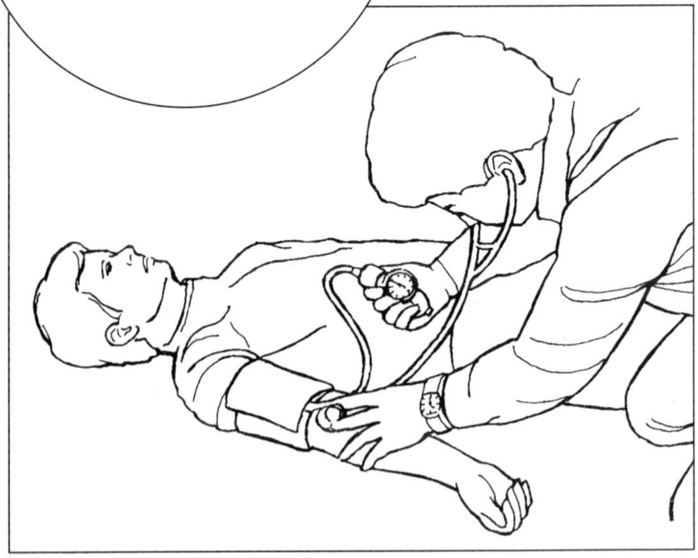

STUDY NOTES

VITAL SIGNS DETERMINATION

Objective: To demonstrate the ability to determine a baseline set of vital signs.

SKILL	YES	NO	NOTATIONS
Pulse			
• Palpates the radial pulse and determines the rate.			
• Verbally describes the rhythm and strength.			
• Palpates the carotid pulse and determines the rate.			
• Demonstrates palpation of the dorsalis pedis pulse.			
Respirations			
• Observes the rise and fall of the chest wall over a 15-second period to determine the rate.			
• Observes chest action for unequal rise, diaphragmatic breathing, flail segments, etc.			
Blood Pressure by Auscultation			
• Applies the blood pressure cuff to the arm above the elbow and centered over the brachial artery.			
• Inflates the cuff while palpating the radial pulse.			
• Inflates the cuff to 30 mm Hg *above the approximate systolic*.			
• Replaces stethoscope over the artery and slowly releases the pressure, noting when sound is first heard (systolic) and again when absent (diastolic). Reports the values.			

Did the trainee or patroller adequately demonstrate the performance criteria of this skill?			

COMMENTS

CHAPTER

4

Introduction to Patient Assessment

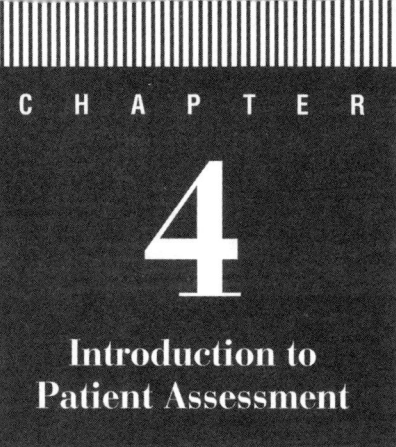

CONCLUDING OBJECTIVES

The learner will:

Content

- Explain the purpose of patient assessment

- Explain the techniques that make up Basic Life Support (BLS)

- Explain the four major parts of patient assessment

- Define key patient assessment terminology

- Explain the methodology and psychology of dealing with patients and the potential reactions of rescuers

- Explain the importance of body substance isolation (BSI) precautions when using equipment and techniques that allow contact with body fluids

- Explain the importance of dealing with and disposing of hazardous materials

- Explain the legal aspects of emergency care

Skill Performance

- Demonstrate BSI precautions with the use and disposal of personal protective equipment and hazardous materials

CHAPTER 4 STUDY QUESTIONS

1. List six objectives of patient assessment.

   _____
   _____
   _____
   _____
   _____
   _____

2. Most mistakes in emergency care are caused by _____ rather than _____.

3. One of the purposes of patient assessment is to care immediately for conditions that threaten life or limb. Assessment may be interrupted periodically while certain emergency care is provided. These interruptions are called _____.

4. List some examples of interventions.

   _____
   _____
   _____
   _____
   _____

5. What are the four major parts of patient assessment?

   _____
   _____
   _____
   _____

6. What mnemonic is used to help remember the first part of the urgent survey. What does each letter stand for?

   _____ : _____
   _____ : _____
   _____ : _____

7. When approaching the scene the rescuer must be cognizant of several things such as safety, mechanism of injury, and witnesses. When approaching the patient, what should the rescuer keep in mind?

8. What should be done when a patient who is rational refuses care?

9. If a patient refuses care, the rescuer must

10. Children require special care in an emergency. What are some things that will help when dealing with a child?

11. List five physical or psychological reactions in rescuers following involvement with patients who are seriously injured.

12. Describe Critical Incident Stress Debriefing (CISD).

13. AIDS is caused by _____.

14. How is HIV transmitted?

15. List four high-risk substances in the transmission of bloodborne pathogens.

16. List some body substance isolation (BSI) precautions.

17. What are the risks for HIV or hepatitis infection for an emergency care provider who does not give injections or start IVs?

18. What is the number one rule for body substance isolation?

19. What personal protective equipment is appropriate for a patroller?

20. What body substance isolation procedures should be followed for cleaning equipment contaminated with blood or other body fluids?

21. List some hazardous materials.

22. The first thing you should do when you identify a possible haz-mat incident is

23. Define emergency care.

24. Define standard of care.

25. Once patient care is started, continue until

26. What are Good Samaritan Laws?

Chapter 4 Local Protocol

1. Describe the location in the aid room for personal protective equipment and the local patrol procedures for use of personal protective equipment.

2. Describe local patrol procedures for cleaning and disposal of contaminated clothing, equipment, and supplies.

3. Describe local patrol procedures for initiating a critical incident stress debriefing.

   _____
   _____
   _____
   _____
   _____

4. Describe local patrol procedures for obtaining the hepatitis B vaccine. What is your patrol requirement for the vaccine?

   _____
   _____
   _____
   _____
   _____

5. Describe local Good Samaritan Laws.

   _____
   _____
   _____
   _____
   _____

CHAPTER 4 SKILL PERFORMANCE REQUIREMENTS

- Demonstrate BSI precautions with the use, cleaning, and disposal of personal protective equipment and hazardous materials

  ➢ Follow local protocols for use and disposal of personal protective equipment

  ➢ Follow local protocols for cleaning of equipment exposed to body substances and hazardous materials

Skill Performance Guidelines

- No skill performance guidelines (SPGs) in this chapter

Chapter 4 Scenarios

1. While conducting an OEC clinic off the slope near the top of the beginner lift, you get called over by the lift operator. He yells, "A little boy is bleeding." You determine the little boy fell and his mother accidentally skied over both of his gloveless hands. Both hands are bleeding profusely. Describe the BSI precautions you should take.

   _____
   _____
   _____
   _____
   _____

2. You respond to an accident on the beginner slope. An 18-year-old male is sitting in the snow holding his knee. You introduce yourself and ask if you can help. He says he twisted his knee but refuses your help. You repeatedly attempt to question the patient and he still refuses any help. Describe what you would do.

   _____
   _____
   _____
   _____
   _____

STUDY NOTES

Table 4.1. Outline of Assessment

First Impression
↓
Urgent Survey
↓
Nonurgent Survey
↓
Ongoing Survey

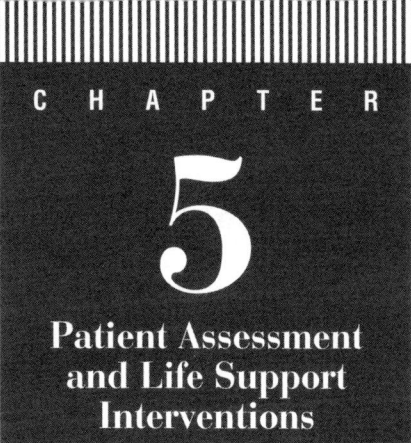

CHAPTER 5
Patient Assessment and Life Support Interventions

CONCLUDING OBJECTIVES

The learner will:

Content

- Explain the basic components of a first impression

- Explain the components and differences of a rapid body survey and a whole body survey

- Explain the basic components of an urgent survey for the unresponsive patient

- Explain the basic components of an urgent survey for the responsive patient (both injured and ill)

- Explain trauma/medical history and focused body survey

- Explain the following mnemonics
  AVPU
  SAMPLE
  DCAP-BTLS
  OPQRST
  CMS

- Explain the significance of interventions

- Explain transport decisions and considerations

- Explain the basic components of the nonurgent and ongoing surveys

Skill Performance

- Demonstrate a complete patient assessment for an unresponsive patient

- Demonstrate a complete patient assessment for a responsive injured (trauma) patient

- Demonstrate a complete patient assessment for a responsive ill (medical) patient

CHAPTER 5 STUDY QUESTIONS

1. List the four components of patient assessment.
   _____
   _____
   _____
   _____

2. What information is gathered in the first impression?
   _____
   _____
   _____
   _____
   _____
   _____

3. To reduce your exposure to possible infection, what should you do before beginning the urgent survey?
   _____

4. Describe the following anatomical terms.
   Prone _____
   Semi-prone _____
   Supine _____

5. What should be the first thing you determine in the urgent survey?
   _____

6. When is the patient considered unresponsive?
   _____

7. If the patient is unresponsive, describe the turning priorities when the patient is prone or semi-prone.

Breathing normal	No neck or back injury
	Possible neck or back injury
Breathing not normal	

8. When you determine that a patient is unresponsive, you should

_____
_____

9. One important concern when dealing with an unresponsive trauma patient is

_____

10. Describe the single-rescuer turning technique.

_____
_____
_____
_____
_____

11. What is the most common cause of airway obstruction in an unresponsive patient?

_____

Why?

_____

12. What is the preferred method of opening the airway in an unresponsive patient where trauma is unlikely?

_____

13. What method should be used for opening an airway if there is suspected neck injury?

_____

14. Once the airway is opened in an unresponsive patient, proceed with the urgent survey by

_____
_____

15. Define gag reflex.

_____
_____

16. If the patient has no gag reflex, the rescuer should

_____

17. If an unresponsive patient is breathing effectively, what should you watch for?

_____

18. If breathing is ineffective or absent, begin _____.

19. Describe rescue breathing.
    _____
    _____

20. Why should you use a pocket face mask or bag-valve mask?
    _____
    _____

21. Once you have determined the patient is breathing (or have given two rescue breaths), you should
    _____
    _____

22. If the patient has no pulse, you should _____

23. What should any patient who is unresponsive due to trauma be assumed to have?
    _____

24. What does the rapid body survey in the unresponsive patient help determine?
    _____

25. During the urgent body survey, severe bleeding is found. What kind of intervention is called for in this situation?
    _____
    _____

26. After the ABCs, the next steps in the urgent survey of the unresponsive patient are
    _____
    _____

27. Define the acronym SAMPLE that helps you remember what a patient history should include
    S _____
    A _____
    M _____
    P _____
    L _____
    E _____

28. List the two types of assessment of the entire body.
    _____

29. What is the rapid body survey?
    _____

30. How is the whole body survey performed?

   _____

31. Describe how the mnemonic DECAP-BTLS is useful in helping you remember things to look for during the rapid body survey.

   D _____
   E _____
   C _____
   A _____
   P _____
   B _____
   T _____
   L _____
   S _____

32. How do you assess CMS?

   Circulation _____
   Motion   _____
   Sensation   _____

33. Describe procedures for conducting the rapid body survey and whole body survey for each part of the body.

   Head _____

   Neck _____

   Chest _____

   Abdomen and pelvis _____

   Lower extremities _____

   Upper extremities _____

   Back _____

34. Describe the techniques for removing contact lenses.

   _____
   _____

35. When should you never remove a contact lens?

36. What is crepitus?

37. What should be checked in the extremity distal to a fracture or injury?
_____, _____, and _____

38. Why should you ask the patient to squeeze both your hands simultaneously?

39. What are interventions?

40. Describe the recovery position (semi-prone and NATO position).

41. What is the Golden Hour?

42. Without hospital care during the Golden Hour, a patient with a serious or life-threatening injury or illness reduces his or her chance of survival for every _____ that passes.

43. Describe the urgent survey techniques of the responsive patient.

44. What does a trauma history include?

45. What two questions should you always ask a trauma patient?

46. List important things to question the injured patient about his or her pain in the following areas.

    General _____

    Head _____

    Neck or Back _____

    Chest _____

    Abdomen _____

    Pelvis _____

    Extremities _____

47. After completing the history in a responsive (injured/trauma) patient, perform the _____.

48. Describe the trauma focused body survey.

49. While you are waiting to transport your responsive patient, perform the _____ and obtain a SAMPLE history.

50. What are the three most important signs and symptoms of an ill patient?

51. List some significant symptoms of variations from normal functions.

    Nonspecific _____

    Respiratory _____

    Circulatory _____

    Digestive _____

    Genitourinary _____

    Musculoskeletal/Neurologic _____

    Cutaneous _____

52. What does the medical history include?

53. Define the mnemonic OPQRST that can be used to remember questions to ask about pain.

O _____

P _____

Q _____

R _____

S _____

T _____

54. Describe the medical focused body survey.

Head _____

Neck _____

Chest _____

Abdomen _____

Skin _____

Extremities _____

Back _____

55. While waiting to transport the responsive ill patient, expand the focused body survey into a complete _____.

56. When should you perform the nonurgent survey?

_____

_____

57. Outline the main steps of the nonurgent survey.

_____

_____

_____

58. When can the nonurgent survey be abbreviated or omitted?

_____

_____

59. What is the purpose of the ongoing survey?

_____

60. How often should patients be monitored?

Stable _____

Unstable _____

61. What does monitoring consist of?

   _____

   _____

   _____

62. List the order in which the following body areas are to be assessed during the body survey.

   ___ Abdomen and pelvis

   ___ Chest

   ___ Lower extremities

   ___ Upper extremities

   ___ Back

   ___ Head

   ___ Neck

Chapter 5 Local Protocol

1. List local patrol procedures for handling the assessment of the unresponsive patient.

   _____

   _____

   _____

   _____

   _____

2. List local patrol procedures for the assessment of a responsive patient.

   _____

   _____

   _____

   _____

   _____

CHAPTER 5 SKILL PERFORMANCE REQUIREMENTS

- Review *Outdoor Emergency Care* scenarios 5.1, 5. 2, 5.3, 5.4, and 5.5

- Demonstrate single-rescuer turning techniques

- Demonstrate the techniques for a rapid body survey and a whole body survey

- Demonstrate the technique for removing contact lenses

- Demonstrate the basic assessment techniques as they pertain to the urgent survey for the unresponsive patient

- Demonstrate the basic assessment techniques as they pertain to the urgent survey for the responsive patient which includes the trauma history and focused body survey

- Demonstrate the basic assessment techniques as they pertain to the urgent survey for the responsive patient which includes the medical history and focused body survey

- Demonstrate the basic assessment techniques as they pertain to the nonurgent and ongoing surveys

- Demonstrate a complete patient assessment for an unresponsive patient

- Demonstrate a complete patient assessment for a responsive injured (trauma) patient

- Demonstrate a complete patient assessment for a responsive ill (medical) patient

Skill Performance Guidelines

- Vital Signs Determination (see Chapter 3)
- Patient Assessment—Body Survey (Rapid and Whole)
- Patient Assessment—Unresponsive Patient
- Patient Assessment—Responsive Patient—Injured (Trauma)
- Patient Assessment—Responsive Patient—Ill (Medical)
- Patient Assessment—Nonurgent and Ongoing Surveys

First Impression

- Notes the presence of dangers or hazards.

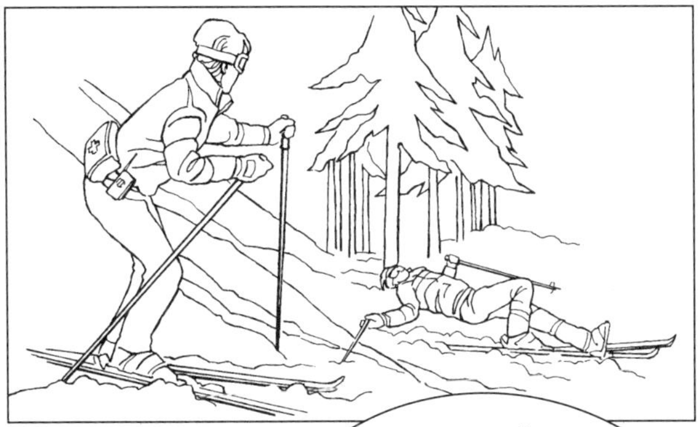

- Notes the number of patient(s) and responsiveness of each

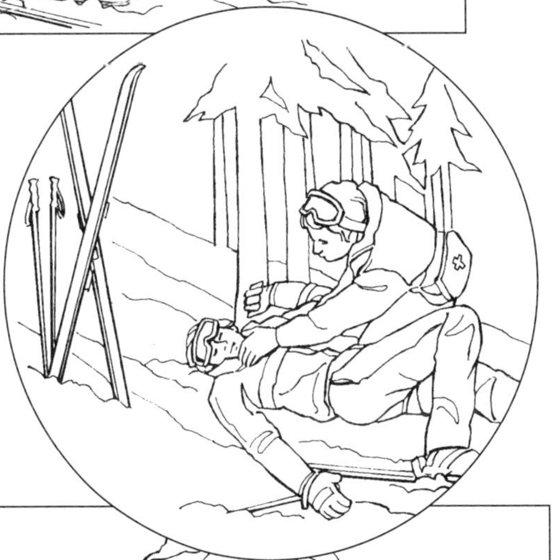

- Determines the nature of the incident and the mechanism of injury (MOI)

- Evaluates the need to access or extricate the patient

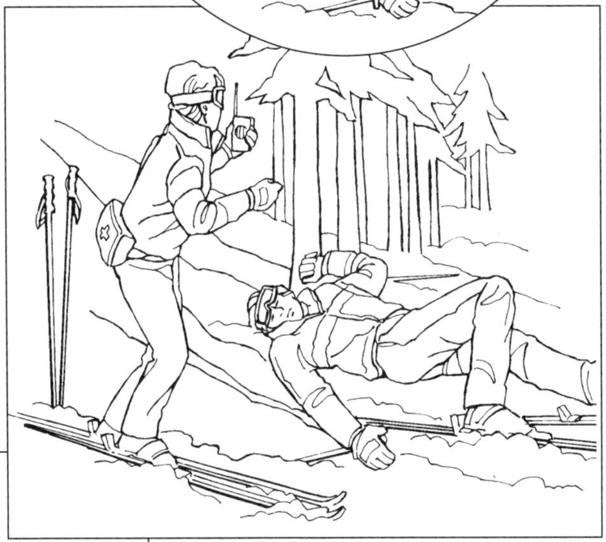

- Notes the need for personnel or equipment

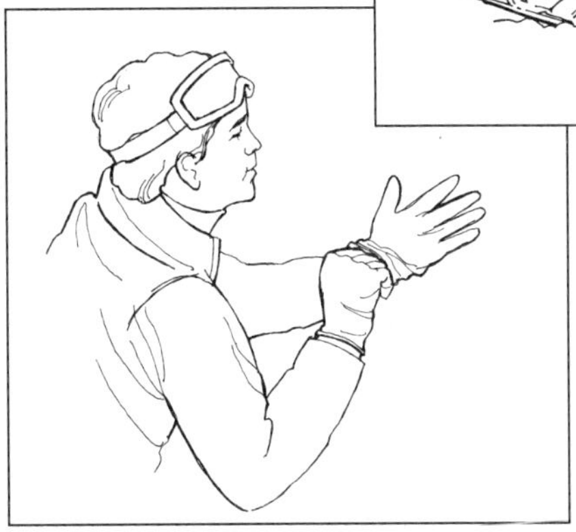

- Initiates BSI precautions

Urgent Survey—Unresponsive Patient

- Determines the level of responsiveness (LOR)

- Calls for transport, equipment, assistance, and/or EMS as needed

- Opens airway

- Guards cervical spine as needed

- Checks breathing: interventions = confirms open airway and/or provides rescue breathing

- Checks carotid pulse: intervention = CPR

- Checks for severe bleeding: intervention = control bleeding

- Obtains SAMPLE history

- Performs rapid body survey: interventions = immediately as needed

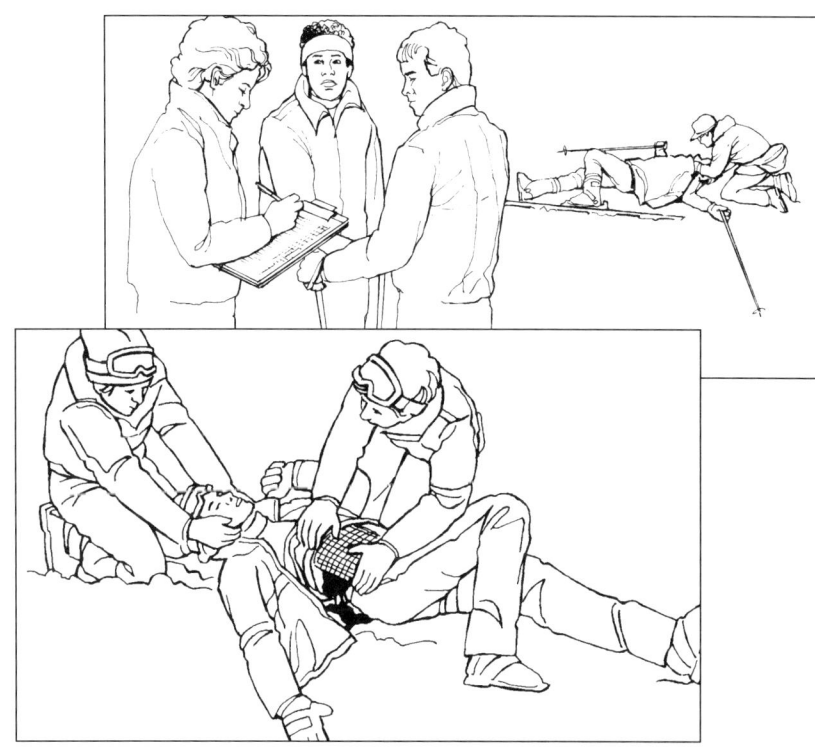

- Determines pulse and respiration rates

- Stabilizes and maintains body temperature

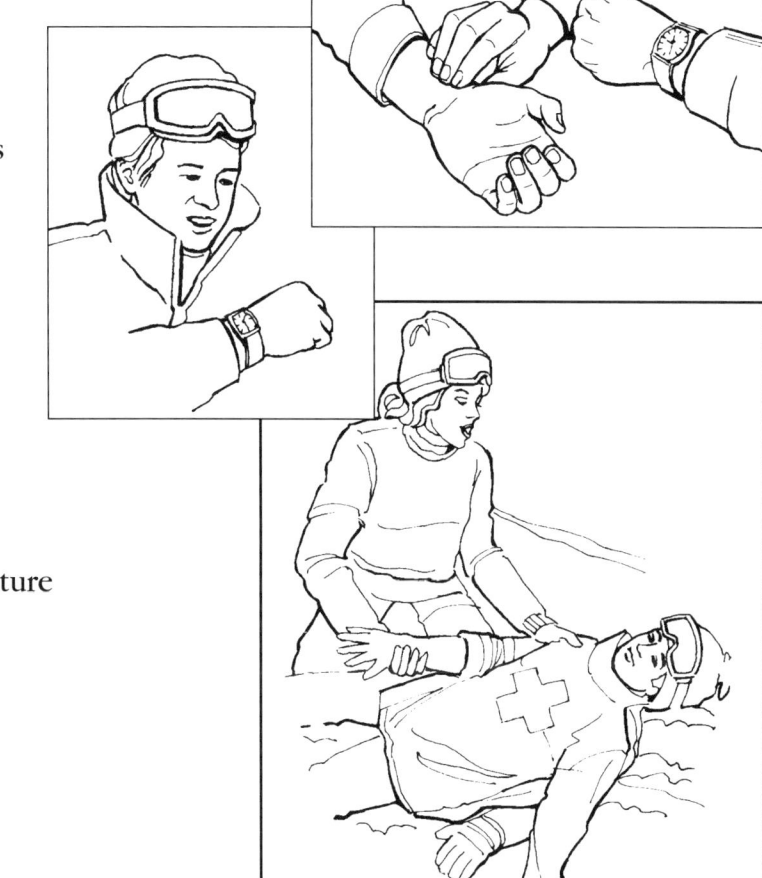

- In a trauma patient, manually and/or mechanically stabilizes the neck, or

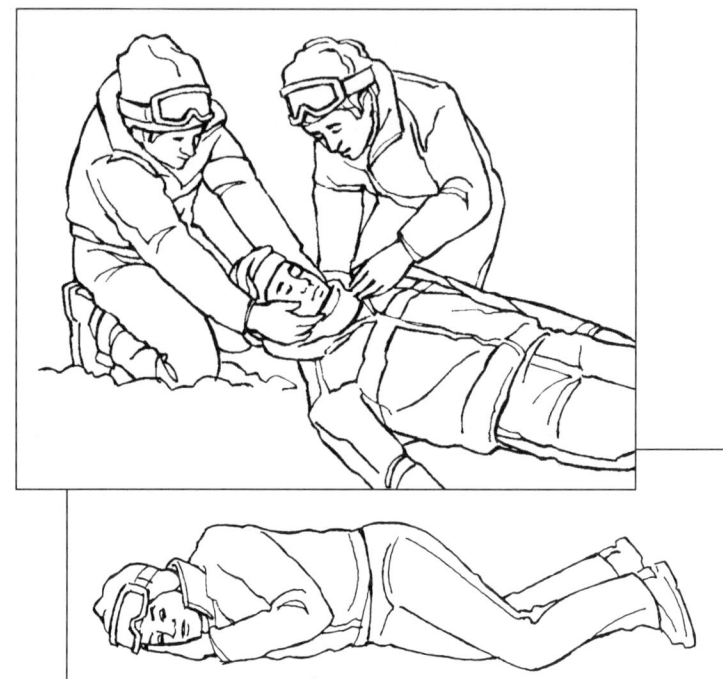

In a non-trauma patient, places the patient in a semi-prone position

- Transports off the hill

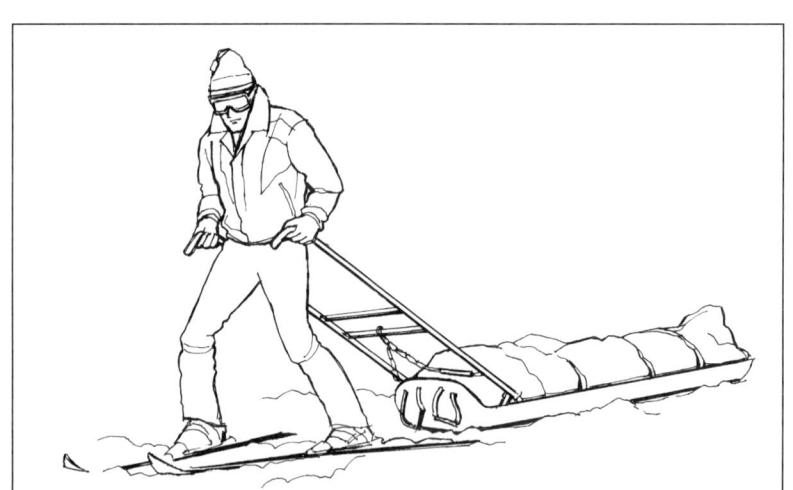

- Performs ongoing survey *while awaiting* transport (if possible)

Urgent Survey: Responsive Patient (Injured And Ill)

- Offers to assist

- Assesses ABCs
  Illustrated in Urgent Survey: Unresponsive Patient

- Checks for severe bleeding:
  intervention = control bleeding
  Illustrated in Urgent Survey: Unresponsive Patient

- Observes patient expression and skin condition

- Obtains chief complaint

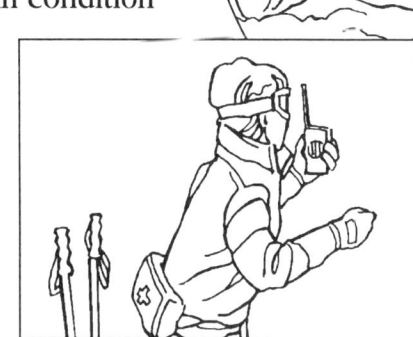

- Calls for transport, equipment, assistance, and/or EMS as needed

- Obtains trauma history (DCAP-BTLS) and confirms MOI
  or
- Obtains medical history (OPQRST)

Trauma History (DCAP-BTLS)	Medical History (OPQRST)
Deformities	Onset – when did the symptoms start?
Contusions	Provocation – what "provokes" the symptoms?
Abraisions	Quality – if pain, what is the pain like?
Punctures, Penetrations	Radiation – does the symptom radiate to another area?
Burns, Bleeding	Severity – how bad is it?
Tenderness	Time – how long has it lasted?
Lacerations	
Swelling	

- Conducts focused body survey of the area of chief complaint, confirms chief complaint

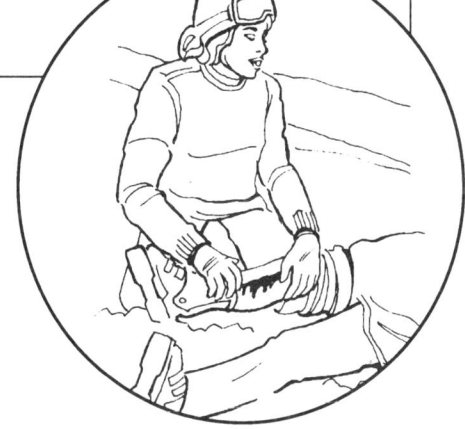

- Stabilizes and maintains body temperature

- Determines pulse and respiration rates

- If **injured (trauma)** patient has *abnormal ABCs, significant MOI, or has poor general impression*, performs rapid body survey, SAMPLE history, interventions, and rapid transport
  or
  If **ill (medical)** patient has *abnormal ABCs* or has *poor general impression*, performs rapid body survey, SAMPLE history, interventions, and rapid transport

- Provides care for chief complaint: interventions = as needed

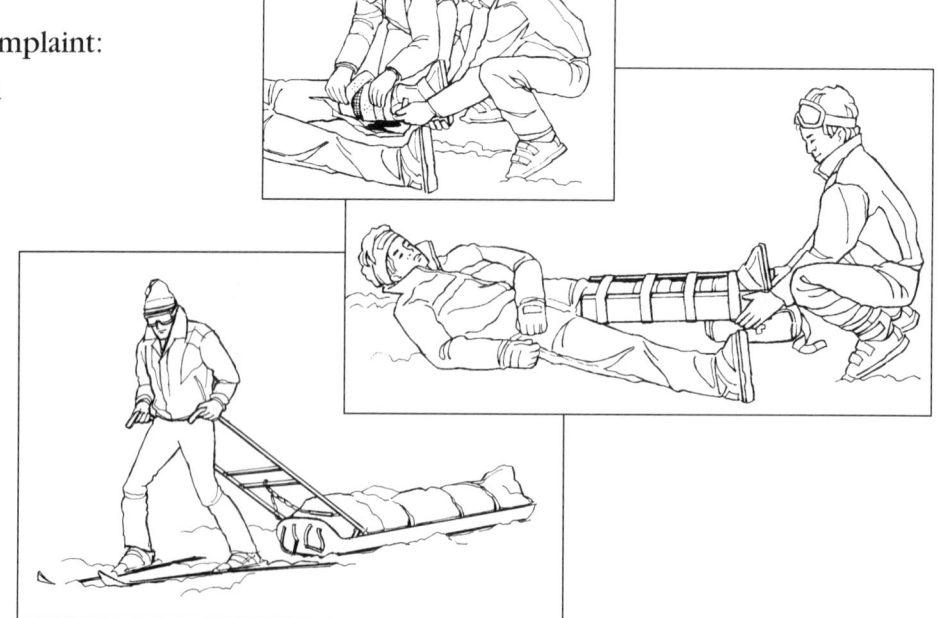

- Transports off the hill

- Performs ongoing survey **while awaiting** transport *(if possible)*

Nonurgent Survey—Patient is in a Warm Shelter

- Assesses and records LOR and vital signs, including pulse, respirations, and blood pressure

- Updates SAMPLE history

- Performs whole body survey (undress as needed for survey)

- Cares for all problems found

- Arranges or provides for transportation

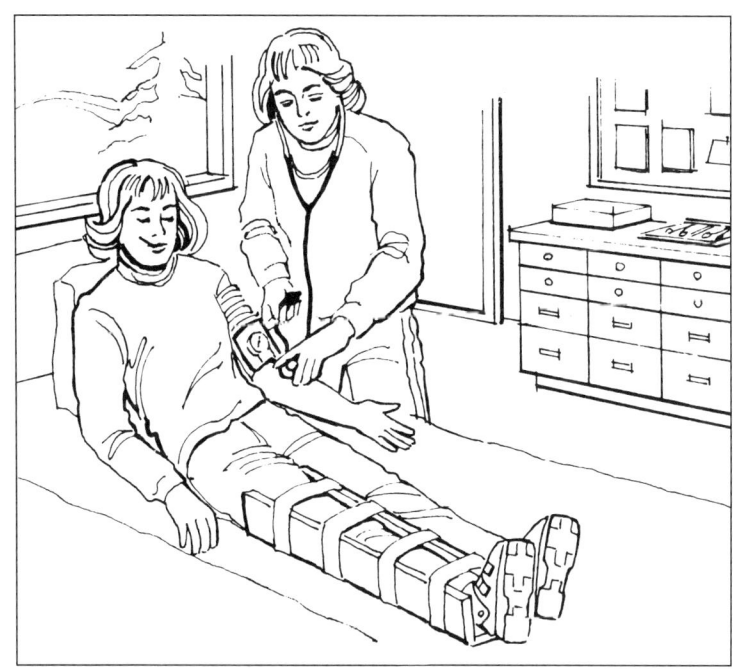

Ongoing Survey—Responsive or Unresponsive Patient

- For responsive patient: How are you feeling now? Has anything changes?

- Rechecks LOR, ABCs, and vital signs = Document

- Rechecks signs and symptoms of conditions found

- Monitors results of care provided and adjusts accordingly

- Documents all aspects completely

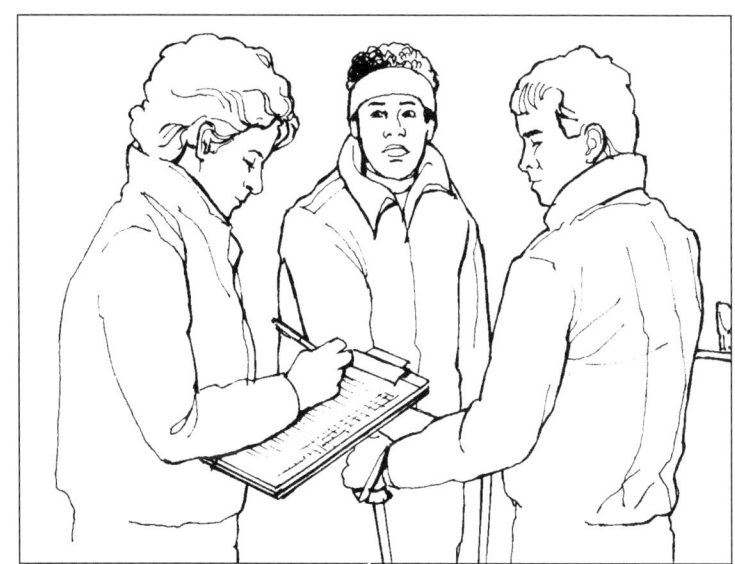

- Repeats at regular intervals until patient is released

Body Survey (to be used during Urgent Survey [*rapid body survey*] and Nonurgent Survey [*whole body survey*])

Note: First five bullets are illustrated in Urgent Survey: Unresponsive Patient

- Assesses level of responsiveness (AVPU)
- Obtains SAMPLE history
- Guards cervical spine as appropriate
- Confirms ABC's
- Confirms control of severe bleeding

- Examines head (skull, facial bones, pupils, ears, nose, mouth)

- Examines and palpates neck (cervical spine, anterior neck, medical-alert tags)

- Examines and palpates chest (abnormality and deformity)

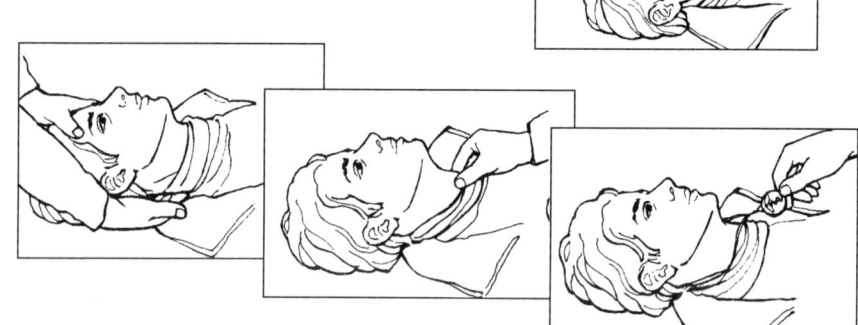

- Examines and palpates abdomen (all quadrants)

- Examines and palpates pelvis

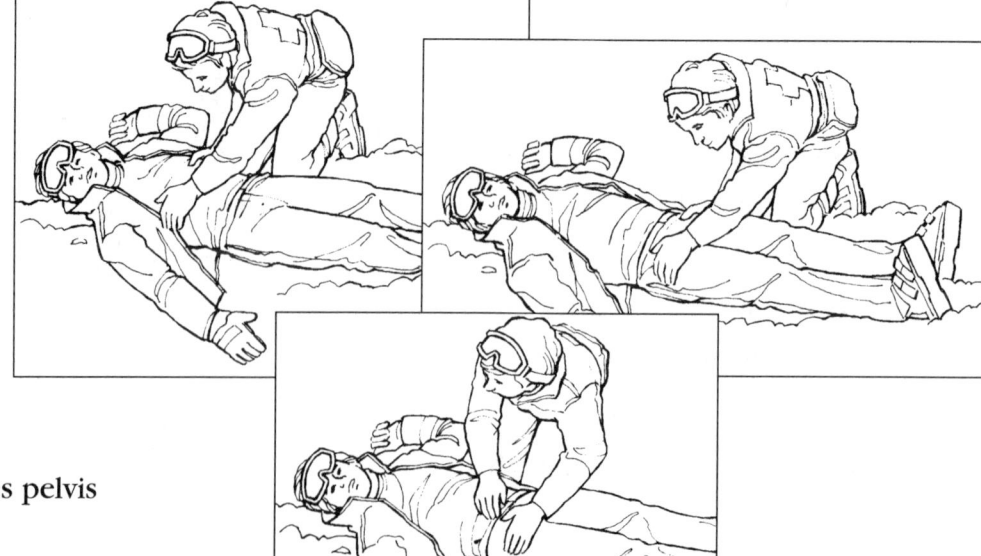

80 OEC Study Book

- Examines and palpates each lower extremity (abnormality, circulatory and neurologic function, medical-alert tags)

- Examines and palpates each upper extremity (abnormality, circulatory and neurologic function, medical-alert tags)

- Examines and palpates back and buttocks

- Determines pulse and respiration rates

- Forms general impression

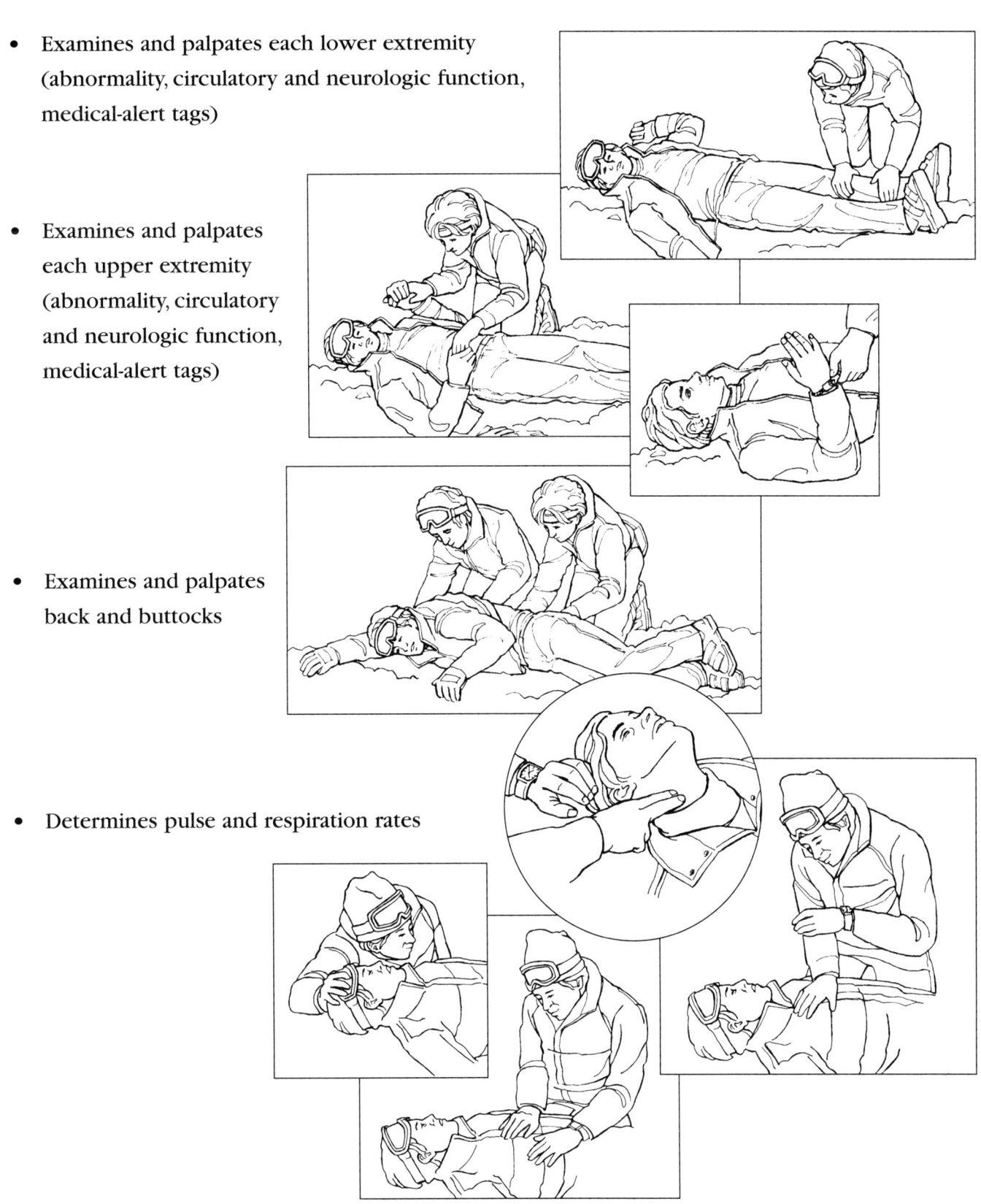

Chapter 5 Scenarios

1. You get called to the scene of an unresponsive patient on the hill who has a facial laceration. Describe your patient assessment from first impression, to urgent survey, to nonurgent survey, to ongoing survey.

   _____
   _____
   _____
   _____
   _____

2. You get called to the cafeteria where a 30-year-old male reportedly fainted and is now responsive and sitting in a chair. Describe your patient assessment.

   _____
   _____
   _____
   _____
   _____

3. You arrive on the scene where there is a 20-year-old snowboarder in the terrain park just below a jump. He complains of an injured shoulder. Describe your patient assessment.

   _____
   _____
   _____
   _____
   _____

STUDY NOTES

PATIENT ASSESSMENT—UNRESPONSIVE PATIENT

Objective: To demonstrate the ability to determine the baseline condition of an unresponsive patient and to make an appropriate transport decision.

SKILL	YES	NO	NA	NOTATIONS
FIRST IMPRESSION				
• Notes the presence of dangers or hazards.				
• Notes the number of patient(s) and responsiveness of each				
• Determines the nature of the incident and the mechanism of injury (MOI)				
• Evaluates the need to access or extricate the patient				
• Notes the need for personnel or equipment				
• Initiates BSI precautions				
URGENT SURVEY—UNRESPONSIVE PATIENT				
• Determines the level of responsiveness (LOR)				
• Calls for transport, equipment, assistance, and/or EMS as needed				
• Opens airway				
• Guards cervical spine as needed				
• Checks breathing: interventions = confirms open airway and/or provides rescue breathing				
• Checks carotid pulse: intervention = CPR				
• Checks for severe bleeding: intervention = control bleeding				
• Obtains SAMPLE history				
• Performs rapid body survey: interventions = immediately as needed				
• Determines pulse and respiration rates				
• Stabilizes and maintains body temperature				
• In a trauma patient, manually and/or mechanically stabilizes the neck, Or				
• In a non-trauma patient, places the patient in a semi-prone position				
• Transports off the hill				
• Performs ongoing survey *while awaiting* transport *(if possible)*				
Did the trainee or patroller adequately demonstrate the performance criteria of these skills?				

COMMENTS

PATIENT ASSESSMENT—RESPONSIVE PATIENT—INJURED (TRAUMA)

Objective: To demonstrate the ability to determine the baseline condition and specific injury(ies) in a responsive injured patient.

SKILL	YES	NO	NA	NOTATIONS
FIRST IMPRESSION				
• Notes the presence of dangers or hazards.				
• Notes the number of patient(s) and responsiveness of each				
• Determines the nature of the incident and the mechanism of injury (MOI)				
• Evaluates the need to access or extricate the patient				
• Notes the need for personnel or equipment				
• Initiates BSI precautions				
URGENT SURVEY—RESPONSIVE PATIENT				
• Offers to assist				
• Assesses ABCs				
• Checks for severe bleeding: intervention = control bleeding				
• Observes patient expression and skin condition				
• Obtains chief complaint (CC)				
• Calls for transport, equipment, assisstance, and/or EMS as needed				
• Obtains trauma history (DCAP-BTLS) and confirms MOI				
• Conducts focused body survey of the area of chief complaint, confirms chief complaint				
• Stabilizes and maintains body temperature				
• Determines pulse and respiration rates				
• If patient has *abnormal ABCs, significant MOI*, or has *poor general impression*, performs **rapid body survey, SAMPLE history, interventions**, and **rapid transport**				
• Provides care for chief complaint: interventions = as needed				
• Transports off the hill				
• Performs ongoing survey *while awaiting* transport (if possible)				
Did the trainee or patroller adequately demonstrate the performance criteria of these skills?				

COMMENTS

PATIENT ASSESSMENT—RESPONSIVE PATIENT—ILL (MEDICAL)

Objective: To demonstrate the ability to determine the baseline condition and specific complaint of a responsive ill patient.

SKILL	YES	NO	NA	NOTATIONS
FIRST IMPRESSION				
• Notes the presence of dangers or hazards.				
• Notes the number of patient(s) and responsiveness of each				
• Determines the nature of the incident and the mechanism of injury (MOI)				
• Evaluates the need to access or extricate the patient				
• Notes the need for personnel or equipment				
• Initiates BSI precautions				
URGENT SURVEY—RESPONSIVE PATIENT				
• Offers to assist				
• Assesses ABCs				
• Checks for severe bleeding: intervention = control bleeding				
• Observes patient expression and skin condition				
• Obtains chief complaint (CC)				
• Calls for transport, equipment, assisstance, and/or EMS as needed				
• Obtains medical (OPQRST) history				
• Conducts focused body survey of the area of chief complaint, confirms chief complaint				
• Stabilizes and maintains body temperature				
• Determines pulse and respiration rates				
• If patient has *abnormal ABCs* or has *poor general impression* performs **rapid body survey, SAMPLE history, interventions**, and **rapid transport**				
• Provides care for chief complaint: interventions = as needed				
• Transports off the hill				
• Performs ongoing survey *while awaiting* transport (if possible)				
Did the trainee or patroller adequately demonstrate the performance criteria of these skills?				

COMMENTS

PATIENT ASSESSMENT—NONURGENT AND ONGOING SURVEYS

Objective: To demonstrate the ability to perform a complete nonurgent and ongoing survey.

SKILL	YES	NO	NA	NOTATIONS
NONURGENT SURVEY—Patient is in a Warm Shelter				
• Assess and records LOR and vital signs, including pulse, respirations, and blood pressure				
• Updates SAMPLE history				
• Performs whole body survey (undress as needed for survey)				
• Cares for all problems found				
• Arranges or provides for transportation				

SKILL	YES	NO	NA	NOTATIONS
ONGOING SURVEY—Responsive or Unresponsive Patient				
• For responsive patient: How are you feeling now? Has anything changed?				
• Rechecks LOR, ABCs, and vital signs = Document				
• Rechecks signs and symptoms found				
• Monitors results of care provided and adjusts accordingly				
• Documents all aspects completely				
• Repeats at regular intervals until patient is released				
Did the trainee or patroller adequately demonstrate the performance criteria of these skills?				

COMMENTS

PATIENT ASSESSMENT—BODY SURVEY (RAPID AND WHOLE)

Objective: Demonstrate the ability to perform a body survey on a patient rapidly on scene or in a comfortable environment.

SKILL	YES	NO	NA	NOTATIONS
FIRST IMPRESSION				
• Assesses level of responsiveness AVPU)				
• Obtains SAMPLE history				
• Guards cervical spine as appropriate				
• Confirms ABCs				
• Confirms control of severe bleeding				
• Examines head (skull, facial bones, pupils, ears, nose, mouith)				
• Examines and palpates neck (cervical spine, anterior neck, medical-alert tags				
• Examines and palpates chest (abnormality and deformity)				
• Examines and palpates abdomen (all quadrants)				
• Examines and palpates pelvis				
• Examines and palpates each lower extremity (abnormality, circulatory and neurologic function, medical-alert tags)				
• Examines and palpates each upper extremity (abnormality, circulatory and neurologic function, medical-alert tags)				
• Examines and palpates back and buttocks				
• Determines pulse and respiration rates				
• Forms general impression				
Did the trainee or patroller adequately demonstrate the performance criteria of these skills?				

COMMENTS

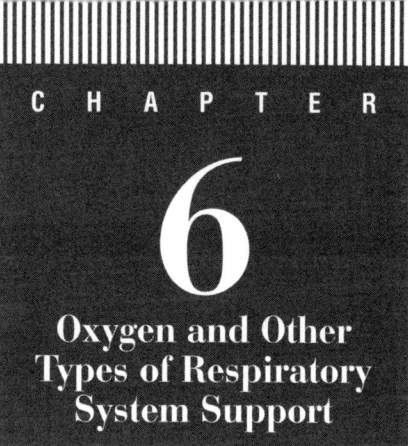

CHAPTER 6
Oxygen and Other Types of Respiratory System Support

CONCLUDING OBJECTIVES

The learner will:

Content

- Recognize the body's need for oxygen

- Explain the use of oxygen systems and other mechanical aids to resuscitation

Skill Performance

- Demonstrate the basic techniques used for oxygen administration

- Demonstrate the use of airway adjuncts: non-rebreather masks, pocket masks, mouth shields, nasal cannulas, bag-valve-masks, oral airways, and suction devices

CHAPTER 6 STUDY QUESTIONS

1. Inhaled air contains _____ oxygen.

2. The lungs extract about _____ of the oxygen in the inhaled air, so that exhaled air contains _____.

3. What does psi stand for?
   _____

4. When full, how many liters of oxygen and how much time does each cylinder of oxygen have at a flow rate of 10 lpm?

   D Cylinder _____

   E Cylinder _____

   M Cylinder _____

5. How do you determine how when a cylinder of oxygen is empty?
   _____

6. Patients who require oxygen can be divided into two general categories. List these categories.
   _____
   _____

7. List the indications for oxygen use.
   _____
   _____
   _____
   _____
   _____

8. Identify the differences between these oxygen devices regarding use and protection.

Non-rebreather mask	
Pocket mask with oxygen inlet	
Mouth shield	
Nasal cannula	
Bag-valve-mask	

OEC Study Book 91

9. Describe the procedure for administering oxygen.

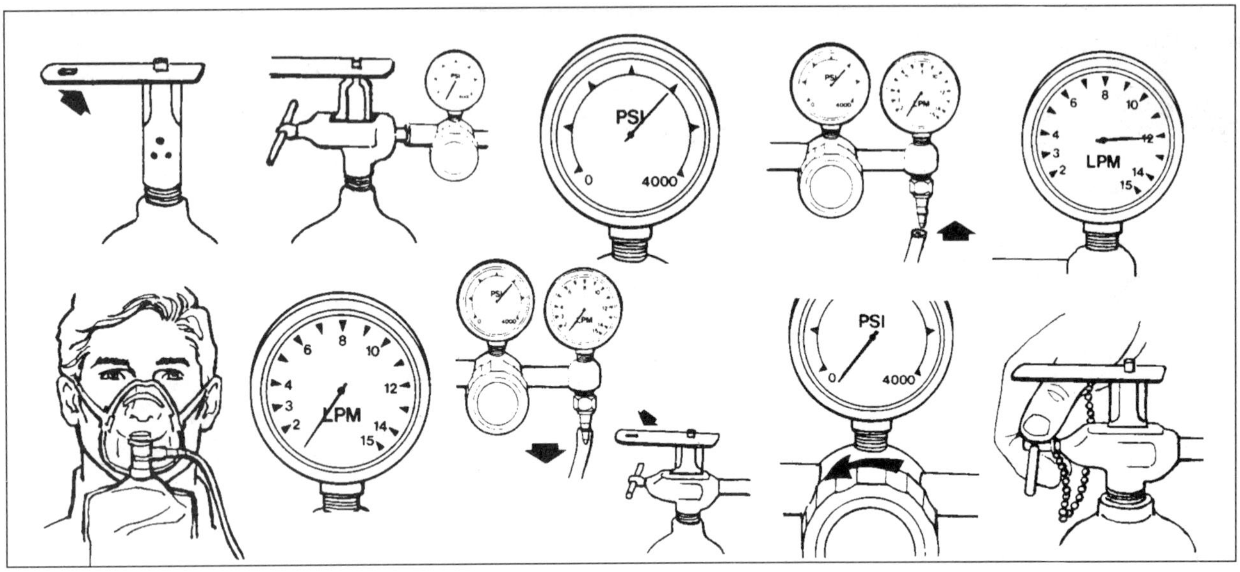

_____
_____
_____
_____
_____
_____
_____
_____

10. How do you clean the tank outlet of debris?
_____
_____

11. List some precautions that should be taken when using an oxygen tank.
_____
_____
_____
_____

12. To decrease the threat of disease transmission from patient to rescuer during rescue breathing, the rescuer should _____.

13. Describe how to measure an oral airway for a proper fit.
_____
_____

92   OEC Study Book

14 List the steps in inserting an oral airway.

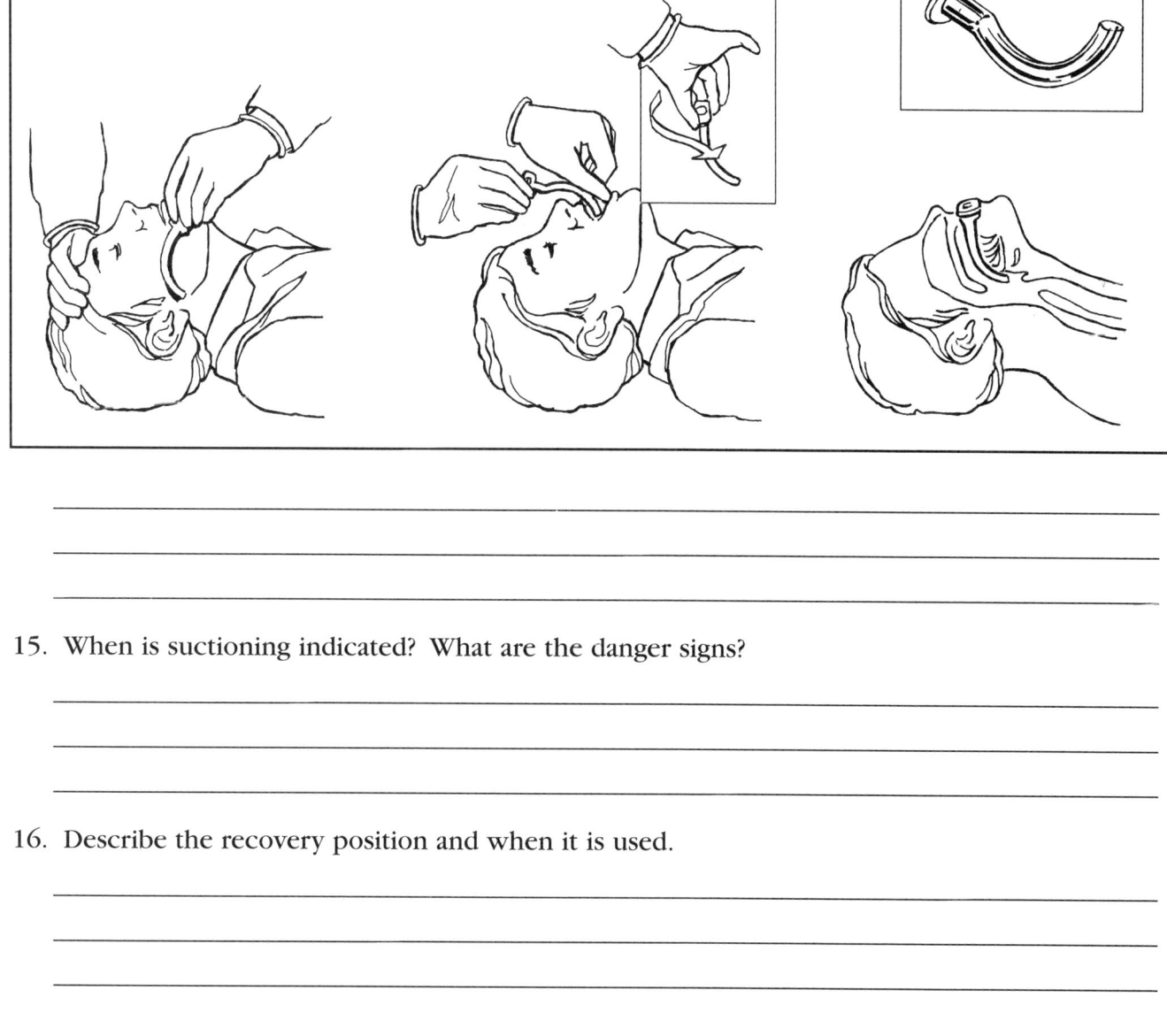

_____
_____
_____

15. When is suctioning indicated? What are the danger signs?

_____
_____
_____

16. Describe the recovery position and when it is used.

_____
_____
_____

Chapter 6 Local Protocol

1. Describe all the equipment contained in your patrol's O_2 pack.

_____
_____
_____
_____
_____

2. Outline local patrol procedures for use of oxygen.

   On-the-hill

   Type

   _____

   Instructions for use

   _____
   _____
   _____

   Local patrol protocols

   _____
   _____
   _____

   In the aid room

   Type(s)

   _____

   Instructions for use

   _____
   _____
   _____

   Local patrol protocols

   _____
   _____
   _____

3. Outline local patrol procedures for each.

   Pocket Masks

   Type(s)

   _____

   Instructions and local patrol procedures for use and care

   _____
   _____

   Mouth Shields

   Type(s)

   _____

Instructions and local patrol procedures for use and care

_____
_____
_____

Oral Airways

    Type(s)

_____

    Instructions and local patrol procedures for use and care

_____
_____
_____

Suction Devices

    Type(s)

_____

    Instructions and local patrol procedures for use and care

_____
_____
_____

Bag-valve-mask

    Type(s)

_____

    Instructions and local patrol procedures for use and care

_____
_____
_____

Other Devices

    Type(s)

_____

    Instructions and local patrol procedures for use and care

_____
_____
_____

CHAPTER 6 SKILL PERFORMANCE REQUIREMENTS

- Demonstrate the basic techniques used for oxygen administration

- Demonstrate the use of airway adjuncts: non-rebreather masks, pocket masks, mouth shields, nasal cannulas, bag-valve masks, oral airways, and suction devices

Skill Performance Guidelines

- Vital Signs Determination (see Chapter 3)
- Patient Assessment—Body Survey (Rapid and Whole) (see Chapter 5)
- Patient Assessment—Unresponsive Patient (see Chapter 5)
- Patient Assessment—Responsive Patient—Injured (Trauma) (see Chapter 5)
- Patient Assessment—Responsive Patient—Ill (Medical) (see Chapter 5)
- Patient Assessment—Nonurgent and Ongoing Surveys (see Chapter 5)
- Use of Oxygen and Airway Adjuncts

Oropharyngeal Airway

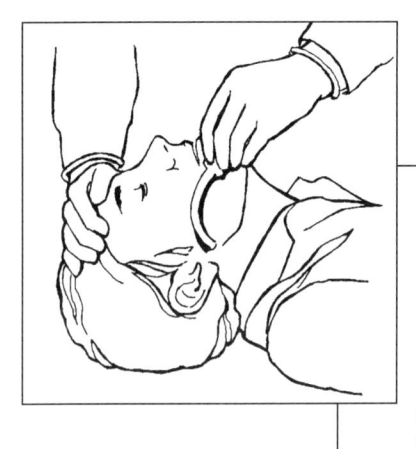
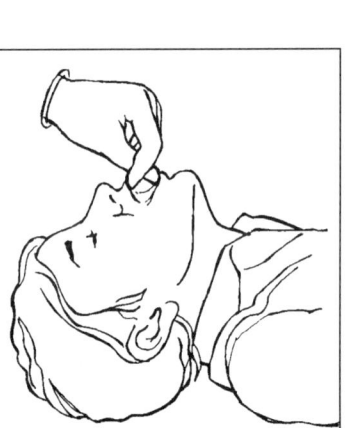

- Selects proper size airway (measures from the corner of the mouth to the angle of the jaw).

- Opens the mouth using an appropriate technique.

- Inserts the airway using an appropriate technique.

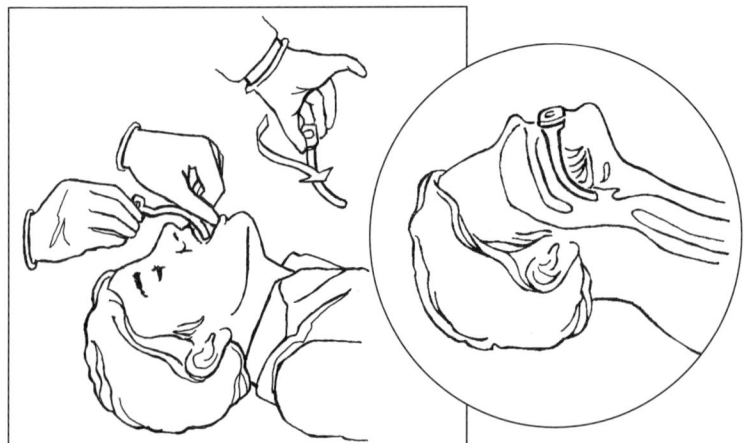

Suctioning of the Oral Cavity

- Assembles, turns on, and tests device.
- Opens the mouth using the crossed-finger technique.
- Inserts rigid tip catheter without suction applied (measures length from corner of mouth to angle of jaw and inserts catheter just until end of tip can be seen).
- Applies suction for no longer than 15 seconds while the rigid catheter is twisted or rotated during withdrawal.

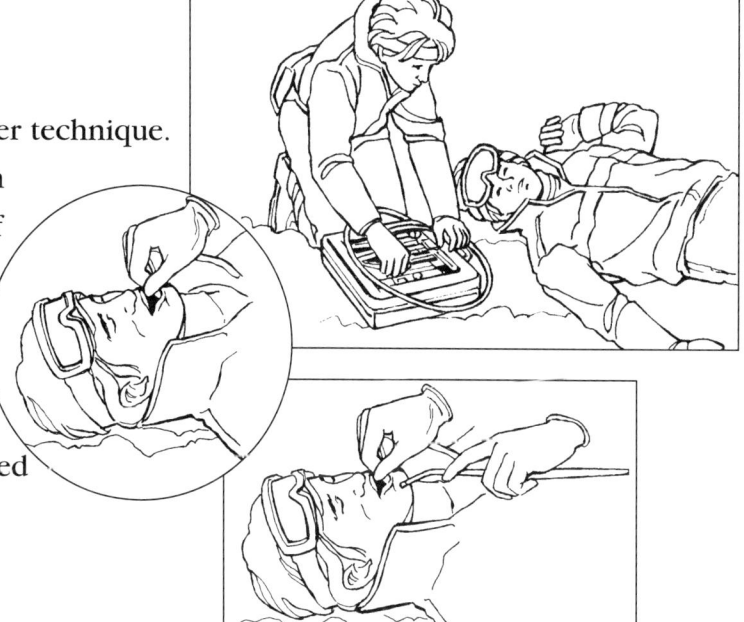

Administration of Oxygen

- Assembles oxygen cylinder and regulator. Checks for leaks.

- Chooses a delivery device by patient need.

    ➤ selects non-rebreather oxygen mask, connects to regulator, initially adjusts oxygen flow to 15 lpm, readjusting to keep bag half-full on inhalation

    ➤ selects nasal cannula, connects to regulator, and adjusts oxygen to 6 lpm maximum

- Applies oxygen delivery device to patient and verifies patient receives oxygen.

- When complete, closes oxygen tank.

- Bleeds regulator device to "0."

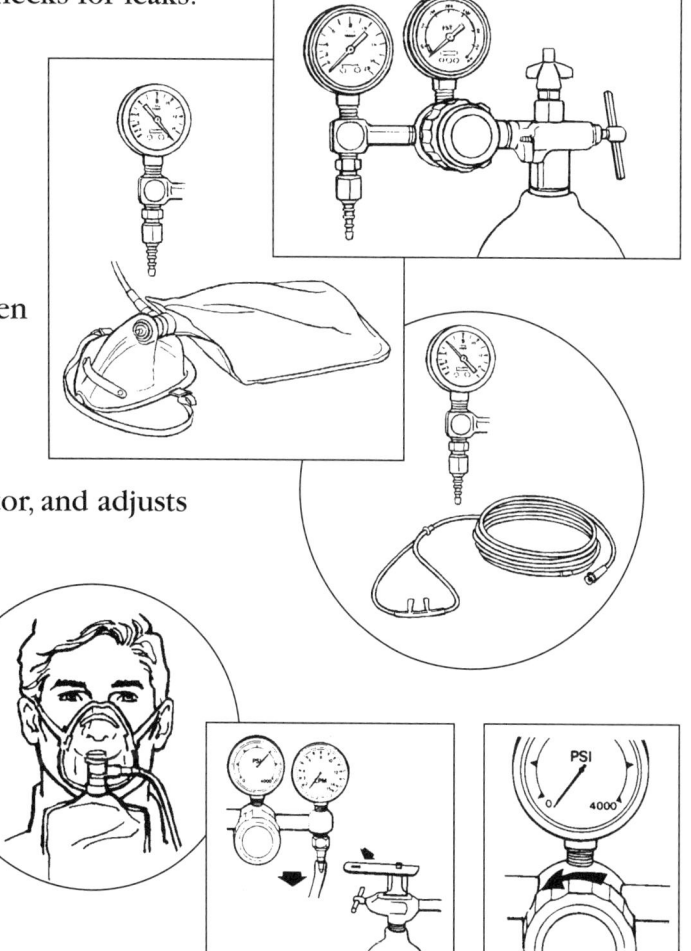

Use of Pocket Mask for Artificial Ventilation

- Assembles mask components as necessary.

- Sizes and inserts airway using appropriate technique.

- Connects oxygen to pocket mask.

- Adjusts oxygen supply to 15 lpm.

- Maintains open airway and mask seal.

- Demonstrates adequate ventilation on a mannequin capable of indicating a minimum 800 cc tidal volume.

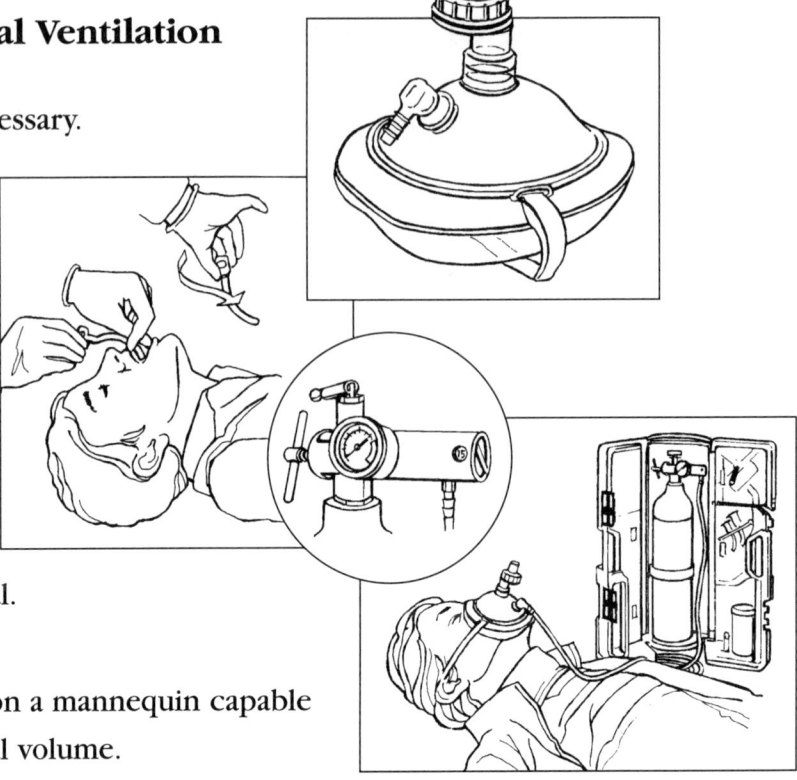

Use of Bag-valve-mask for Artificial Ventilation (Optional Skill)

- Assembles bag-valve mask components, including reservoir.

- Sizes and inserts an airway using appropriate technique.

- Connects oxygen supply to bag-valve mask.

- Adjusts oxygen supply to 15 lpm.

- Maintains open airway and mask seal.

- Demonstrates adequate ventilation on a mannequin capable of indicating a minimum 800 cc tidal volume.

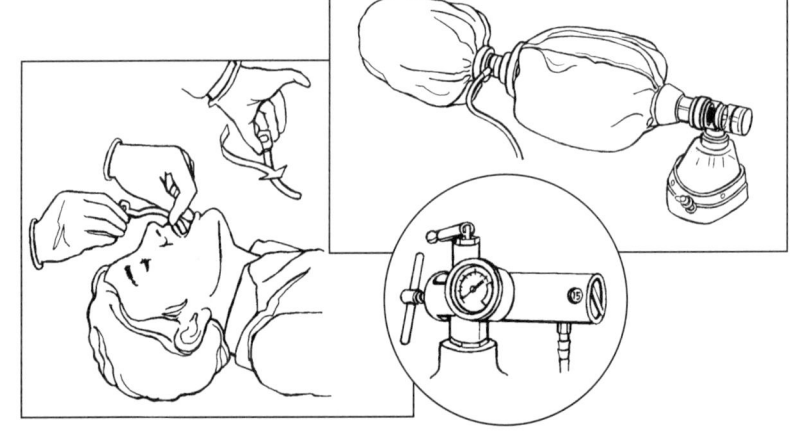

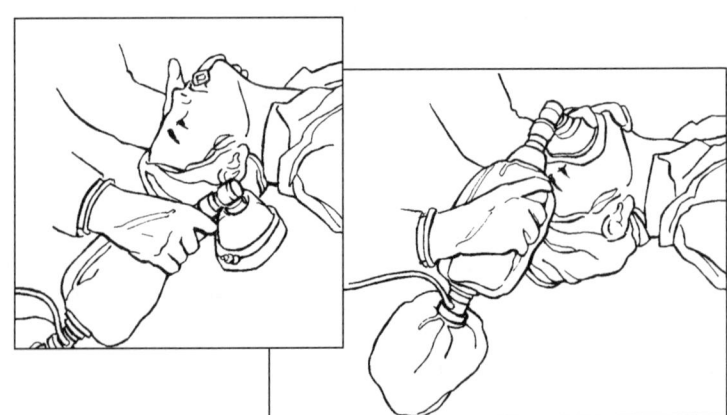

Chapter 6 Scenarios

1. You and another patroller are called to the lodge to examine a woman approximately 65 years old who is having problems breathing. You take with you a pack containing one D cylinder of oxygen, the wrench, and the regulator valve that includes a graduated glass flowmeter, the delivery tubing, a mask, and a cannula. Upon arrival, the patient tells you that she has a history of emphysema. She has come to the area to watch her granddaughter ski.

    1) Which delivery system of oxygen would you use and why?
    2) At what rate would you give this patient oxygen and why?

    _____
    _____
    _____
    _____
    _____

2. Your oxygen cylinder gauge reads pressure 200 or less psi. What do you do?

    _____
    _____
    _____
    _____
    _____

3. You are called to help a 9-year-old male skier who fell 15 feet out of the chair lift. The child is unresponsive and not breathing so you begin rescue breathing. Soon, another patroller comes with the oxygen pack that contains, in addition to the oxygen tank and regulator, a pocket mask, nasal cannula, and a bag-valve-mask.
    1) Which system would you use on this patient and why?
    2) What is the rate of ventilation to be used on this patient, and at what rate should you set the flow of oxygen?

    _____
    _____
    _____
    _____
    _____

STUDY NOTES

USE OF OXYGEN AND AIRWAY ADJUNCTS—OROPHARYNGEAL AIRWAY

Objective: To demonstrate the correct use of oropharyngeal airway

SKILL	YES	NO	NOTATIONS
• Selects proper size airway (measures from the corner of the mouth to the angle of the jaw).			
• Opens the mouth using an appropriate technique.			
• Inserts the airway using an appropriate technique.			
Did the trainee or patroller adequately demonstrate the performance criteria of this skill?			

COMMENTS

USE OF OXYGEN AND AIRWAY ADJUNCTS—SUCTIONING OF THE ORAL CAVITY

Objective: To demonstrate the correct use of suctioning equipment

SKILL	YES	NO	NOTATIONS
• Assembles, turns on, and tests device.			
• Opens the mouth using the crossed-finger technique.			
• Inserts rigid tip catheter without suction applied (measures length from corner of mouth to angle of jaw and inserts the catheter just until end of tip can be seen).			
• Applies suction for no longer than 15 seconds while the rigid catheter is twisted or rotated during withdrawal.			
Did the trainee or patroller adequately demonstrate the performance criteria of this skill?			

COMMENTS

USE OF OXYGEN AND AIRWAY ADJUNCTS—ADMINISTRATION OF OXYGEN

Objective: To demonstrate the correct use of oxygen equipment

SKILL	YES	NO	NOTATIONS
• Assembles oxygen cylinder and regulator and checks for leaks.			
• Chooses a delivery device by patient need. ➢ selects non-rebreather oxygen mask, connects to regulator, initially adjusts oxygen flow to 15 lpm, readjusting to keep bag half-full on inhalation ➢ selects nasal cannula, connects to regulator, and adjusts oxygen to 6 lpm maximum			
• Applies oxygen delivery device to patient and verifies patient receives oxygen			
• When complete, closes oxygen tank.			
• Bleeds regulator device to "0".			
Did the trainee or patroller adequately demonstrate the performance criteria of this skill?			

COMMENTS

USE OF OXYGEN AND AIRWAY ADJUNCTS—USE OF POCKET MASK FOR ARTIFICIAL VENTILATION

Objective: To demonstrate the correct use of oxygen equipment for artificial ventilation

SKILL	YES	NO	NOTATIONS
• Assembles mask components as necessary.			
• Sizes and inserts an airway using appropriate technique.			
• Connects oxygen to pocket mask.			
• Adjusts oxygen supply to 15 lpm.			
• Maintains open airway and mask seal.			
• Demonstrates adequate ventilation on a mannequin capable of indicating a minimum 800cc tidal volume.			
Did the trainee or patroller adequately demonstrate the performance criteria of this skill?			

COMMENTS

USE OF OXYGEN AND AIRWAY ADJUNCTS—USE OF BAG-VALVE-MASK FOR ARTIFICIAL VENTILATION (OPTIONAL SKILL)

Objective: To demonstrate the correct use of oxygen equipment for artificial ventilation

SKILL	YES	NO	NOTATIONS
• Assembles bag-valve-mask components, including reservoir.			
• Sizes and inserts an airway using appropriate technique.			
• Connects oxygen to bag-valve-mask.			
• Adjusts oxygen supply to 15 lpm.			
• Maintains open airway and mask seal.			
• Demonstrates adequate ventilation on a mannequin capable of indicating a minimum 800cc tidal volume.			
Did the trainee or patroller adequately demonstrate the performance criteria of this skill?			

COMMENTS

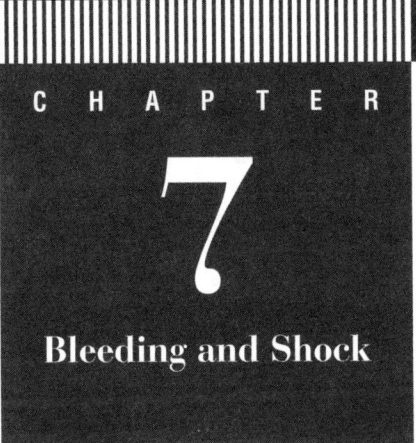

CHAPTER 7
Bleeding and Shock

CONCLUDING OBJECTIVES

The learner will:

Content

- Describe the types and causes of bleeding

- Describe the types of shock

Skill Performance

- Demonstrate the emergency care techniques for controlling external bleeding

- Demonstrate the emergency care techniques for managing internal bleeding

- Demonstrate the appropriate care for shock

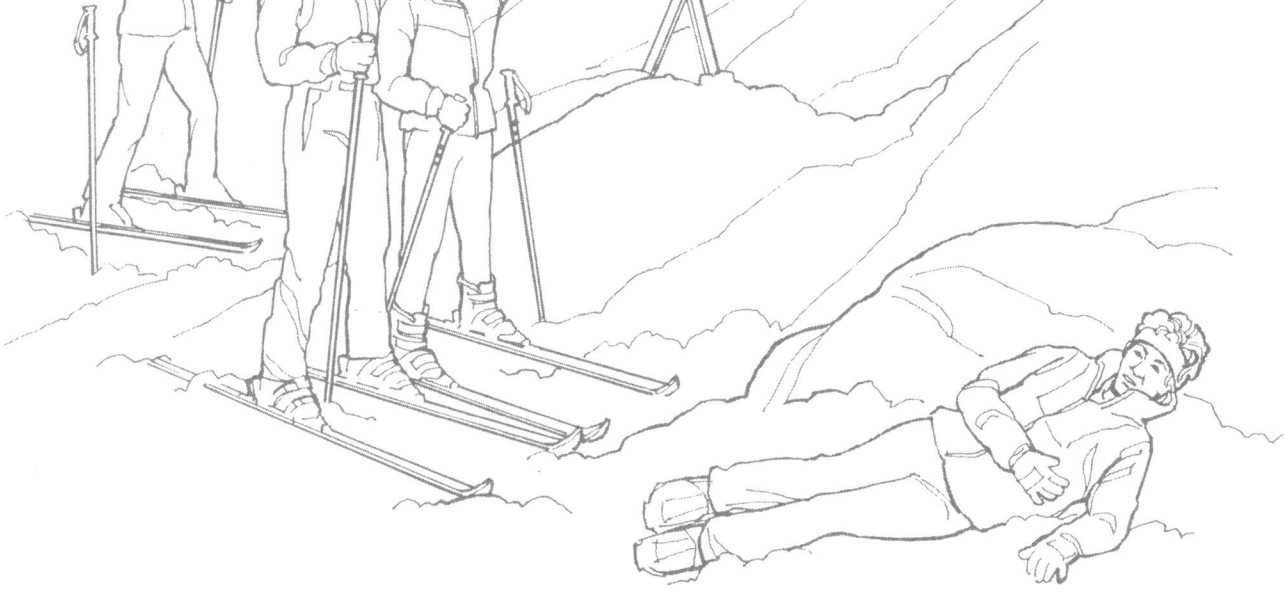

CHAPTER 7 STUDY QUESTIONS

1. Most external bleeding can be controlled with what method?
   A. Direct pressure
   B. Pressure points
   C. Tourniquet
   D. Cold compresses

2. Describe techniques for controlling external bleeding.

Direct Pressure
Pressure Points
Pneumatic Counterpressure Devices
Tourniquet

3. List the signs and symptoms of internal bleeding.

   _____
   _____
   _____
   _____
   _____
   _____
   _____

4. What is the emergency care for a patient with internal bleeding?

   _____
   _____
   _____
   _____

5. Identify three major types of shock and their causes.

Types	Causes

6. Match each type of shock to an appropriate medical condition.
   ___ Severe laceration, loss of more than 1,000 ml of blood   A. Hypovolemic shock
   ___ Heart attack   B. Vascular shock
   ___ Severe infections, metabolic illnesses,   C. Cardiogenic shock
   severe allergic reactions

7. List the common signs and symptoms of shock, regardless of type, in a patient.

   _____
   _____
   _____
   _____
   _____
   _____

8. Describe compensated shock

   _____
   _____

   Describe decompensated shock

   _____
   _____

9. List the key steps for emergency care of shock.

   _____
   _____
   _____
   _____
   _____
   _____
   _____

10. Unless contraindicated by cardiogenic shock or type of injury, the patient with shock should be positioned
    A. On his or her back with the legs raised 12 inches
    B. Flat on his or her back
    C. Flat on his or her stomach
    D. On his or her side

11. The correct position for a patient with shock who is also experiencing breathing difficulty is
    A. Head raised and knees bent
    B. Head and shoulders raised, hips flexed, knees bent
    C. Feet raised
    D. On the side

12. What emergency care is required for a person who has fainted?

13. What will a patient experience if suffering from an allergic reaction?

14. What is the emergency antidote for anaphylactic shock and how must it be administered?

Chapter 7 Local Protocol

1. Outline the local procedures for managing a patient experiencing anaphylactic shock.

2. Outline the local body substance isolation procedures for handling external bleeding incidents.

CHAPTER 7 SKILL PERFORMANCE REQUIREMENTS

- Review *Outdoor Emergency Care* scenario 7.1
- Demonstrate the emergency care for the patient exhibiting external bleeding
- Demonstrate the emergency care for the patient exhibiting signs of internal bleeding
- Demonstrate the appropriate care for shock

Skill Performance Guideline

- Vital Signs Determination (see Chapter 3)
- Patient Assessment—Body Survey (Rapid and Whole) (see Chapter 5)
- Patient Assessment—Unresponsive Patient (see Chapter 5)
- Patient Assessment—Responsive Patient—Injured (Trauma) (see Chapter 5)
- Patient Assessment—Responsive Patient—Ill (Medical) (see Chapter 5)
- Patient Assessment—Nonurgent and Ongoing Surveys (see Chapter 5)
- Use of Oxygen and Airway Adjuncts (see Chapter 6)
- Control of Severe Bleeding in a Wound

Control of Severe Bleeding in a Wound

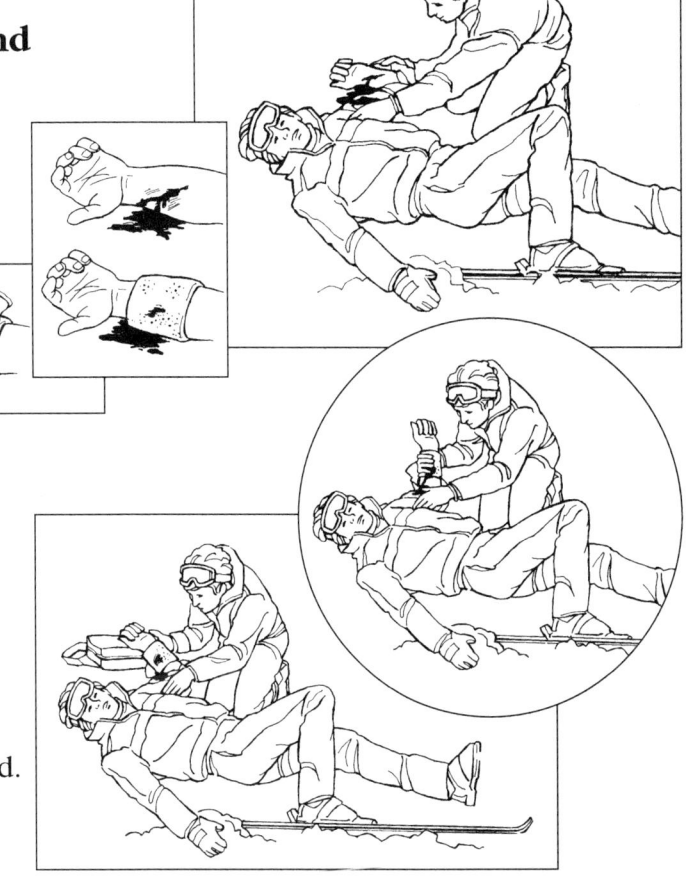

- Uses body substance isolation precautions according to protocols.
- Recognizes the severity of the bleeding and gives it proper priority.
- Exposes the wound site.
- Applies direct pressure.
- Elevates the wound site above the level of the heart.
- Maintains direct pressure and elevation.
- Applies direct pressure to the appropriate pressure point if bleeding has not been controlled.
- Checks that the bleeding has been controlled.
- Immobilizes as necessary.

Chapter 7 Scenario

1. You are called to an accident by a person who had been skiing powder just out of bounds in the trees. He was skiing with a friend who hit a tree. When you arrive, the patient is complaining of severe pain in the pelvic area. You see no obvious bleeding. He says he has been there about 20 minutes waiting for help. He is very upset and thirsty, and somewhat nauseous. His pulse is 110 and relatively weak. His face is white to gray. He repeats that he has been there about an hour waiting for help. What do you suspect? Why? How do you respond?

STUDY NOTES

CONTROL OF SEVERE BLEEDING IN A WOUND

Objective: To demonstrate the ability to control severe bleeding.

SKILL	YES	NO	NOTATIONS
• Uses BSI precautions according to protocols.			
• Recognizes the severity of the bleeding and gives it proper priority.			
• Exposes the wound site.			
• Applies direct pressure.			
• Elevates the wound site above the level of the heart.			
• Maintains direct pressure and elevation.			
• Applies direct pressure to the appropriate pressure point if bleeding has not been controlled.			
• Checks that the bleeding has been controlled.			
• Immobilizes as necessary.			
Did the trainee or patroller adequately demonstrate the performance criteria of this skill?			

COMMENTS

CHAPTER 8

Skin and Soft Tissue Injuries, Burns, and Bandaging

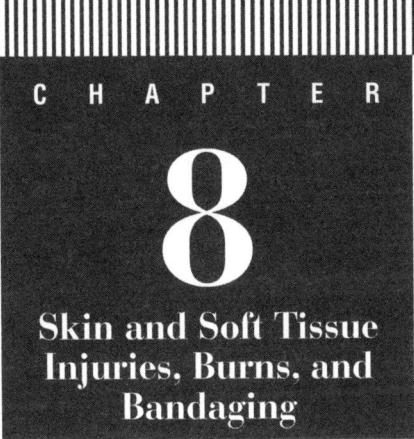

CONCLUDING OBJECTIVES

The learner will:

Content

- List and describe closed soft-tissue injuries

- List and describe open soft-tissue injuries

- Describe the three degrees and three classifications of thermal burns and their significance

- Describe the characteristics of chemical and electrical burns

- List and describe types of dressings and bandages

- Describe special techniques for problem surfaces

Skill Performance

- Demonstrate basic emergency care techniques for open soft-tissue injuries

- Demonstrate basic emergency care techniques for closed soft-tissue injuries

- Demonstrate basic emergency care techniques for burns

- Demonstrate basic techniques of applying dressings and bandages

- Demonstrate basic techniques of applying special types of and improvised dressings and bandages

CHAPTER 8 STUDY QUESTIONS

1. Describe various injuries classified as closed wound injuries.

Contusion	
Hematoma	
Muscle strain	

2. List the key steps of emergency care for contusions and strains.

_____
_____
_____
_____
_____

3. As an aid in remembering the emergency care for closed soft-tissue injuries, list the meaning of the mnemonic RICE.

   R _____
   I _____
   C _____
   E _____

4. Describe the different types of open wounds.

   Abrasion
   _____
   _____

   Laceration
   _____
   _____

   Incision
   _____
   _____

   Avulsion
   _____
   _____

Amputation
_____
_____

Puncture
_____
_____

Impaled object
_____
_____

5. List the key points to follow in the emergency care of open soft-tissue injuries.

_____
_____
_____
_____
_____
_____

6. With an avulsion, the flap should be _____.

7. Describe the technique for cleaning open, contaminated wounds.

_____
_____
_____
_____
_____
_____
_____
_____

8. Identify and describe the signs and symptoms of burns.

Types	Signs and Symptoms
Superficial	
Partial thickness	
Full thickness	

9. What is the general emergency care of burns?

_____
_____
_____
_____
_____
_____
_____

10. Describe thermal burns.

Critical	
Moderate	
Minor	
Minimal	

11. The severity of a thermal burn depends on
    A. The severity, extent, and depth of the wound, and the age and condition of the patient
    B. Location of the wound, heat source, and time until medical attention is reached
    C. Extent and depth of the wound, heat source, and the age and condition of the patient
    D. Time until medical attention is reached and the age and condition of the patient

12. With what type of chemical burn should an emergency care provider avoid the immediate use of water?

_____

_____

13. Identify the "rule of nines" percentage of burned body area on the illustration.

14. When caring for a wet or liquid chemical burn, the most essential emergency care step is
    A. Treating with counteractive chemical
    B. Removal of clothing
    C. Getting the patient to a hospital immediately.
    D. Immediate washing with large quantities of water

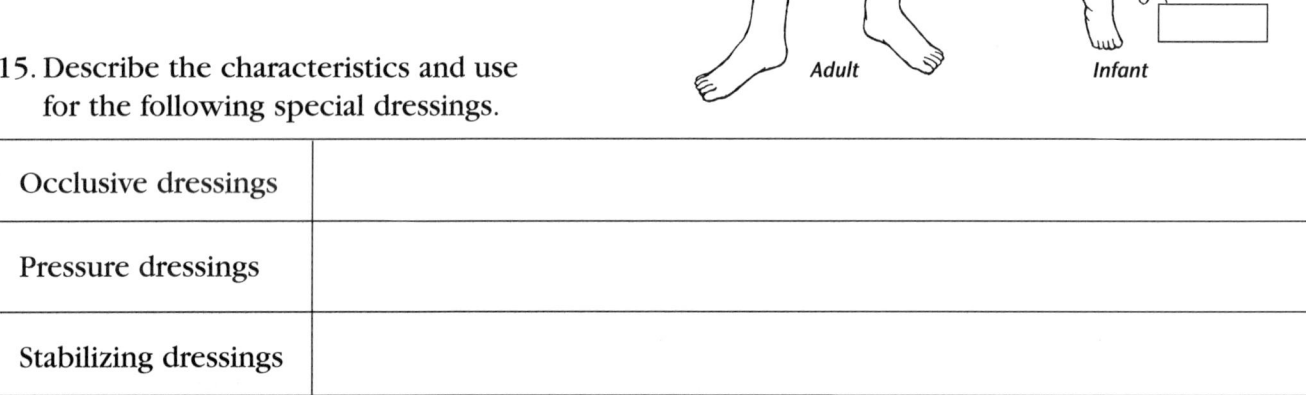

a Adult   b Infant

15. Describe the characteristics and use for the following special dressings.

Occlusive dressings	
Pressure dressings	
Stabilizing dressings	

16. What could be used for improvised bandages and dressings?

Dressings	
Bandages	
Cravats and triangular bandages	
Occlusive dressings	

17. A joint should be bandaged in _____ position.

18. A dressing should not be secured with tape wrapped completely around an extremity because
    A. It is difficult to remove completely
    B. It is too difficult to change the dressing if serious bleeding occurs
    C. Blood vessels may become constricted as swelling occurs
    D. It looks unprofessional

19. Why are self-adhering roller bandages preferred over elastic or rubberized bandages?
    _____

20. Describe the special bandaging techniques for problem surfaces.

Moving joints
Tapering cones

Chapter 8 Local Protocol

1. List local patrol supplies and procedures for handling bleeding, burns, and bandaging.

    _____
    _____
    _____
    _____
    _____

2. List supplies and procedures used at your area for cleaning a wound.

    _____
    _____
    _____
    _____
    _____

CHAPTER 8 SKILL PERFORMANCE REQUIREMENTS

- Review *Outdoor Emergency Care* scenario 8.1

- Demonstrate basic emergency care techniques for open soft-tissue injuries

- Demonstrate basic emergency care techniques for closed soft-tissue injuries

- Demonstrate basic emergency care techniques for burns

- Demonstrate basic techniques of applying dressings and bandages

- Demonstrate basic techniques of applying special types and improvised dressings and bandages

Skill Performance Guidelines

- Vital Signs Determination (see Chapter 3)
- Patient Assessment—Body Survey (Rapid and Whole) (see Chapter 5)
- Patient Assessment—Unresponsive Patient (see Chapter 5)
- Patient Assessment—Responsive Patient—Injured (Trauma) (see Chapter 5)
- Patient Assessment—Responsive Patient—Ill (Medical) (see Chapter 5)
- Patient Assessment—Nonurgent and Ongoing Surveys (see Chapter 5)
- Use of Oxygen and Airway Adjuncts (see Chapter 6)
- Control of Severe Bleeding in a Wound (see Chapter 7)

Chapter 8 Scenarios

1. You are sitting in the aid room when one of the kitchen crew comes in holding his arm. He says that he has spilled the contents of the french fry cooker on his arm and on his body. His arm and hand have large blisters and are very red. Upon examination, it is clear that he has also been saturated in his groin area. His genitals are also blistered and red. How would you classify these burns? What emergency care would you recommend?

   _____
   _____
   _____
   _____

2. A skier has fallen on the lodge steps and is complaining of a very painful shin. Your examination reveals heavy bruising and an abrasion on his shin, but no evidence of a broken bone. What is your emergency care of this injury?

_____
_____
_____
_____
_____

3. A 26-year-old male lift attendant is in the lift house at the top of the slope. The past three days have been extremely cold, so for added warmth he brought a small kerosene heater to work. He is kneeling in an attempt to light the heater when it explodes with a burst of flame. When you arrive, the attendant has a painful redness of the face and anterior neck. His eyebrows are singed and his nose and right cheek quickly develop multiple small blisters. The patient is frightened, anxious, and complaining of a raspy feeling in his throat when he tries to breathe deeply. His lips show signs of early edema and his breathing is somewhat labored.

   Please include the answers to the following questions in your response.
   1. What problem(s) does your overall assessment indicate?
   2. What factors caused you to reach this conclusion?
   3. What BSI precautions are appropriate in this circumstance?
   4. Is oxygen administration appropriate?
   5. Explain the emergency care steps you would take in the order you would take them in handling this situation.
   6. What common problems and complications might develop?
   7. Describe the transportation decisions you would make.

_____
_____
_____
_____
_____
_____
_____
_____

STUDY NOTES

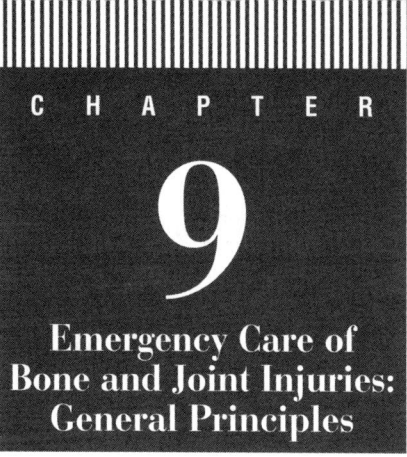

CHAPTER 9
Emergency Care of Bone and Joint Injuries: General Principles

CONCLUDING OBJECTIVES

The learner will:

Content

- Describe the general characteristics of fractures, dislocations, and sprains

- Explain the general principles of emergency care for musculoskeletal injuries

- Name the types of splints and explain the general principles of their application

Skill Performance

- Demonstrate techniques for long spineboard immobilization

- Demonstrate techniques for traction splint immobilization

CHAPTER 9 STUDY QUESTIONS

1. Identify and describe the general characteristics of fractures.

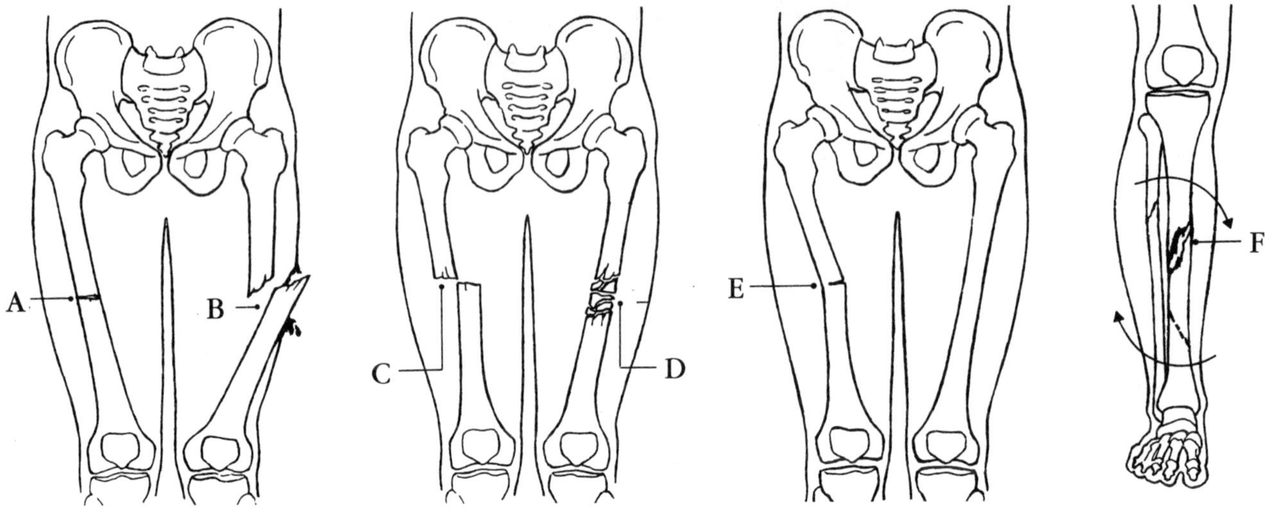

A. _____

B. _____

C. _____

D. _____

E. _____

F. _____

2. A comminuted fracture
   A. Involves a bone broken into more than two fragments
   B. Involves bones that break and commute to different places
   C. Is life threatening because of contamination
   D. Rarely results in misalignment of a limb

3. Tenderness at the site of a sprain can be determined by _____.

4. Swelling and ecchymosis are signs of a sprain and are caused by
_____

5. An injury that forces a joint beyond its range is called a
   A. Sprain
   B. Dislocation
   C. Strain
   D. Fracture

6. A sprain is _____.

7. How does a sprain differ from a dislocation?
_____
_____
_____

8. Describe the signs and symptoms for fractures, dislocations, and sprains.

Signs and Symptoms		
Fractures	**Dislocations**	**Sprains**

9. Before and after aligning or splinting, what should be checked?
_____

10. Identify six steps in the assessment of musculoskeletal injuries.
_____
_____
_____
_____
_____

11. List the major purposes of splinting.

12. What fracture locations usually are splinted without attempting alignment?

13. Generally speaking, fractures of the _____ can be safely aligned.
    A. knee, neck, midfemur, or wrist
    B. hand, spine, ankle, or elbow
    C. shoulder, toes, midfemur, or midhumerus
    D. ankle, lower leg, midfemur, or midhumerus

14. Dislocations of the knee and ankle present what special problem?

14. Special care for an open wound with exposed bone ends that will not receive definitive medical care within the first couple hours includes

16. Patients with an open fracture should not be given _____ because they will be taken to surgery upon reaching the hospital.

17. Describe the process used to align a deformed fracture.

124 OEC Study Book

18. List the signs and symptoms that indicate the loss of circulation or nerve supply in an extremity.

19. List the emergency care for musculoskeletal injuries.

20. Describe types of splints and additional supplies that are most effectively used for splinting various types of injuries.

Type of Splint	Additional Supplies Required	Types of Injuries Used
FIXATION		
Quick Splint		
Cardboard Splint		
Wire, Ladder Splint		
Malleable Metal Splint		
Air Splint		
Vacuum Splint		
Sling and Swathe		
TRACTION		
Hare		
Sager or Kendrick Traction Device		
Thomas (modified)		
Improvised (several variations)		

21. The best way to splint a suspected midshaft femur fracture is with
    A. A spineboard
    B. An airplane splint
    C. A traction splint
    D. A quick splint

22. Describe the sequence of long spineboard immobilization.

23. Why must a patient wearing a cervical collar be manually stabilized until fully immobilized on a spineboard?

Chapter 9 Local Protocol

1. Describe the local patrol procedures required for traction splinting.

    Type of equipment

    Location of equipment

    Splinting procedures

    Transportation procedures

2. Identify general patrol procedures for working with bone and joint injuries.

	Fractures	**Dislocations**	**Sprains**
Types of equipment			
Location of equipment			
Splinting procedures			
Positions on toboggan			

3. Describe procedures for using spinal immobilization devices at your area.

   Type(s) of immobilization devices available.

   _____
   _____
   _____

   Describe or illustrate the strapping procedures.

   _____
   _____
   _____

   Detail the specific instructions for the rigid collars used for immobilization at your area.

   _____
   _____
   _____

CHAPTER 9 SKILL PERFORMANCE REQUIREMENTS

- Review *Outdoor Emergency Care* scenario 9.1

- Demonstrate technique(s) for long spineboard immobilization
  Note: This skill does not involve assessment or care of injuries

- Demonstrate technique(s) for traction splint immobilization
  Note: This skill does not involve assessment or care of injuries

Skill Performance Guidelines

- Traction Splinting
- Spinal Immobilization

Spinal Immobilization

Note: Learn to use a spinal immobilization device in accordance with the manufacturer's instructions.

- Assesses mechanism of injury and neurological functions to determine nature and extent of injury
- Uses manual stabilization techniques to firmly stabilize the head and neck.
  Note: Continuous manual stabilization must be maintained until the head is mechanically immobilized and secured.
- Applies a rigid collar (or equivalent) without excessive movement of the head/neck.
- Transfers the patient as a unit onto spinal immobilization device without excessive movement, maintains spinal integrity, and properly positions patient on spinal immobilization device.
- Fills any voids present under the neck or along the spine as necessary.
- Adequately secures the torso and pelvis to the spinal immobilization device.
  Note: The torso must be mechanically secured before the head and neck.
- Secures the patient's head and neck to the spinal immobilization device.
- Secures the patient's extremities.
- Correctly applies the spinal immobilization device without further aggravation of injury or compromising the cervical spine integrity.

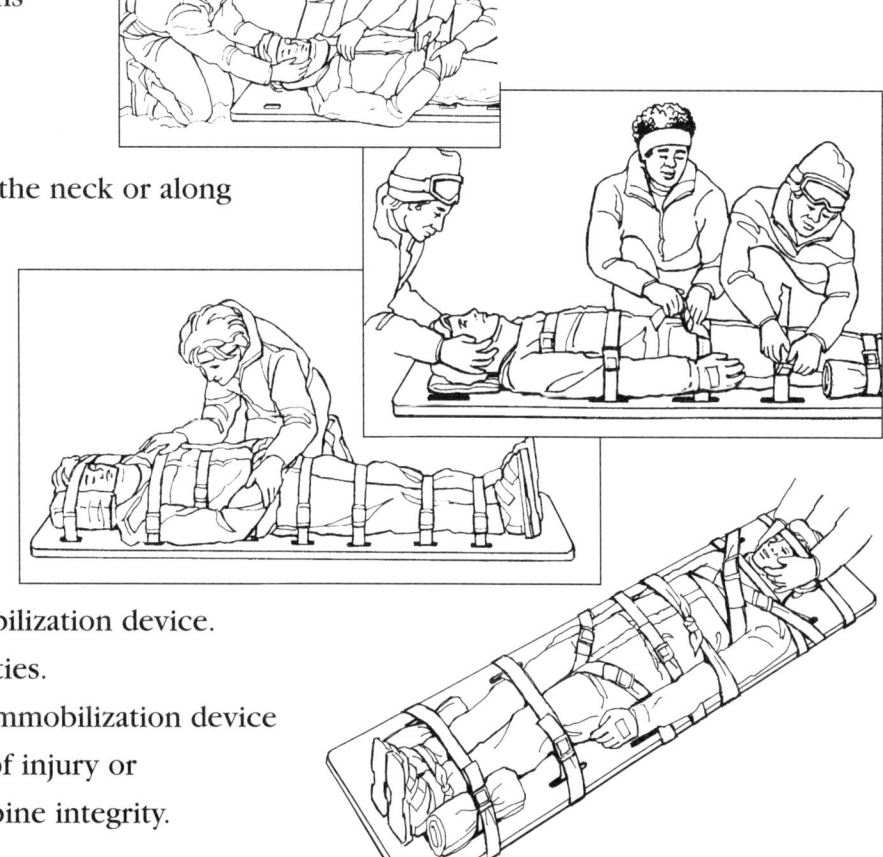

Traction Splinting

Note: Learn to apply a traction-splinting device in accordance with manufacturer's instructions.

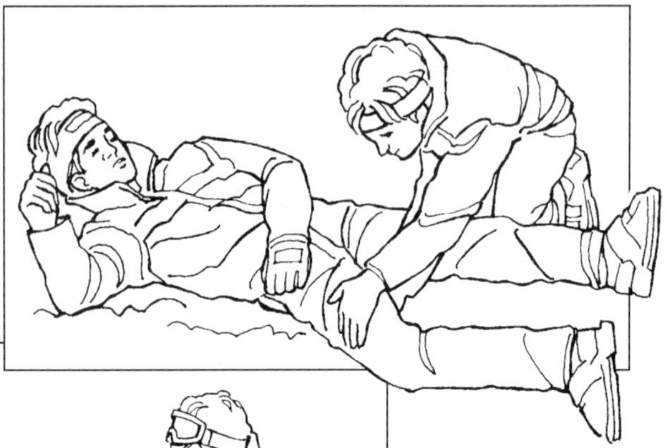

- Assess the limb and mechanism of injury to determine the presence and location of a fracture
- Manually stabilizes the fracture site and limb.
  Note: This must be continually maintained until the splint device is applied and completely secured.
- Assesses the circulatory and neurological function of the limb 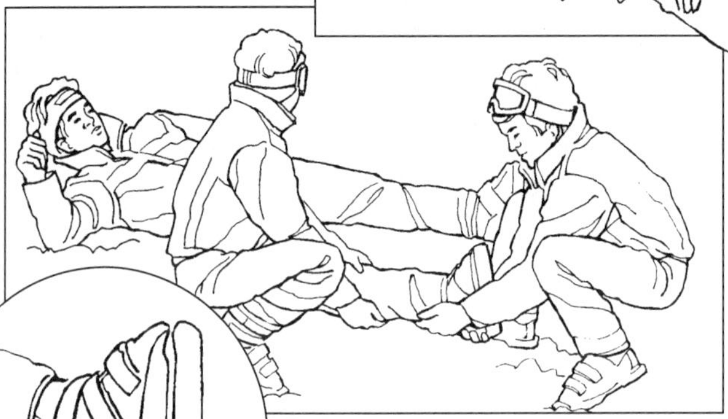
- Applies an ankle hitch.
- Prepares the immobilization device and materials to be used. 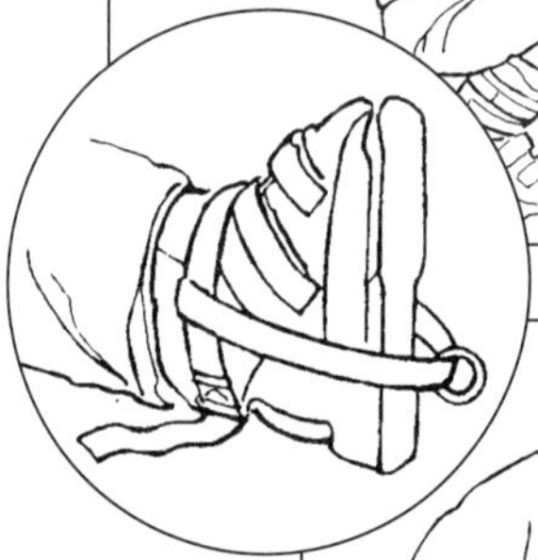
- Applies and maintains traction to the entire limb for the duration of splint application. 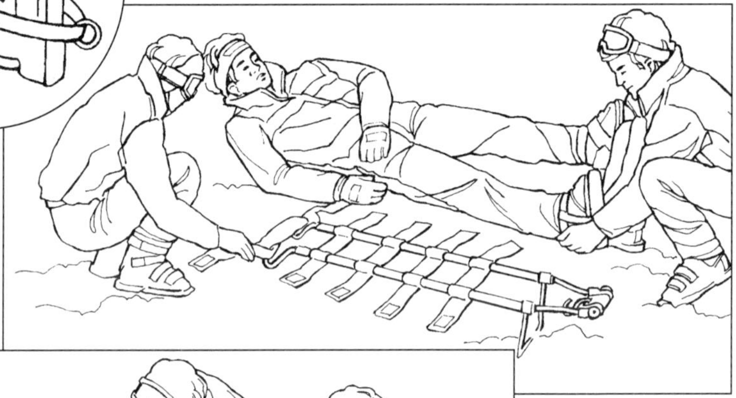
- Positions the splint properly under the limb and against the ischial tuberosity or pelvic bone (depending on the splint type) without excessive movement or elevation of the limb.
- Applies the splint, including any necessary cradles, supports, etc. 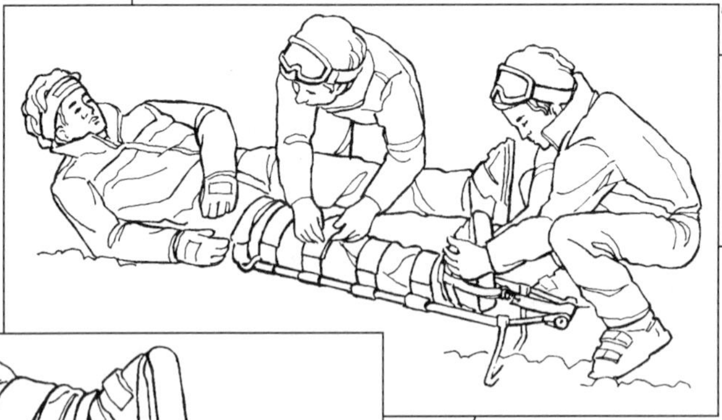
- Applies mechanical traction at the ankle, using hitch assembly.
- Secures the limb properly in the splint.

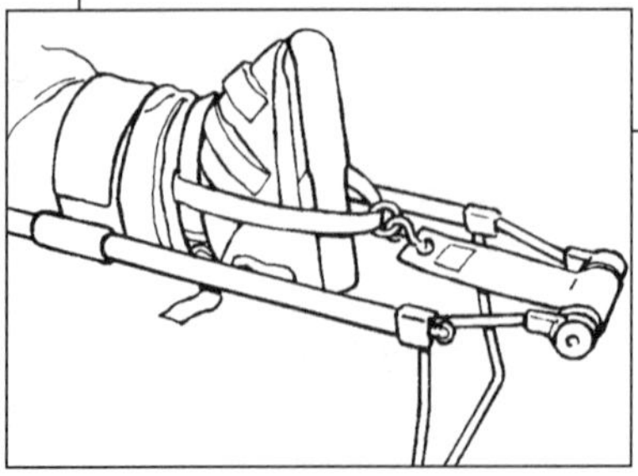

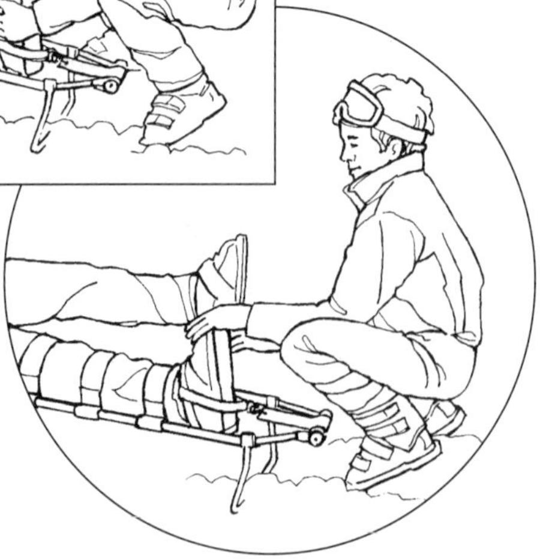

Chapter 9 Scenario

1. An injured skier has a fractured elbow. A normal radial pulse and normal sensation in the fingers are present before immobilizing the elbow. After immobilizing the elbow with a padded board splint and cravats, the radial pulse is weak and numbness is present in the fingers. How do you respond?

STUDY NOTES

TRACTION SPLINTING

Objective: To immobilize a fracture of the femur using a traction-splinting device.

SKILL	YES	NO	NOTATIONS
• Assesses the limb and mechanism of injury to determine the presence and location of a fracture.			
• Manually stabilizes the fracture site and limb. *Note: Continuous manual stabilization must be maintained until a splint device is applied and completely secured.*			
• Assesses the circulatory and neurological function of the limb.			
• Realigns the limb if needed. *Note: Manual stabilization/traction should be applied at the knee initially until the limb is straightened and the ankle hitch is applied.*			
• Applies an ankle hitch.			
• Prepares the immobilization device and materials to be used.			
• Applies and maintains traction to the entire limb for the duration of splint application.			
• Positions the splint properly under the limb and against the ischial tuberosity or pelvic bone (depending on the splint type) without excessive movement or elevation of the limb.			
• Applies the splint, including any necessary cradles, supports, etc.			
• Applies mechanical traction at the ankle, using hitch assembly.			
• Secures the limb properly in the splint.			
• Reassesses the circulatory and neurological function of the limb.			
Did the trainee or patroller adequately demonstrate the performance criteria of this skill?			

COMMENTS

SPINAL IMMOBILIZATION

Objective: To demonstrate spinal immobilization techniques using a long or short spinal immobilization device.

Note: The use of a web strap system is the method of choice to allow immobilizing "bone-to-board." Any device chosen must be applied correctly and in accordance with the manufacturer's instructions.

SKILL	YES	NO	NOTATIONS
• Assesses mechanism of injury and neurological functions to determine nature and extent of injury.			
• Uses manual stabilization techniques to firmly stabilize the head and neck. *Note: Continuous manual stabilization must be maintained until the head is mechanically immobilized and secured.*			
• Applies a rigid collar (or equivalent) without excessive movement of the head/neck.			
• Transfers the patient as a unit onto spinal immobilization device without excessive movement, maintaining spinal integrity, and properly positions patient on spinal immobilization device.			
• Fills any voids present under the neck or along the spine as necessary.			
• Adequately secures the torso and pelvis to the spinal immobilization device. *Note: The torso must be mechanically secured before the head and neck.*			
• Secures the patient's head and neck to the spinal immobilization device.			
• Secures the patient's extremities.			
• Reassesses the circulatory and neurological function in the patient's extremities.			
• Correctly applies the spinal immobilization device without further aggravation of injury or compromising the cervical spine integrity.			
Did the trainee or patroller adequately demonstrate the performance criteria of this skill?			

COMMENTS

CHAPTER 10

Mechanisms and Patterns of Injury

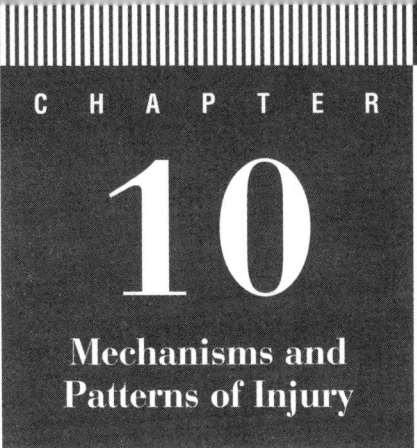

CONCLUDING OBJECTIVES

The learner will:

Content

- Describe how trauma is influenced by laws of physics
- Distinguish between various types of trauma and their implications

Skill Performance

- Inspect an accident scene and reconstruct the probable sequence of events

CHAPTER 10 STUDY QUESTIONS

1. List two forms of energy.

   _____

   _____

2. List the five types of trauma caused by changes in speed or direction.

   _____

   _____

   _____

   _____

3. Describe the characteristics of the following types of trauma. It is important to develop the ability to predict potential internal injuries from various trauma.

Penetration	
Compression	
Bending	
Rotational	
Distraction	

4. Match the types of trauma to their possible causes.
   - ___ Compression   A. Landing on a ski pole tip
   - ___ Stretching   B. Hitting a lift tower at great speed
   - ___ Potential   C. Falling forward over ski tips
   - ___ Penetration   D. Catching a ski edge

5. The skier catching an edge and falling to the ground is an example of _____ energy.

6. Trauma caused by bullets, ice, axes, ski poles, and other sharp objects is called _____.

7. Identify the types of injuries that could be produced by a collision.

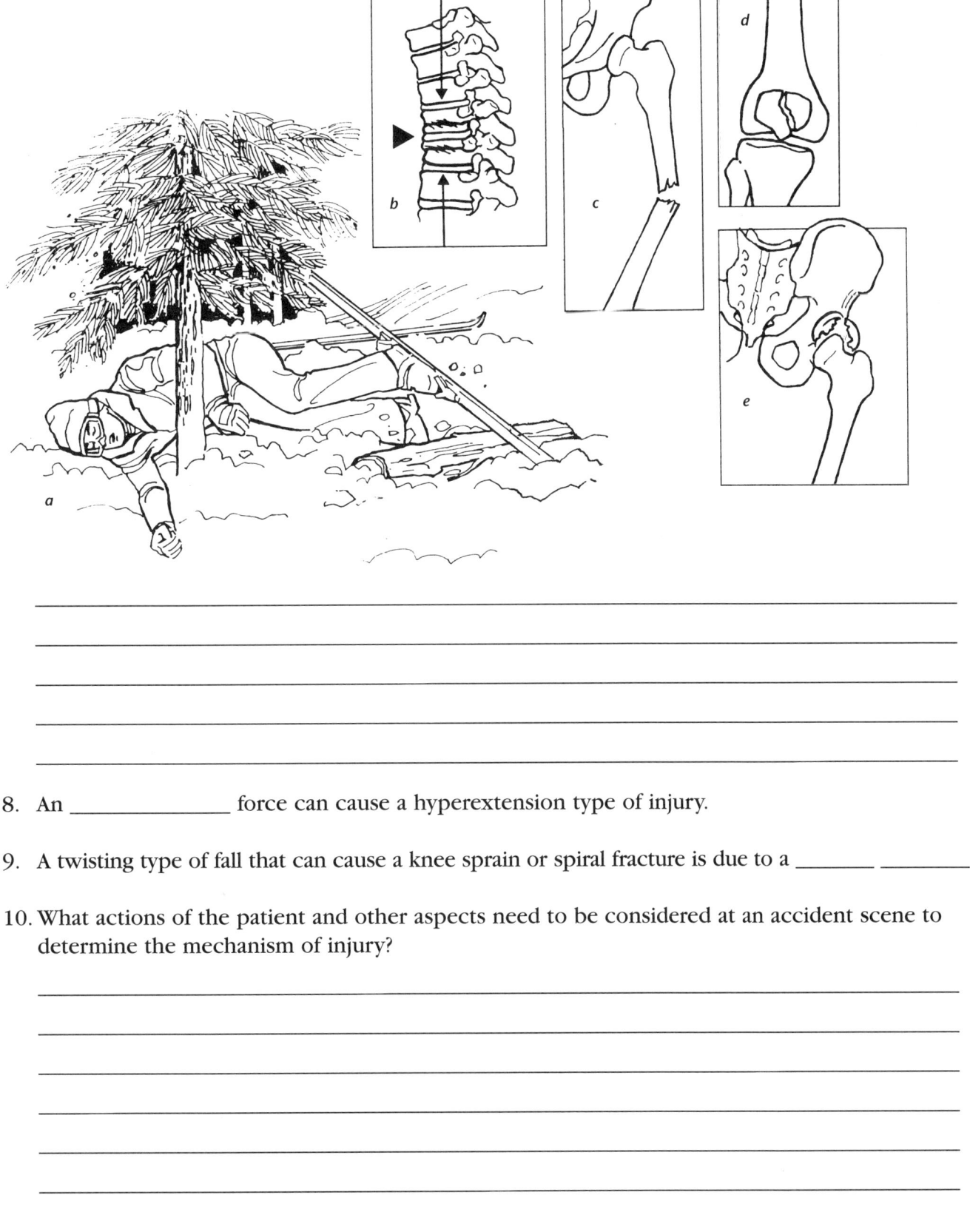

_____
_____
_____
_____
_____

8. An _____ force can cause a hyperextension type of injury.

9. A twisting type of fall that can cause a knee sprain or spiral fracture is due to a _____ _____.

10. What actions of the patient and other aspects need to be considered at an accident scene to determine the mechanism of injury?

_____
_____
_____
_____
_____
_____

11. Identify the mechanisms of injury in the illustrations below. Also identify whether these are rotational or nonrotational injuries.

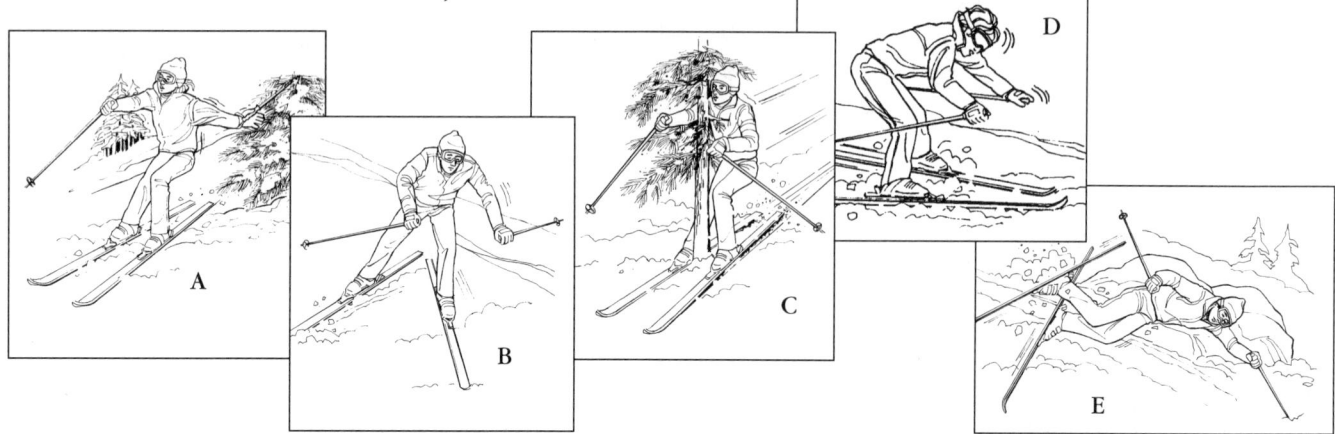

A. _____
B. _____
C. _____
D. _____
E. _____

12. Damage to the body caused by an external force is
    A. Force
    B. Trauma
    C. Energy
    D. Mass

13. List at least eight cases where multiple and/or serious injuries should be suspected.

_____
_____
_____
_____
_____
_____
_____
_____

Chapter 10 Local Protocol

1. Outline local patrol procedures for accident site investigation.

CHAPTER 10 SKILL PERFORMANCE REQUIREMENTS

- Inspect an accident scene and reconstruct the probable sequence of events

Chapter 10 Scenario

1. While watching a GS race, you observe a racer miss the gate at a tremendous rate of speed. He spins and swirls in a cloud of snow, striking his head on the left side two times. You ski over to him and find that he has collided with a horizontal, rigid metal pipe and is doubled over on it. One ski released and the other is still on. This injury will be severe.
   1) Both legs are broken. What kind of trauma should you suspect?
   2) Seeing the patient doubled over a pipe tells you he may have suffered what kind of injury?
   3) The pipe that the skier struck has caused what kind of trauma to the pelvic area?

_____
_____
_____
_____
_____

STUDY NOTES

CHAPTER 11

Specific Injuries to the Upper Extremity

CONCLUDING OBJECTIVES

The learner will:

Content

- Describe the general characteristics of sprains, fractures, and dislocations of the upper extremities

- Describe the principles of emergency care for upper extremity injuries

Skill Performance

- Demonstrate the appropriate assessment and emergency care for sprains, fractures, and dislocations of the upper extremities

CHAPTER 11 STUDY QUESTIONS

1. Detail the signs and symptoms of various types of fractures, sprains, and dislocations to the upper extremity.

Types	Signs and Symptoms
FRACTURES	
Clavicle	
Scapula	
Upper Arm	
Above the Elbow	
Forearm and Wrist	
Hand	
SPRAINS	
Shoulder	
AC Separations	
Elbow	
Wrist	
Hand and Finger	
DISLOCATIONS	
Shoulder	
Elbow	
Wrist	
Finger	

2. Describe the general emergency care of specific injuries to the upper extremity.

Types	Emergency Care
FRACTURES	
Clavicle	
Scapula	
Upper Arm	
Above the Elbow	
Forearm and Wrist	
Hand	
SPRAINS	
Shoulder	
AC Separations	
Elbow	
Wrist	
Hand and Finger	
DISLOCATIONS	
Shoulder	
Elbow	
Wrist	
Finger	

3. Describe the differences between posterior and anterior shoulder dislocation.

_____

_____

4. Fractures of the clavicle are best treated using a
   A. Sling and swathe
   B. Blanket roll in the armpit to hold the arm away from body
   C. Traction splint
   D. Cardboard splint

5. A patient with a dislocated shoulder will usually be most comfortable when transported in a toboggan in which of the following positions? (Circle one)
   A. In the supine position
   B. In the prone position
   C. In the fetal position, injured side up
   D. In a sitting position and supported from behind

6. When the splinting process for upper extremities is completed, what must be reassessed and why?

   _____
   _____
   _____
   _____

7. In what position is a fracture or dislocation generally best treated and transported?

   _____

8. Describe the possible injury that could occur if the patient falls with the arm in these positions.
   Adducted _____
   Abducted _____

Chapter 11 Local Protocol

1. Outline types of equipment and local patrol procedures used for upper extremity injuries.

   _____
   _____
   _____
   _____
   _____

CHAPTER 11 SKILL PERFORMANCE REQUIREMENTS

- Review *Outdoor Emergency Care* scenario 11.1

- Demonstrate the appropriate technique(s) for splinting sprains:
  Shoulder
  AC separations
  Elbow
  Wrist
  Hand and finger

- Demonstrate the appropriate technique for splinting fractures:
  Clavicle
  Scapula
  Upper arm
  Forearm and wrist
  Hand

- Demonstrate the appropriate technique for splinting dislocations:
  Shoulder
  Elbow
  Wrist
  Finger

Skill Performance Guidelines

- Vital Signs Determination (see Chapter 3)
- Patient Assessment (see Chapter 5)
- Use of Oxygen and Airway Adjuncts (see Chapter 6)
- Control of Severe Bleeding in a Wound (see Chapter 7)
- General Management of Long Bone Fractures
- General Management of a Fracture or Dislocation At or Near a Joint
- Alignment of Angulated or Displaced Fracture

Focused Body Survey—Extremity Injury
Examine and palpate each extremity for abnormality
Question the injured patient about • Pain on motion • Inability to move or use extremity • Weakness • Numbness or tingling
Assess circulatory and neurologic function in the extremity
Look for medical-alert tags.

General Management of Long Bone Fractures

- Assesses the limb and mechanism of injury to determine the presence and location of a fracture.

- Assesses the circulatory and neurological function of the limb.

- Manually stabilizes the fracture site.
  Note: Continuous manual stabilization must be maintained until mechanical device is applied and completely secured.

- Aligns the limb to a near-anatomically correct position.

- Prepares the immobilization device to be used.

- Positions the device without excessive movement of the limb.

- Applies and secures the device to the limb without excessive movement, ensures that all voids are filled, and checks that the fracture site and the adjacent joints are immobilized.

- Reassesses the circulatory and neurological function of the limb.

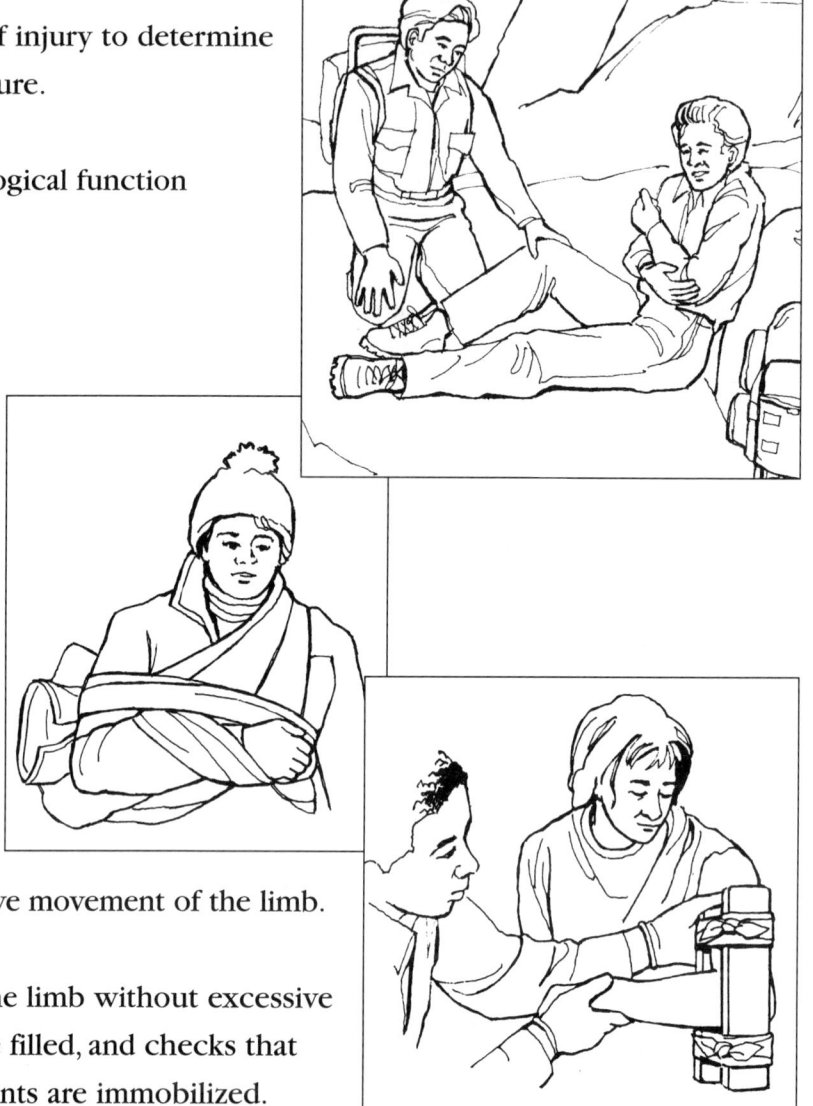

General Management of a Fracture or Dislocation At or Near a Joint

- Assesses the limb, joint, and mechanism of injury to determine the presence and location of a fracture and/or dislocation.

- Assesses the circulatory and neurological function of the limb.

- Manually stabilizes the fracture site and the limb.
  Note: Continuous manual stabilization must be maintained until mechanical device is applied and completely secured.

- Moves the limb toward a nearer-anatomically-correct position, if possible, with the assistance of the patient.

- *If there is no distal circulation*, aligns limb until resistance is met or circulation returns.

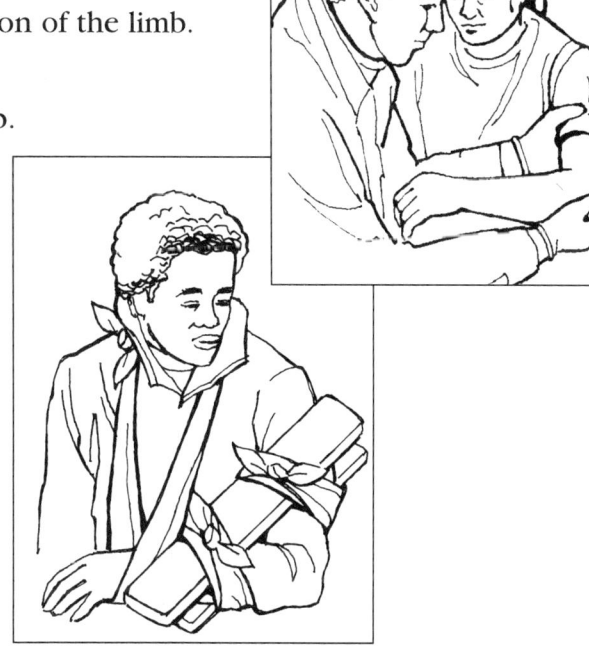

- Prepares the immobilization device for use, taking into account any unusual anatomical positioning of the limb.

- Positions the device without any excessive movement of the limb.

- Applies and secures the device to the limb and body without excessive movement, ensuring all voids are filled, and checks the fracture site, the adjacent joints, and the limb are immobilized.

- Reassesses the circulatory and neurological function of the limb.

Alignment of Angulated or Displaced Fracture

- Assesses the limb and mechanism of injury to determine the presence and location of a fracture.

- Assesses the circulatory and neurological function of the limb.

- Manually stabilizes the fracture site and the limb. *Note: Continuous manual stabilization must be maintained until mechanical device is applied and completely secured.*

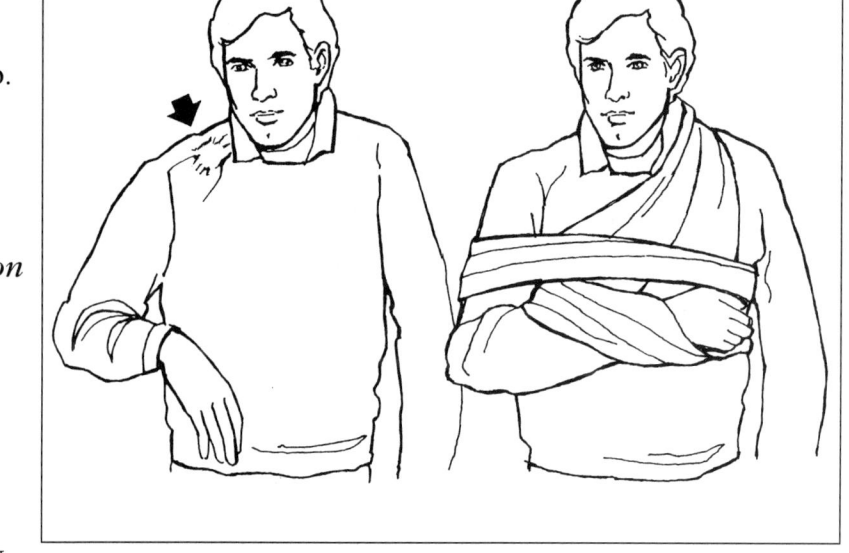

- Begins straightening the limb by moving each joint individually and applies axial traction at the nearest distal joint or the end of the limb as needed to complete the straightening process.

- Rotates the limb as necessary to approximately normal anatomical position.

- Monitors patient for indications of resistance or excessive pain during alignment.

Chapter 11 Scenarios

1. A skier skis very fast through the trees and loses control trying to avoid a collision with a blue spruce. The skier crashes into the tree and dislocates her right shoulder. The skier is in a supine position with her right arm above her head. During assessment, she will not allow you to bring the arm to near-normal position. What equipment will be needed for emergency care and transport?

   _____
   _____
   _____
   _____
   _____
   _____
   _____

2. You are dispatched to a call for help from a guest who says, "I saw a snowboarder catch air and land hard on her shoulder." Upon your arrival at the incident site, you find a 14-year-old female lying supine with her left arm completely abducted. She is in great pain and firmly states that she cannot and will not move her arm. The girl has a weak grip, faint distal pulse, and complains of *numbness and tingling* in her fingers.

   Please include the answers to the following questions in your response:
   1. What problem(s) does your overall assessment indicate?
   2. Explain the emergency care steps you would take in the order you would take them in handling this situation.
   3. What common problems and complications might develop?
   4. Describe the transportation decisions you would make.

   _____
   _____
   _____
   _____
   _____
   _____
   _____
   _____
   _____
   _____

3. A skier has fallen very hard and landed on his shoulder. When you arrive, he is lying face down with his arm outstretched and is complaining of severe pain in his shoulder. The patient has a good pulse in both wrists. He is unwilling to move his arm.

   Please include the answers to the following questions in your response:
   1. What problem(s) does your overall assessment indicate?
   2. What factors caused you to reach this conclusion?
   3. What body substance isolation precautions are appropriate in this circumstance?
   4. Is oxygen administration appropriate?
   5. Explain the emergency care steps you would take in the order you would take them in handling this situation.
   6. What common problems and complications might develop?
   7. Describe the transportation decisions you would make.

STUDY NOTES

GENERAL MANAGEMENT OF LONG BONE FRACTURES

Objective: To immobilize the fracture site and adjacent joints for a long bone fracture in an extremity.

NOTE: *Any device chosen must be applied correctly and in accordance with its manufacturer's instructions. If the device choden for the upper extremity is "soft" (e.g., sling and swathe), all of the objectives must be met.*

SKILL	YES	NO	NOTATIONS
• Assesses the limb and mechanism of injury to determine the presence and location of a fracture.			
• Assesses the circulatory and neurological function of the limb.			
• Manually stabilizes the fracture site. *(Note: Continous manual stabilization must be maintained until mechanical device is applied and completely secured.)*			
• Aligns the limb to a near-anatomically correct position.			
• Prepares the immobilization device to be used.			
• Positions the device without excessive movement of the limb.			
• Applies and secures the device to the limb without excessive movement, ensures that all voids are filled, and checks that the fracture site and the adjacent joints are immobilized.			
• Reassesses the circulatory and neurological function of the limb.			
Did the trainee or patroller adequately demonstrate the performance criteria of this skill?			

COMMENTS

GENERAL MANAGEMENT OF A FRACTURE OR DISLOCATION AT OR NEAR A JOINT

Objective: To demonstrate the immobilization of a fracture site, the adjacent joints, and the extremity for a fracture or dislocation in or near a joint.

SKILL	YES	NO	NOTATIONS
• Assesses the limb, joint, and mechanism of injury to determine the presence and location of a fracture and/or dislocation.			
• Assesses the circulatory and neurological function of the limb.			
• Manually stabilizes the fracture site and the limb. *(Note: Continous manual stabilization must be maintained until mechanical device is applied and completely secured.)*			
• Moves the limb toward a nearer-anatomically correct position, if possible, with the assistance of the patient.			
• *If there is no distal circulation*, aligns limb until resistance is met or circulation returns.			
• Prepares the immobilization device for use, taking into account any unusual anatomical positioning of the limb.			
• Positions the device without excessive movement of the limb.			
• Applies and secures the device to the limband body without excessive movement, ensuring all voids are filled, and checks that the fracture site, the adjacent joints, and the limb are immobilized.			
• Reassesses the circulatory and neurological function of the limb.			
Did the trainee or patroller adequately demonstrate the performance criteria of this skill?			

COMMENTS

ALIGNMENT OF ANGULATED OR DISPLACED FRACTURE

Objective: To return a fractured limb to a near-normal position, thereby improving circulatory and neurological function, the limb's stability, and ability to function.

SKILL	YES	NO	NOTATIONS
• Assesses the limb and mechanism of injury to determine the presence and location of a fracture.			
• Assesses the circulatory and neurological function of the limb.			
• Manually stabilizes the fracture site and the limb. *(Note: Continous manual stabilization must be maintained until mechanical device is applied and completely secured.)*			
• Begins straightening the limb by moving each joint individually, and applies axial traction at the nearest distal joint or the end of the limb as needed to complete the straightening process.			
• Rotates the limb as necessary to approximately normal anatomical position.			
• Monitors patient for indications of resistance or excessive pain during alignment.			
Did the trainee or patroller adequately demonstrate the performance criteria of this skill?			

COMMENTS

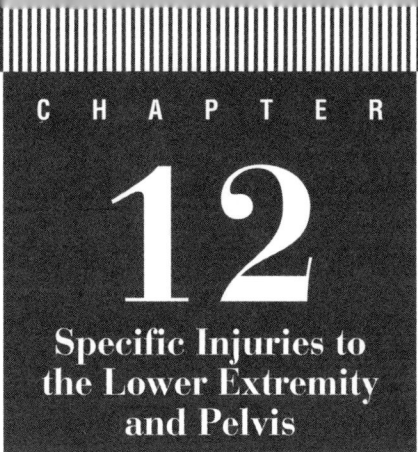

CHAPTER 12
Specific Injuries to the Lower Extremity and Pelvis

CONCLUDING OBJECTIVES

The learner will:

Content

- Describe the features of sprains, fractures, and dislocations of the lower extremities

- Describe the principles of emergency care for lower extremity injuries

Skill Performance

- Demonstrate the appropriate assessment and emergency care for sprains, fractures, and dislocations of the lower extremities

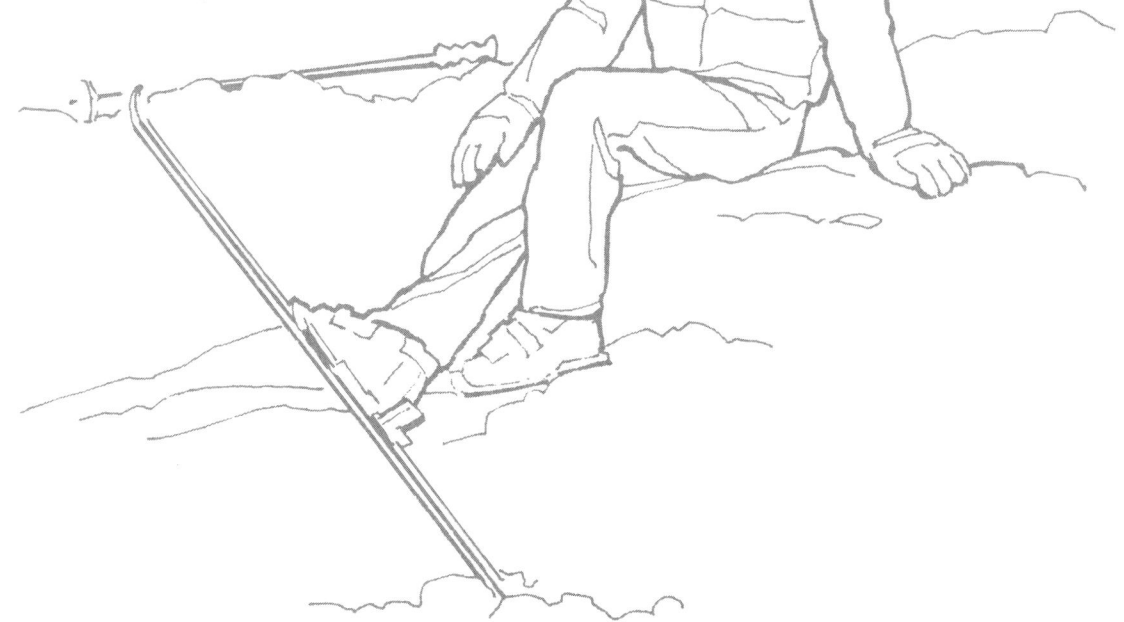

CHAPTER 12 STUDY QUESTIONS

1. Detail the signs and symptoms of various types of sprains, fractures, and dislocations.

Types	Signs and Symptoms
SPRAINS	
Knee	
Ankle	
FRACTURES	
Pelvic	
Hip	
Femoral Shaft	
Above-knee Femur	
Lower Leg	
Ankle	
Foot	
DISLOCATIONS	
Hip	
Knee	
Patella	
Ankle	

2. The position of the knee when it is strongest and most stable is

   A. Slightly flexed
   B. Fully extended
   C. Greatly flexed
   D. Hyperextended

3. Label the major components of the knee.

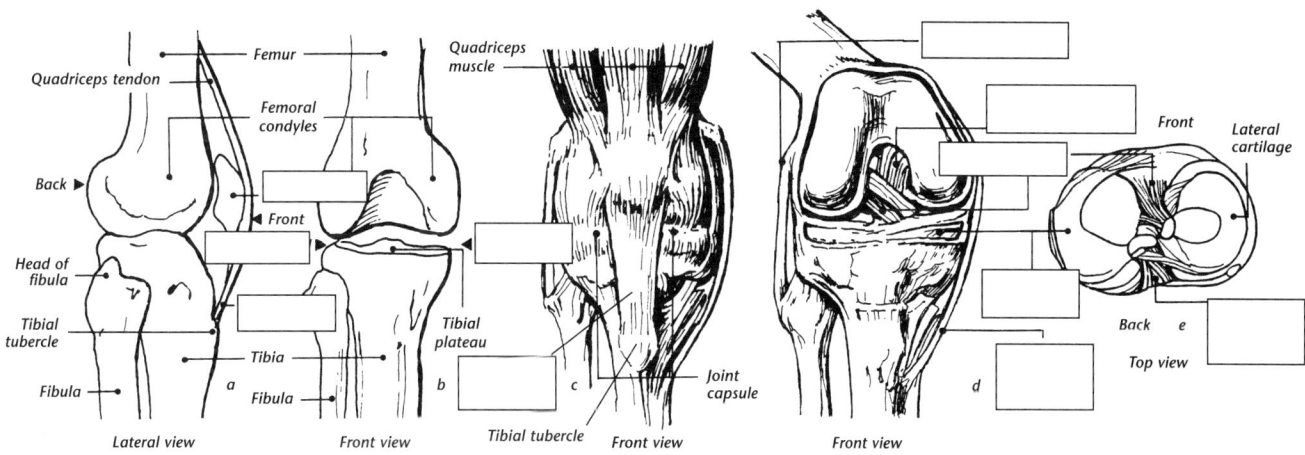

4. The knee ligament that is most frequently injured by skiers is the
   A. anterior cruciate
   B. lateral collateral
   C. medial collateral
   D. posterior cruciate

5. List three symptoms of a pelvic fracture

   _____
   _____
   _____

6. Downward pressure and then inward pressure on the iliac crests is a test for injury to the
   A. Spine
   B. Femur
   C. Abdomen
   D. Pelvis

7. A patient with a suspected knee sprain should be encouraged to consult an orthopedic surgeon if symptoms do not subside in
   A. Three to four days
   B. One week
   C. 24 hours
   D. Two weeks

8. Detail the emergency care for various types of sprains, fractures, and dislocations.

Types	Emergency Care
SPRAINS	
Knee	
Ankle	
FRACTURES	
Pelvic	
Hip	
Femoral Shaft	
Above-knee Femur	
Lower Leg	
Ankle	
Foot	
DISLOCATIONS	
Hip	
Knee	
Patella	
Ankle	

9. Why shouldn't a subtrochanteric fracture be splinted with a traction splint? What emergency care should be provided?

___
___
___
___

10. Emergency care of a suspected midshaft femur fracture consists of

___

11. Describe the emergency care for an angulated or rotated tibia/fibula fracture?

___

12. When the splinting process for lower extremities is completed, what must be reassessed and why?

___

Chapter 12 Local Protocol

1. Describe your local patrol assessment procedures when evaluating a suspected lower extremity injury.

___

2. Identify types of equipment and local patrol procedures for handling lower extremity injuries.

Types	Local Equipment	Patrol Procedures
SPRAINS		
Knee		
Ankle		
FRACTURES		
Pelvic		
Hip		
Femoral Shaft		
Above-knee Femur		
Lower Leg		
Ankle		
Foot		
DISLOCATIONS		
Hip		
Knee		
Patella		
Ankle		

CHAPTER 12 SKILL PERFORMANCE REQUIREMENTS

- Review *Outdoor Emergency Care* scenario 12.1

- Demonstrate the appropriate assessment and emergency care for splinting pelvic and hip fractures and hip dislocations

- Demonstrate the appropriate assessment and emergency care for splinting a femoral shaft fracture

- Demonstrate the appropriate technique for splinting a knee or patella dislocation and an above-knee femur fracture

- Demonstrate the appropriate assessment and emergency care for splinting knee and ankle sprains; lower leg, ankle, and foot fractures; and ankle dislocations

Skill Performance Guidelines

- Vital Signs Determination (see Chapter 3)
- Patient Assessment (see Chapter 5)
- Use of Oxygen and Airway Adjuncts (see Chapter 6)
- Control of Severe Bleeding in a Wound (see Chapter 7)
- Traction Splinting (see Chapter 9)
- Spinal Immobililization (see Chapter 9)
- General Management of Long Bone Fractures
- General Management of a Fracture or Dislocation At or Near a Joint
- Alignment of Angulated or Displaced Fracture
- Managment of an Open Fracture

Focused Body Survey
Extremity injury
Examine and palpate each extremity for abnormality
Question the injured patient about • Pain on motion • Inability to move or use extremity • Weakness • Numbness or tingling • Inability to bear weight
Assess circulatory and neurologic function in the extremity
Look for medical-alert tags
Pelvic injury
Examine and palpate the pelvic area
Questions the injured patient about • Trouble urinating • Blood in urine • Blood coming from urethra, vagina, or rectum • Pregnancy
Back and Buttocks
If *not* contraindicated, roll the patient over and examines and palpates the back, spine, and buttocks.
Question the injured patient about • Numbness, tingling, weakness, inability to move • Difficulty breathing

General Management of Long Bone Fractures

- Assesses the limb and mechanism of injury to determine the presence and location of a fracture.

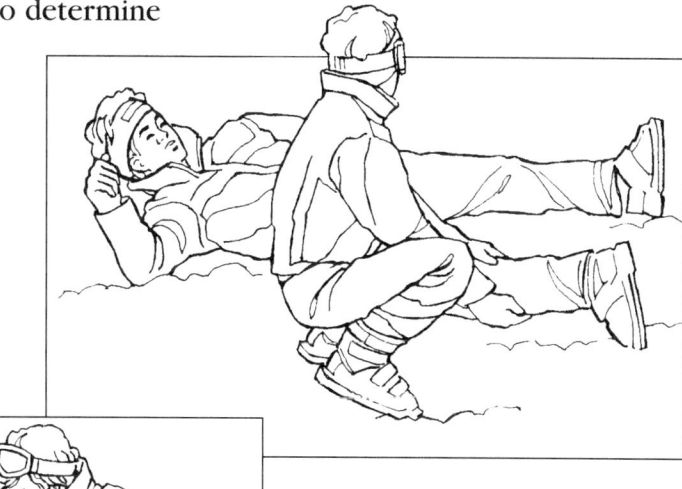

- Assesses the circulatory and neurological function of the limb.

- Manually stabilizes the fracture site. *Note: Continuous manual stabilization must be maintained until mechanical device is applied and completely secured.*

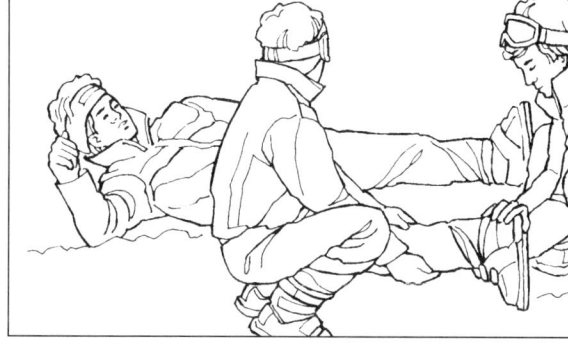

- Aligns the limb to a near-anatomically correct position.

- Prepares the immobilization device to be used.

- Positions the device without excessive movement of the limb.

- Applies and secures the device to the limb without excessive movement, ensures that all voids are filled, and checks that the fracture site and the adjacent joints are immobilized.

- Reassesses the circulatory and neurological function of the limb.

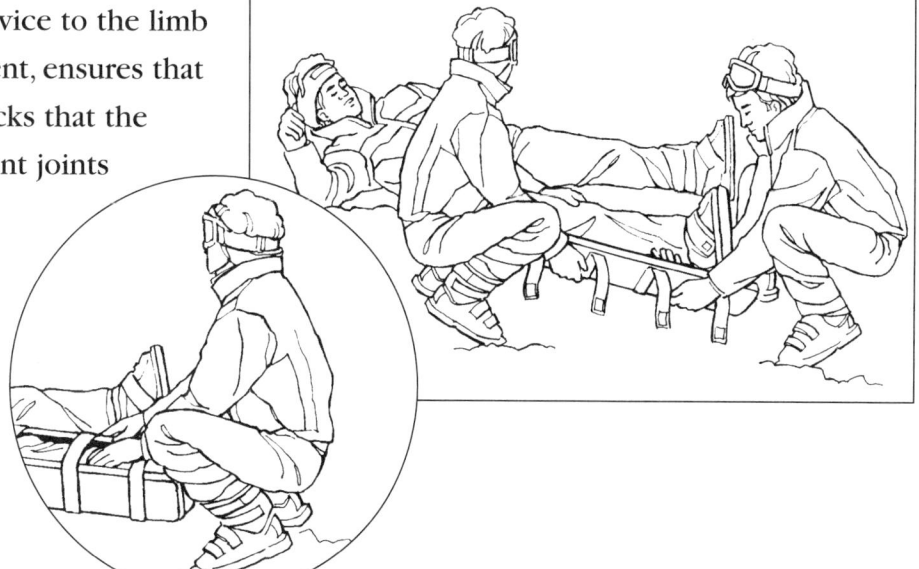

General Management of a Fracture or Dislocation At or Near a Joint

- Assesses the limb, joint, and mechanism of injury to determine the presence and location of a fracture and/or dislocation.

- Assesses the circulatory and neurological function of the limb.

- Manually stabilizes the fracture site and the limb. *Note: Continuous manual stabilization must be maintained until mechanical device is applied and completely secured.*

- Moves the limb toward a nearer-anatomically correct position, if possible, with the assistance of the patient.

- *If there is no distal circulation,* aligns limb until resistance is met or circulation returns.

- Prepares the immobilization device for use, taking into account any unusual anatomical positioning of the limb.

- Positions the device without any excessive movement of the limb.

- Applies and secures the device to the limb and body without excessive movement, ensuring all voids are filled, and checks the fracture site, the adjacent joints, and the limb are immobilized.

- Reassesses the circulatory and neurological function of the limb.

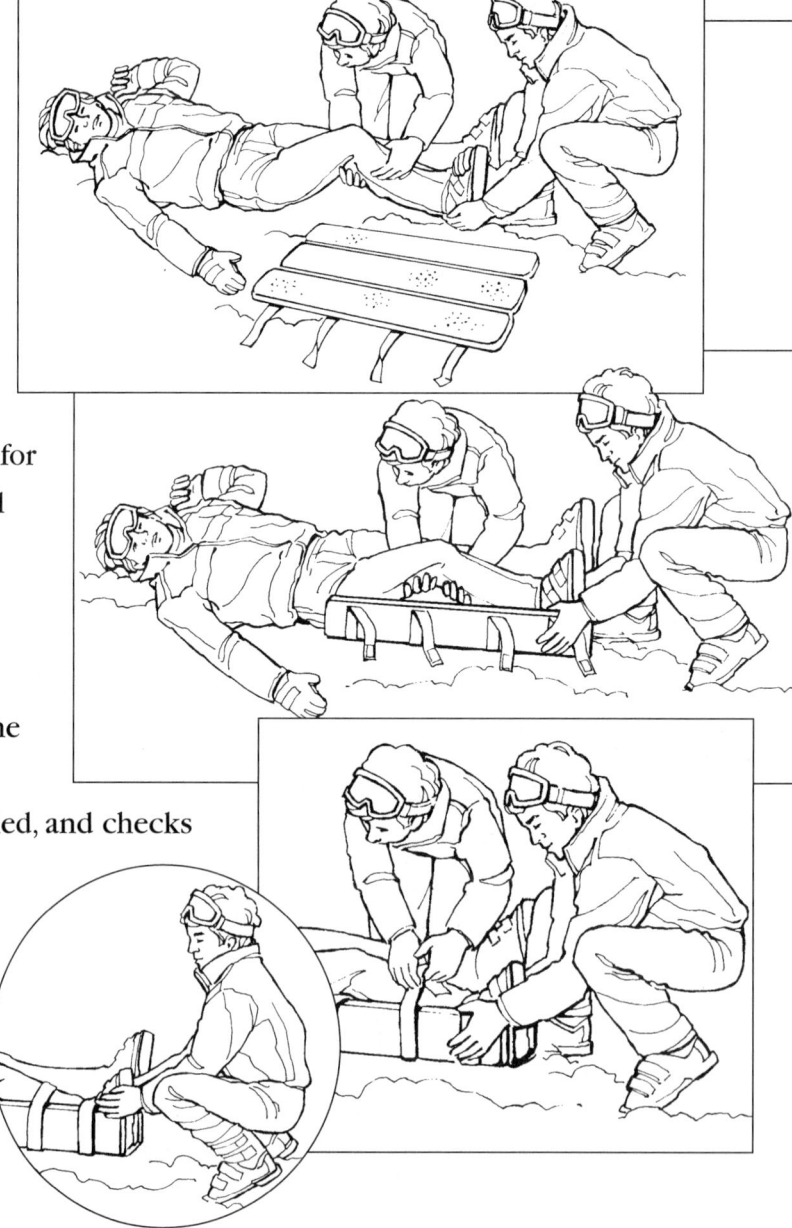

Alignment of Angulated or Displaced Fracture

- Assesses the limb and mechanism of injury to determine the presence and location of a fracture.

- Assesses the circulatory and neurological function of the limb.

- Manually stabilizes the fracture site and the limb.
  Note: Continuous manual stabilization must be maintained until mechanical device is applied and completely secured.

- Begins straightening the limb by moving each joint individually and applies axial traction at the nearest distal joint or the end of the limb as needed to complete the straightening process.

- Rotates the limb as necessary to approximately normal anatomical position.

- Monitors patient for indications of resistance or excessive pain during alignment.

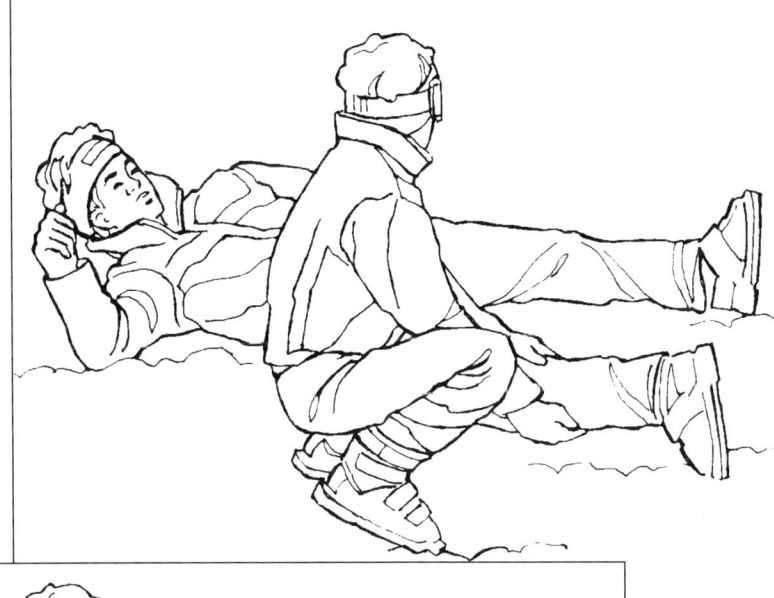

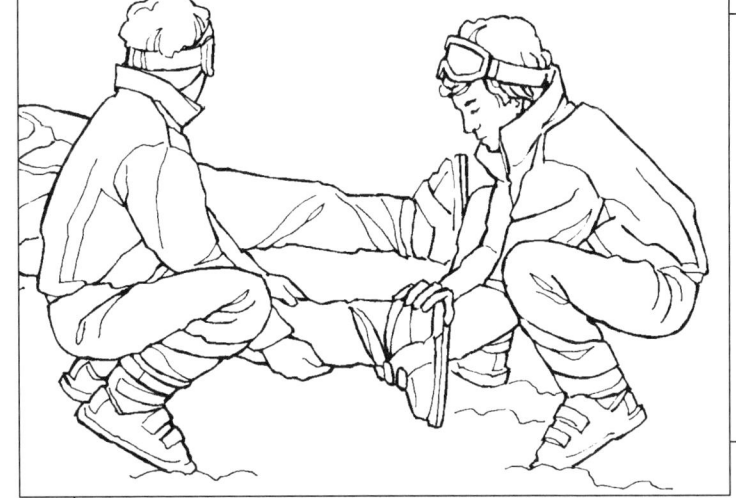

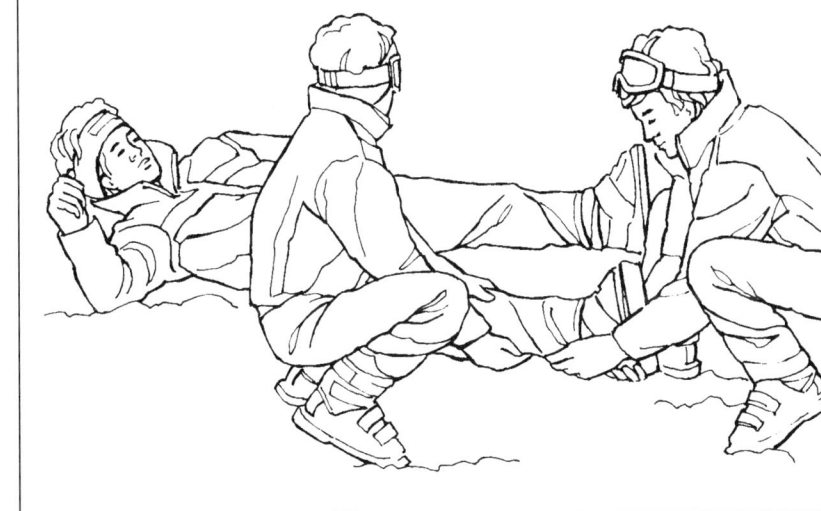

Management of an Open Fracture

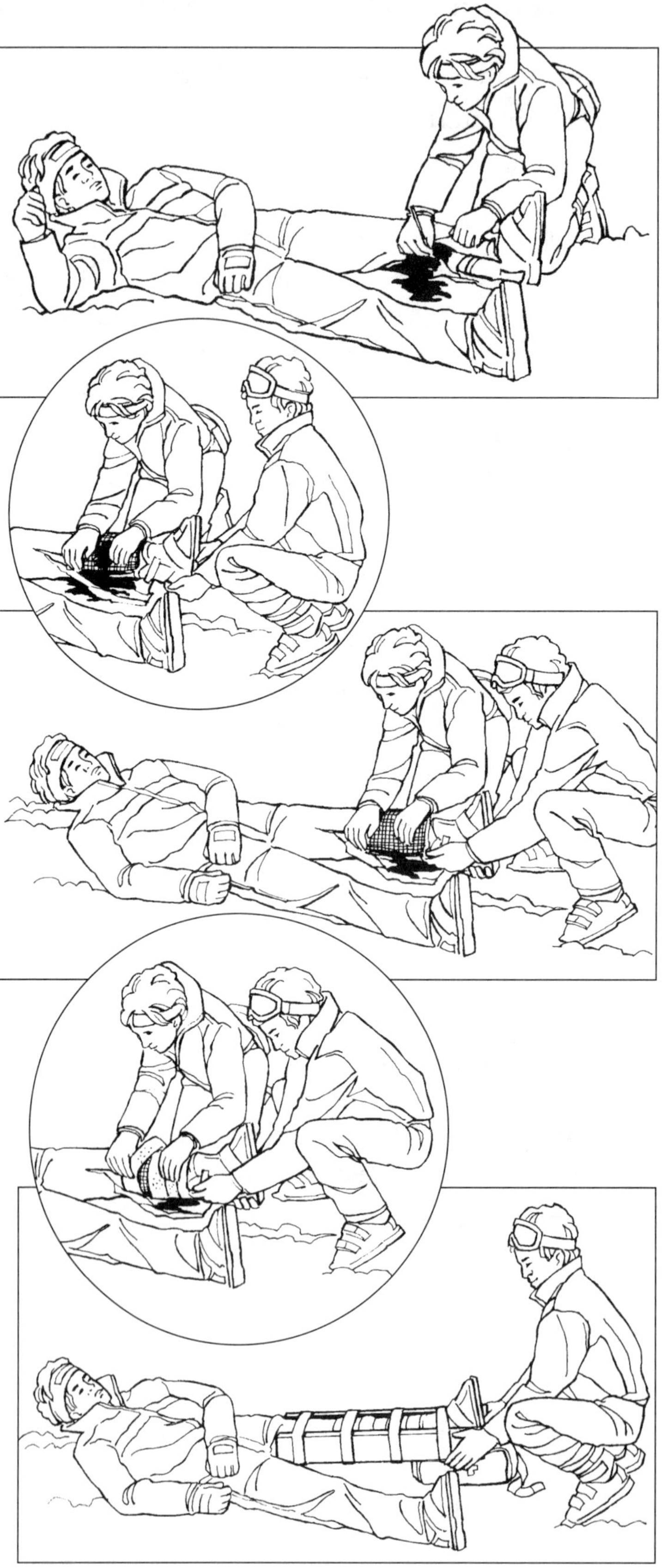

- Uses body substance isolation precautions according to protocols.

- Assesses the limb, identifying the presence of an open fracture, its severity and stability.

- Assesses the circulatory and neurological function of the extremity, if not contraindicated by bleeding severity.

- Begins to control any severe bleeding.

- Manually stabilizes the fracture site and the limb.

- Aligns the limb to near-anatomically correct position

- Controls any bleeding that is present.
    - Exposes the fracture site.
    - Uses direct and indirect pressure.
    - Uses the pressure point if necessary.
    - Applies a dressing over the wound.

- Cleans and irrigates the wound (determined by local protocol).

- Dresses and initially bandages the wound with pressure as needed.

- Immobilizes the limb and adjacent joints, maintaining elevation, if possible.

- Applies final bandaging of the wound after immobilization.

- Reassesses the circulatory and neurological function of the extremity.

Chapter 12 Scenarios

1. You come upon a skier in his mid-20s who, while telemarking, went into a twisting fall as he crossed a section of ice on the advanced slope. His fall carried him into the trees, where he sustained an open fracture of the ankle with deformity and exposed bone. The skier is wearing low ankle boots. Vital signs are pulse: 100; respirations: 24. Based on possible mechanisms of injury, describe the potential and anticipated problems with this scenario. What equipment would be needed? What type of emergency care should you provide?

   _____
   _____
   _____
   _____

2. An 18-year-old man becomes airborne on a steep, moguled slope; loses control; and hits a tree on the edge of the trail. He lands on his left leg in soft snow. Your assessment indicates that there is no head or upper body impact point or injury and no altered level of responsiveness. The patient is fully responsive and complains of severe pain in the middle of his left thigh, where you note there is obvious angular deformity. Your assessment further reveals good neurological and circulatory function in all four extremities, a pulse of 88, and respirations of 18. What do you suspect? What is the emergency care for the victim?

   _____
   _____
   _____
   _____

3. A 20-year-old female, skiing for the first time, catches an inside edge and falls of the T-bar lift. The patient complains of severe pain in her right leg just above the top of her ski boot. She says she can move her toes. Her pulse is 100 beats per minute, and her respirations are 20 per minute. What do you suspect? What is the emergency care for the victim?

   _____
   _____
   _____
   _____

GENERAL MANAGEMENT OF LONG BONE FRACTURES

Objective: To immobilize the fracture site and adjacent joints for a long bone fracture in an extremity.

NOTE: *Any device chosen must be applied correctly and in accordance with its manufacturer's instructions. If the device choden for the upper extremity is "soft" (e.g., sling and swathe), all of the objectives must be met.*

SKILL	YES	NO	NOTATIONS
• Assesses the limb and mechanism of injury to determine the presence and location of a fracture.			
• Assesses the circulatory and neurological function of the limb.			
• Manually stabilizes the fracture site. *(Note: Continous manual stabilization must be maintained until mechanical device is applied and completely secured.)*			
• Aligns the limb to a near-anatomically correct position.			
• Prepares the immobilization device to be used.			
• Positions the device without excessive movement of the limb.			
• Applies and secures the device to the limb without excessive movement, ensures that all voids are filled, and checks that the fracture site and the adjacent joints are immobilized.			
• Reassesses the circulatory and neurological function of the limb.			
Did the trainee or patroller adequately demonstrate the performance criteria of this skill?			

COMMENTS

GENERAL MANAGEMENT OF A FRACTURE OR DISLOCATION AT OR NEAR A JOINT

Objective: To demonstrate the immobilization of a fracture site, the adjacent joints, and the extremity for a fracture or dislocation in or near a joint.

SKILL	YES	NO	NOTATIONS
• Assesses the limb, joint, and mechanism of injury to determine the presence and location of a fracture and/or dislocation.			
• Assesses the circulatory and neurological function of the limb.			
• Manually stabilizes the fracture site and the limb. *(Note: Continous manual stabilization must be maintained until mechanical device is applied and completely secured.)*			
• Moves the limb toward a nearer-anatomically correct position, if possible, with the assistance of the patient.			
• *If there is no distal circulation*, aligns limb until resistance is met or circulation returns.			
• Prepares the immobilization device for use, taking into account any unusual anatomical positioning of the limb.			
• Positions the device without excessive movement of the limb.			
• Applies and secures the device to the limband body without excessive movement, ensuring all voids are filled, and checks that the fracture site, the adjacent joints, and the limb are immobilized.			
• Reassesses the circulatory and neurological function of the limb.			
Did the trainee or patroller adequately demonstrate the performance criteria of this skill?			

COMMENTS

ALIGNMENT OF ANGULATED OR DISPLACED FRACTURE

Objective: To return a fractured limb to a near-normal position, thereby improving circulatory and neurological function, the limb's stability, and ability to function.

SKILL	YES	NO	NOTATIONS
• Assesses the limb and mechanism of injury to determine the presence and location of a fracture.			
• Assesses the circulatory and neurological function of the limb.			
• Manually stabilizes the fracture site and the limb. *(Note: Continous manual stabilization must be maintained until mechanical device is applied and completely secured.)*			
• Begins straightening the limb by moving each joint individually, and applies axial traction at the nearest distal joint or the end of the limb as needed to complete the straightening process.			
• Rotates the limb as necessary to approximately normal anatomical position.			
• Monitors patient for indications of resistance or excessive pain during alignment.			
Did the trainee or patroller adequately demonstrate the performance criteria of this skill?			

COMMENTS

MANAGEMENT OF AN OPEN FRACTURE

Objective: To demonstrate the control of severe bleeding associated with an open fracture.

SKILL	YES	NO	NOTATIONS
• Uses BSI precautions according to protocols.			
• Assesses the limb, identifying the presence of an open fracture, its severity and stability.			
• Assesses the circulatory and neurological function of the extremity, if not contraindicated by bleeding severity.			
• Begins to control any severe bleeding.			
• Manually stabilizes the fracture site and the limb.			
• Aligns the limb to near-anatomically correct position			
• Controls any bleeding that is present			
• Exposes the fracture site			
• Uses direct and indirect pressure			
• Uses the pressure point if necessary			
• Applies a dressing over the wound			
• Cleans and irrigates the wound (determined by local protocol).			
• Dresses and initially bandages the wound with pressure as needed.			
• Immobilizes the limb and adjacent joints, maintaining elevation, if possible.			
• Applies final bandaging of the wound after immobilization.			
• Reassesses the circulatory and neurological function of the extremity.			
Did the trainee or patroller adequately demonstrate the performance criteria of this skill?			

COMMENTS

TRACTION SPLINTING

Objective: To immobilize a fracture of the femur using a traction-splinting device.

SKILL	YES	NO	NOTATIONS
• Assesses the limb and mechanism of injury to determine the presence and location of a fracture.			
• Manually stabilizes the fracture site and limb. *(Note: Continuous manual stabilization must be maintained until a splint device is applied and completely secured.)*			
• Assesses the circulatory and neurological function of the limb.			
• Realigns the limb if needed. *(Note: Manual stabilization/traction should be applied at the knee initially until the limb is straightened and the ankle hitch is applied.)*			
• Applies an ankle hitch.			
• Prepares the immobilization device and materials to be used.			
• Applies and maintains traction to the entire limb for the duration of splint application.			
• Positions the splint properly under the limb and against the ischial tuberosity or pelvic bone (depending on the splint type) without excessive movement or elevation of the limb.			
• Applies the splint, including any necessary cradles, supports, etc.			
• Applies mechanical traction at the ankle, using hitch assembly.			
• Secures the limb properly in the splint.			
• Reassesses the circulatory and neurological function of the limb.			
Did the trainee or patroller adequately demonstrate the performance criteria of this skill?			

COMMENTS

STUDY NOTES

CHAPTER 13

Injuries to the Head, Eye, Face, and Soft Tissues of the Neck

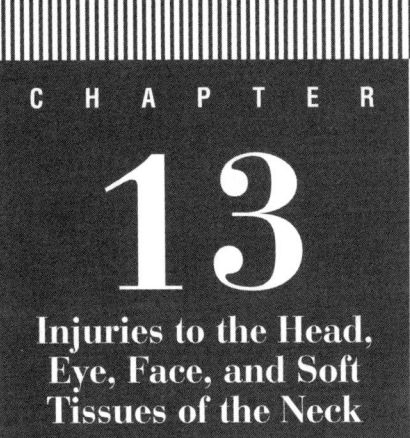

CONCLUDING OBJECTIVES

The learner will:

Content

- List possible causes of unresponsiveness and appropriate emergency care

- Describe appropriate emergency care for a responsive patient with injuries to the head, eye, face, throat and soft tissues of the neck

Skill Performance

- Demonstrate assessment techniques for a patient with a head injury

- Demonstrate basic techniques of emergency care for an unresponsive patient

- Demonstrate basic techniques of emergency care for injuries to the head, eye, face, and soft tissues of the neck

CHAPTER 13 STUDY QUESTIONS

1. Name the injury with each illustration.

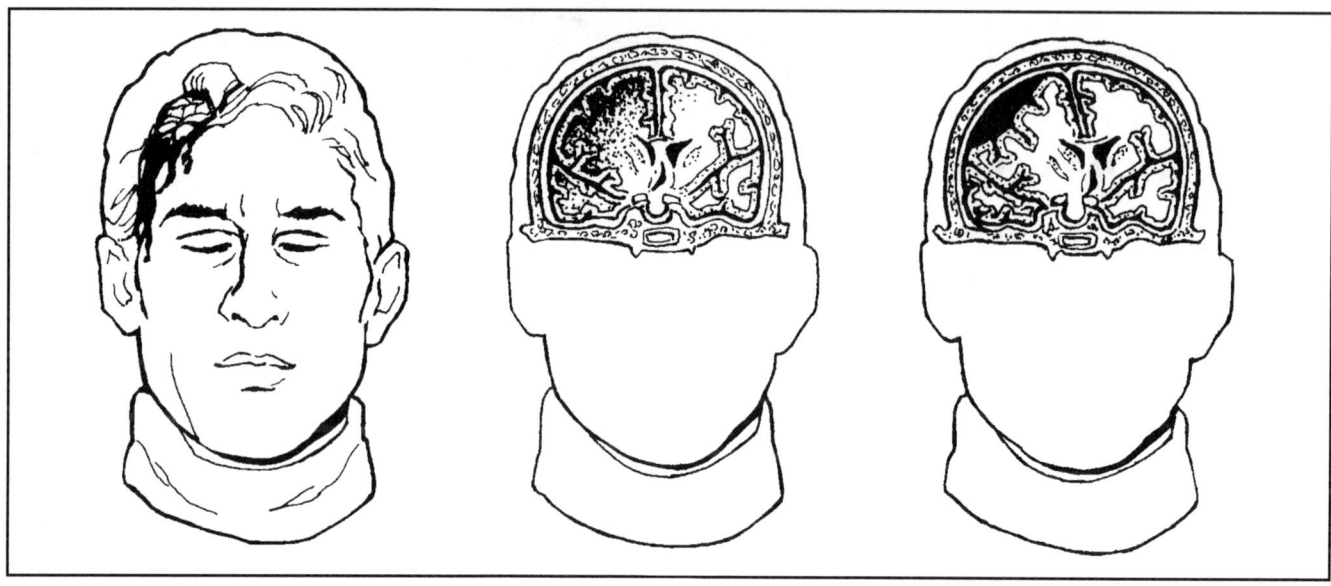

    A. _____   B. _____   C. _____

2. What is a sign (or symptom) in any significant head injury?
   _____

3. What tool is available to assess the level of responsiveness in a patient?
   _____

4. What is the main cause of secondary injury to the brain?
   _____

5. A head injury by itself rarely causes shock.
   ☐ True   ☐ False

6. Every unresponsive patient or every patient with a head injury must be considered to have _____.

7. Describe the signs and symptoms of increased intracranial pressure (ICP) associated with a head injury.

176 OEC Study Book

8. What two things can rescuers do that may slow the process of ICP?

9. List the assessment summary of an unresponsive patient.

10. List the major components of the emergency care for the unresponsive patient.

11. Describe the recovery position and how to place an unresponsive, non-trauma patient in this position.

12. Match the following emergency care problems with the proper characteristics.

    ___ Scalp lacerations   A. Bruise in brain
    ___ Concussions   B. Excess pressure is serious
    ___ Brain contusions   C. Temporary loss of responsiveness from bump on head
    ___ Bleeding inside skull   D. Caused by penetrating object or brain damage
    ___ Skull fractures   E. Bleeds freely, requires dressing

13. Fill in the appropriate boxes with signs and symptoms of and emergency care for specific types of head injuries.

Types	Signs and Symptoms	Emergency Care
Scalp Lacerations		
Concussions		
Brain Contusions		
Bleeding Inside the Skull		
Skull Fractures		

14. Describe the specific assessment procedures for the patient with head injuries who is unresponsive when discovered.

_____
_____
_____
_____
_____

What signs and symptoms indicate that a patient should be transported to the hospital without delay?

_____
_____
_____
_____
_____

15. Name the parts of the eye.

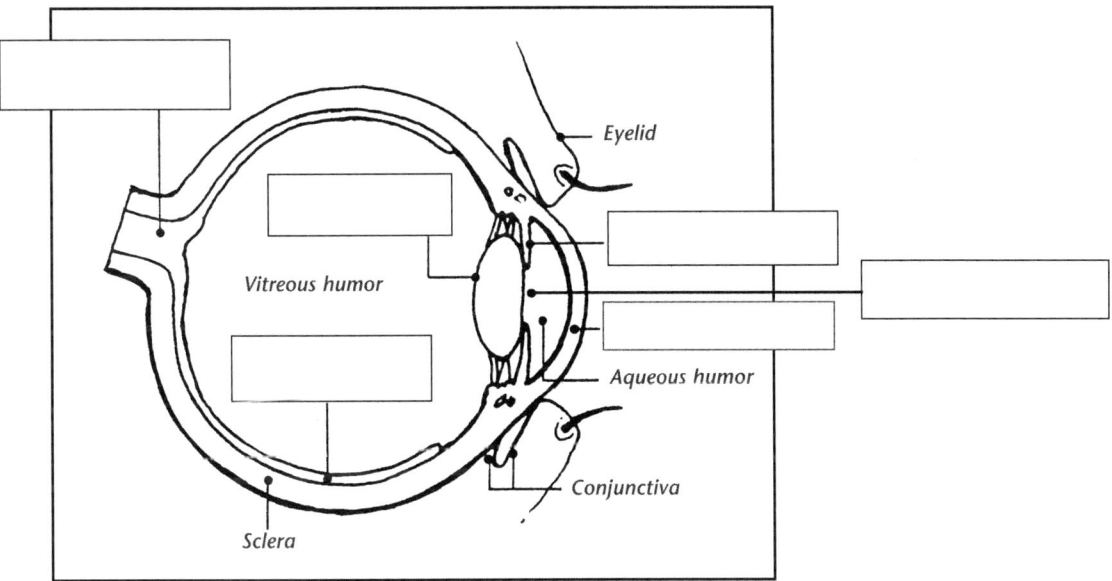

16. Patients with blunt trauma to the eye should have an eye shield applied, and the opposite eye should be
    A. Left uncovered
    B. Covered
    C. Watched for movement
    D. Taped tightly shut

17. When caring for a patient who has been splashed in the eye with a chemical, an emergency care provider should
    A. Cover it to prevent any light from entering it
    B. Wash the eye with a large amount of tap water
    C. Only wash the eye with sterile water to prevent contamination
    D. Not do anything because only a physician should treat eye injuries

18. List the important factors of emergency care of a patient with a facial fracture.

    _____
    _____
    _____
    _____
    _____
    _____

19. Your first concern for a patient with an injury to the mouth should be to
    A. Stop the bleeding
    B. See that the patient does not swallow any blood
    C. Maintain an open airway
    D. Pack the mouth with gauze

20. A laceration completely through the cheek and into the mouth will require a pressure dressing
    A. On both sides
    B. On the outside only
    C. On the inside only
    D. No dressing should be used

21. Describe the methods for stopping or slowing a nosebleed.

22. Match the following emergency problems with the proper characteristics.
    ___ Eye injury   A. Give oxygen in high concentration
    ___ Head injury   B. Cover bilaterally
    ___ Oral/dental injury   C. Protect from cold air
    ___ Facial fracture   D. Maintain upper airway
    ___ Throat injury   E. Care same as for unresponsive

23. Vomiting is common in unresponsive patients. What precautions should be taken?

Chapter 13 Local Protocol

1. Describe local patrol protocols for a patient with head injuries.

2. Describe local patrol protocols for injuries to the head, eye, face, and soft tissues of the neck.
   _____
   _____
   _____
   _____
   _____

CHAPTER 13 SKILL PERFORMANCE REQUIREMENTS

- Review *Outdoor Emergency Care* scenario 13.1

- Demonstrate assessment techniques for a patient with a head injury

- Demonstrate basic techniques of emergency care for an unresponsive patient

- Demonstrate basic techniques of emergency care for injuries to the head, eye, face, and soft tissues of the throat

Skill Performance Guidelines

- Vital Signs Determination (see Chapter 3)
- Patient Assessment (see Chapter 5)
- Use of Oxygen and Airway Adjuncts (see Chapter 6)
- Control of Severe Bleeding in a Wound (see Chapter 7)

Focused Body Survey
Check head, skull, and facial bones.
Check pupils for reaction, unequalness.
Check ears, nose, and mouth for blood, fluids, or foreign objects.
Question the injured patient about • Headache • Dizziness • Loss of responsiveness, even momentary • Double vision or inability to see normally

Chapter 13 Scenarios

1. A skier loses control while skiing in trees. The skier is sitting on the snow between trees with a portion of the branch protruding from his eye and goggles. He is in a panic and in a great deal of pain. He complains of pain in his face and neck but is so disoriented and shaken up that he has a difficult time articulating specifics. A rapid body survey indicate no further injury. Vital signs: Pulse, 130, Respirations, 30 and jerky. Explain the emergency care steps you would take in handling this situation. Based on possible mechanisms of injury, describe the potential and anticipated problems of this scenario. What equipment would be needed? What type of emergency care should you provide?

2. On a very busy holiday weekend, a 46-year-old woman is skiing late in the day on an intermediate slope that was machine-groomed early that morning. She loses edge control and takes a very hard fall. When you arrive on the scene about 4 minutes later, the skier is sitting on the edge of the trail talking to her companion. You begin your assessment by asking the patient what happened. You quickly realize the patient does not know where she is and cannot recall what has happened in the last 10 minutes. The skier does remember all other events of the day and the trip to the ski area. Your assessment determines a pulse of 88 and respirations of 16. What questions would you ask her to ascertain the nature and degree of the injury? What problems does your overall assessment indicate?

3. You are patrolling your usual shift when called to a serious head injury situation. You arrive first, and during the urgent survey you find an unresponsive male in his late 20s. He obviously has impacted a lift tower, and his head is resting against the concrete tower base. His initial vital signs are a pulse of 86 and shallow respirations of 32. You notice that the intensity of the breathing is cycling from adequate to almost none over one-minute periods. Another patroller arrives immediately after you. What do you suspect? What is the emergency care for the patient?

STUDY NOTES

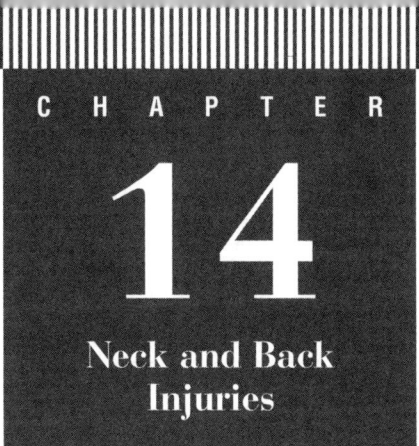

CHAPTER 14

Neck and Back Injuries

CONCLUDING OBJECTIVES

The learner will:

Content

- Describe characteristics of spine and spinal cord injuries

Skill Performance

- Demonstrate the appropriate emergency care of a patient with suspected spine or spinal cord injuries

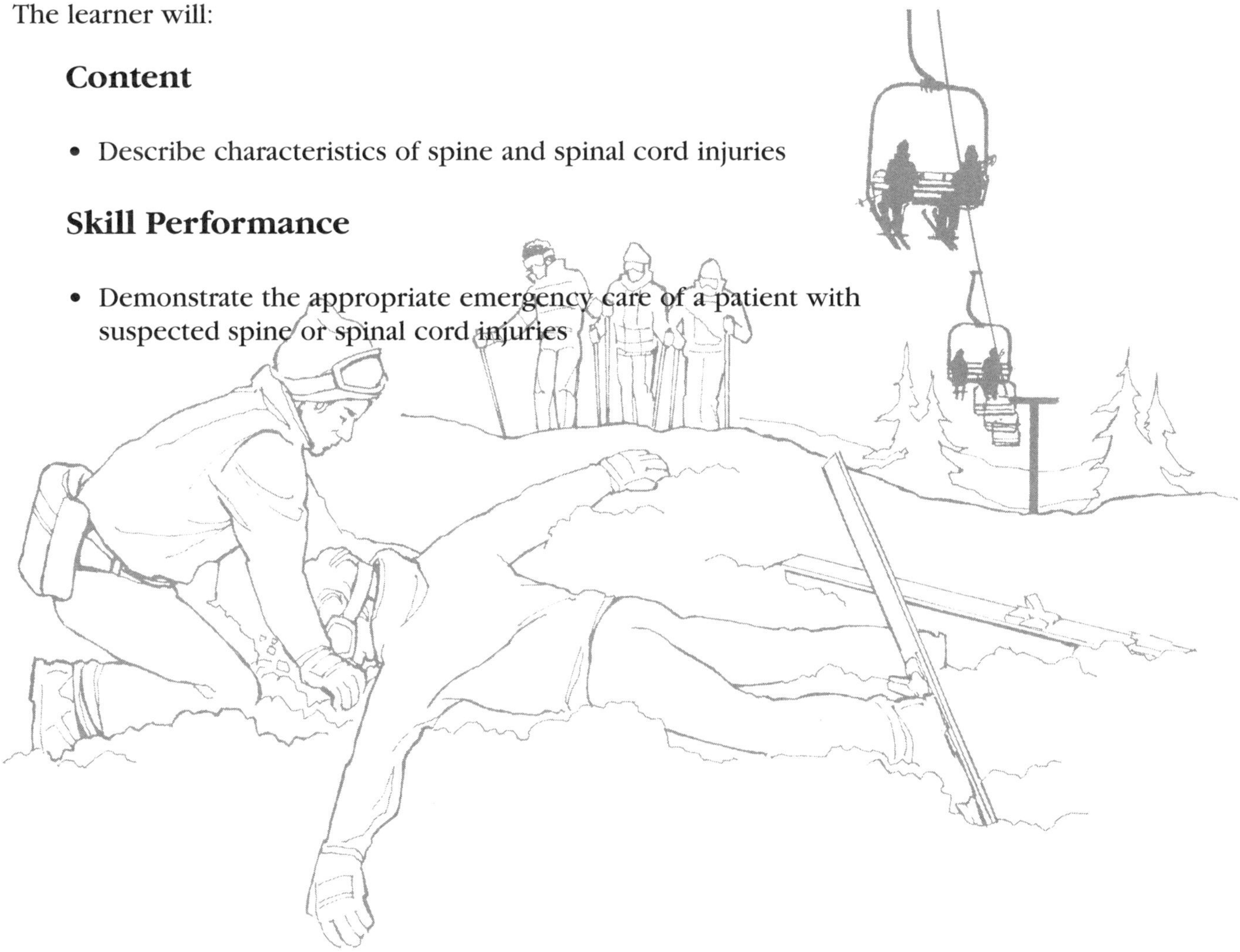

CHAPTER 14 STUDY QUESTIONS

1. Identify the four types of spinal injuries illustrated below.

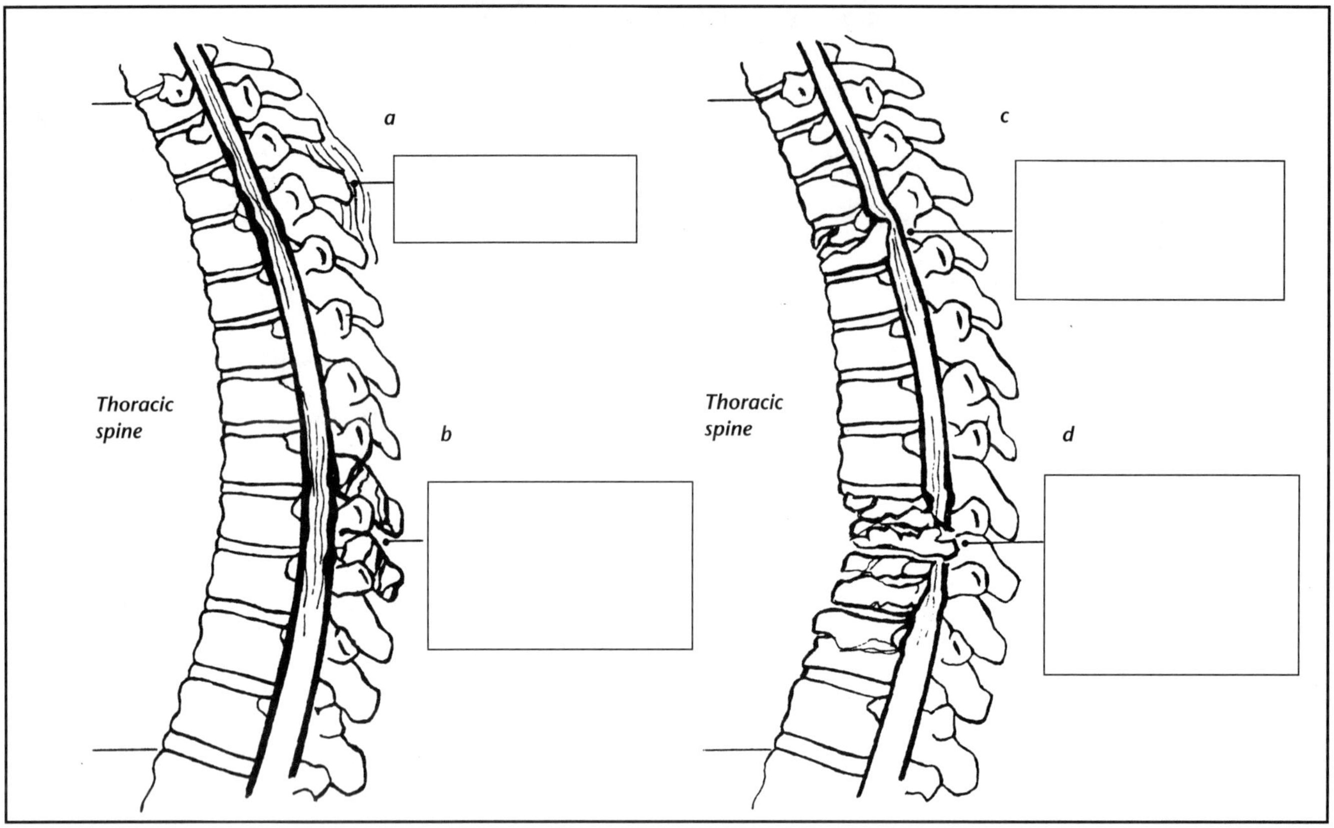

2. What is the major goal of emergency care for a patient with a spinal cord injury?
   _____

3. A patient with spinal cord injury may have shortness of breath because
   A. The pain is extremely intense.
   B. Heart action may be irregular.
   C. Nerve damage fails to regulate oxygen and carbon dioxide exchange.
   D. Chest muscles, or the chest muscles plus the diaphragm, may be paralyzed.

4. Summarize the signs and symptoms of spine and spinal cord injuries.

Spine	Spinal Cord

5. What at least six mechanisms and patterns of injury would make you suspect significant neck and/or back injuries?

6. List the procedures for assessment of a patient with a neck or back injury.

7. What types of assessment tests can you conduct on a patient with a spinal injury to document the presence or lack of circulation, motion, and sensation?

8. Summarize the emergency care of a patient with a neck or back injury.

9. Which of the following methods of establishing an airway is preferable if a cervical spine injury is suspected?
    A. Head-tilt/neck-lift
    B. Head-tilt/chin-lift
    C. Jaw-thrust maneuver
    D. Abdominal thrusts

10. Describe the technique of logrolling a patient from the prone to the supine position.

11. Summarize the steps used in the bridge lift.

12. Explain the procedure for helmet removal.

13. Summarize the steps to immobilize a patient on a long spineboard.

14. When would it be appropriate to immobilize a patient on a short spineboard?

    On a standing spineboard?

Chapter 14 Local Protocol

1. Describe local patrol procedures, equipment, and techniques used in handling suspected neck and back injuries.

   _____
   _____
   _____
   _____
   _____

2. What is your resort's policy on helmet removal?

   _____
   _____

CHAPTER 14 SKILL PERFORMANCE REQUIREMENTS

- Review *Outdoor Emergency Care* scenario 14.1

- Demonstrate the appropriate care of a patient with suspected spine or spinal cord injuries

- Demonstrate the procedure for logrolling

- Demonstrate the procedure for helmet removal

- Demonstrate the procedures for the long-axis drag

- Demonstrate the procedure for multi-person direct ground lift

- Demonstrate the procedure for bridge lift

- Demonstrate the procedure for immobilizing a patient on a long spineboard

- Demonstrate the procedure for immobilizing a patient on a standing spineboard

Skill Performance Guidelines

- Vital Signs Determination (see Chapter 3)
- Patient Assessment (see Chapter 5)
- Use of Oxygen and Airway Adjuncts (see Chapter 6)
- Control of Severe Bleeding in a Wound (see Chapter 7)
- Spinal Immobililization (see Chapter 9)
- Lifting Techniques—Long -Axis Drag
- Lifting Techniques—Logroll
- Lifting Techniques—Multiple-Person Direct From the Ground
- Lifting Techniques—Bridge Lift
- Helmet Removal
- Application of a Standing Spineboard

Focused Body Survey—Neck and Back
Checks head, skull, facial bones
Checks pupils for reaction, unequalness
Checks ears, nose, mouth for blood, fluids, or foreign objects
Questions the injured patient on the following: • Numbness, tingling • Weakness • Inability to move • Difficulty breathing
Examine and palpate the cervical spine
Examine and palpate the anterior neck
Look for medical-alert tags

Lifting Techniques—Long-Axis Drag

- Maintains manual stabilization of the body throughout maneuver.

- Headward drag: supports or cradles the upper torso

- Footward drag: supports or cradles the ankles and lower torso

- Moves in a crouched position, pulling the patient slowly and smoothly about 12 inches at a time.

- Repositions, and repeats drag until reaching the desired location.

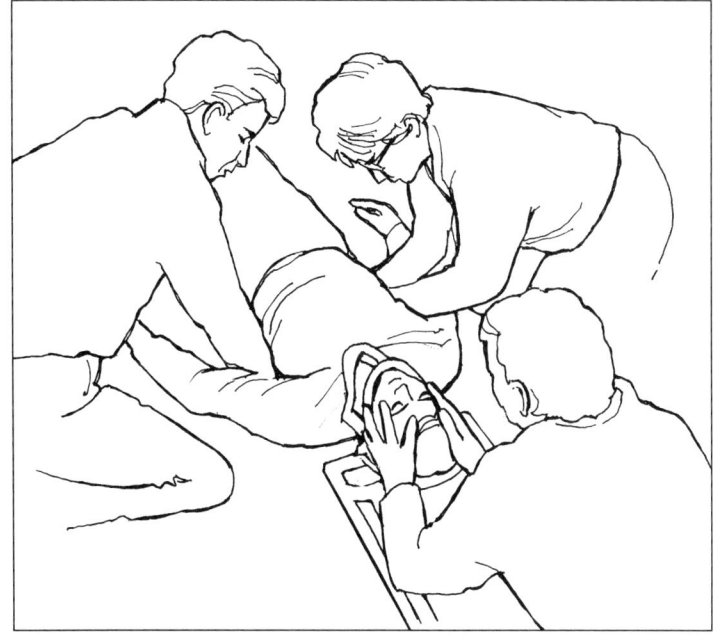

Lifting Techniques—Logroll

- Manually stabilizes the head and neck.

- Positions sufficient rescuers on the same side of the patient. Moves the patient as a unit while monitoring vital signs.

- Positions hands on the far side, takes body mass into consideration.

- Rolls the patient toward the rescuers on command from the leader (at the head), keeping the body in line. (The patient's arm may be alongside the body or elevated at local option.)

- Places the stretcher, litter, or board alongside the patient and underneath as far as possible without excessive movement.

- Rolls the patient onto the device on command from the leader, keeping the body in line.

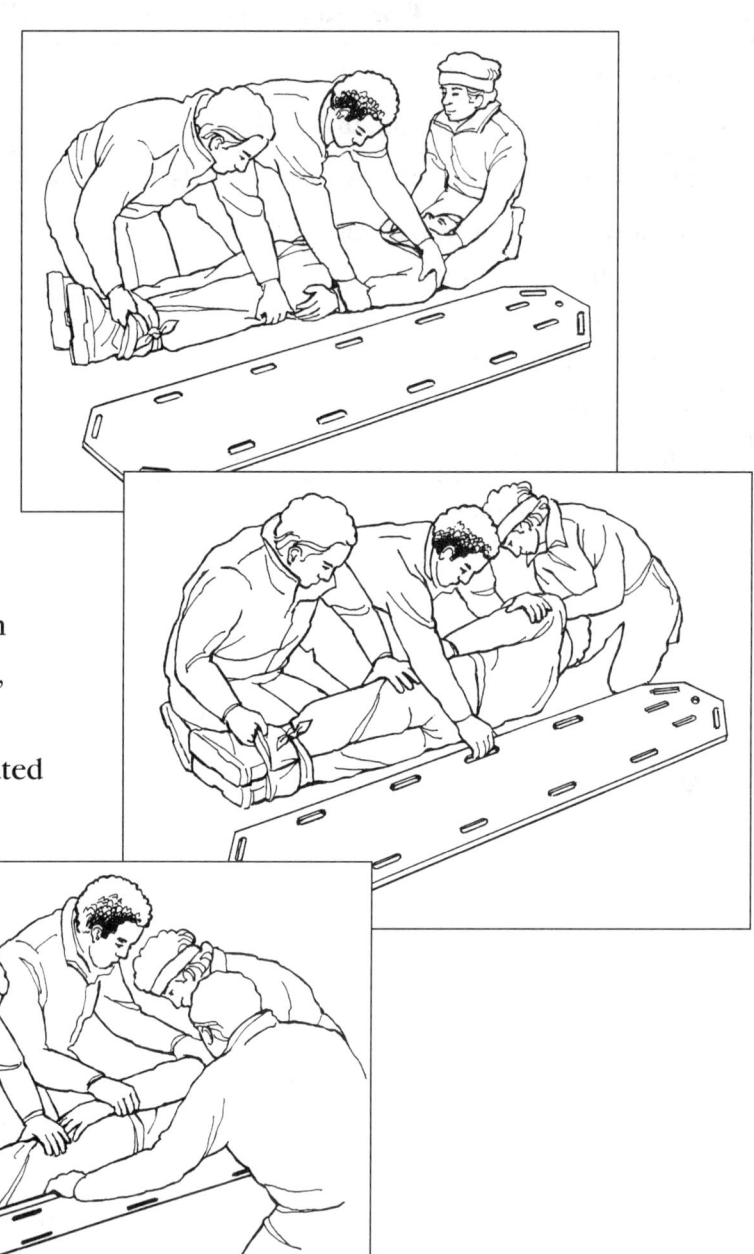

Lifting Techniques—Multiple-Person Direct From The Ground

- Manually stabilizes the head/neck as necessary for the injury.

- Determines the people pattern needed and available:
  5 people—3 to lift, 1 at head, 1 to move the device.
  6 people—4 to lift, 1 at head, 1 to move the device.

- Prepares all of the equipment needed for the lift or the device.

- Explains the commands and procedures, and demonstrates the hand positions.

- Executes the lift and slides the device into place, lifting the body as a unit.

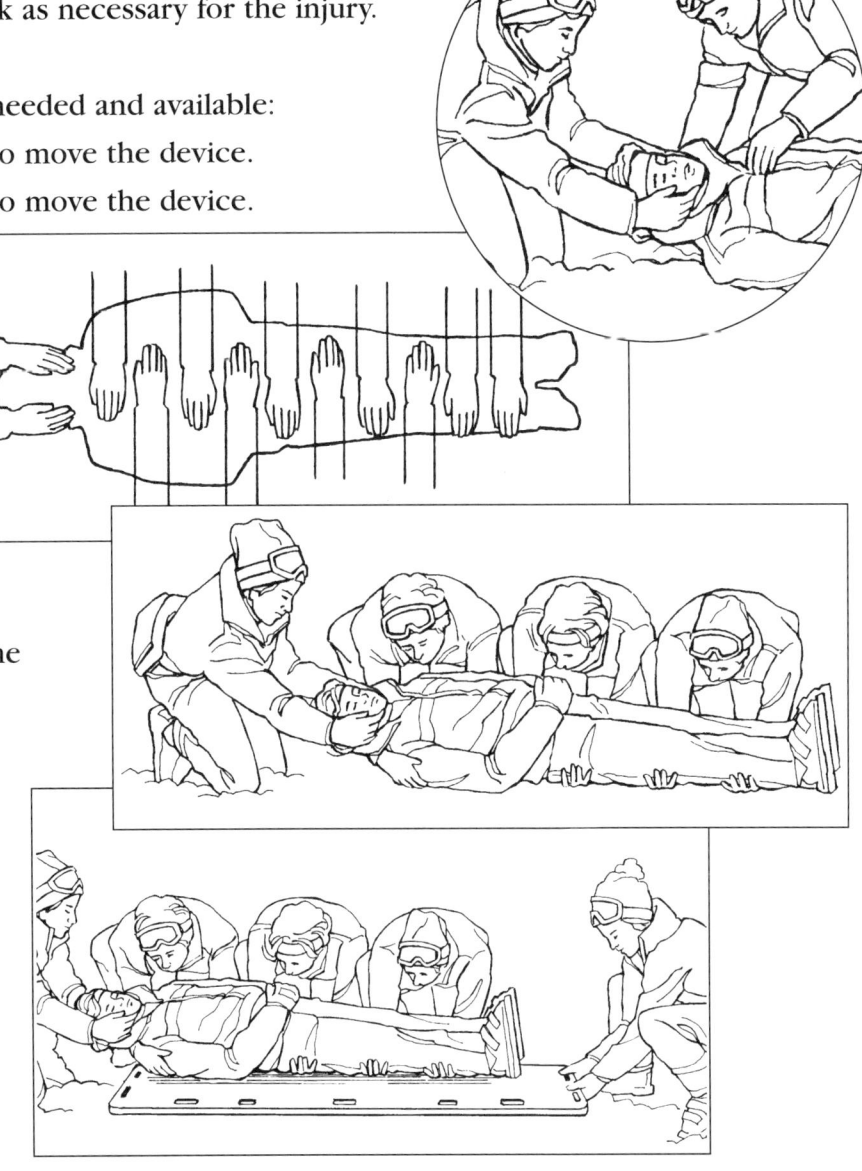

Lifting Techniques—Bridging

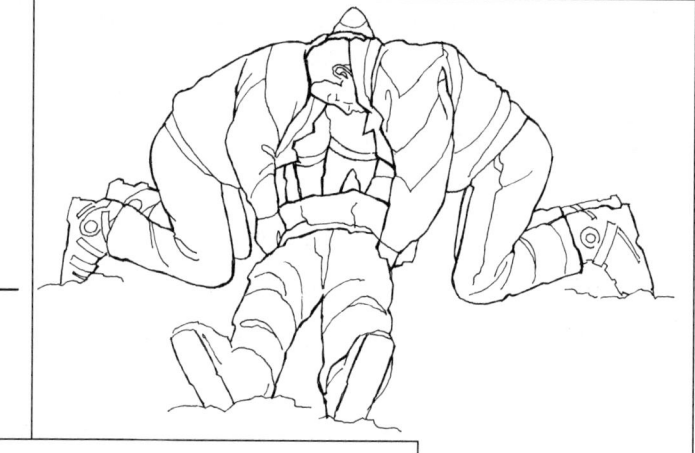

- Manually stabilizes the head and neck.

- Determines the number of lifters available and, therefore, the people pattern: 5 people— 3 to lift, 1 at head, 1 to move the device; 6 people—4 to lift, 1 at head, 1 to move the device.

- Positions the lifters and has them form a bridge over the patient, head-to-shoulder or shoulder-to-shoulder.
  Note: All lifters must use the same configuration whether it be head-to-shoulder or shoulder-to-shoulder.

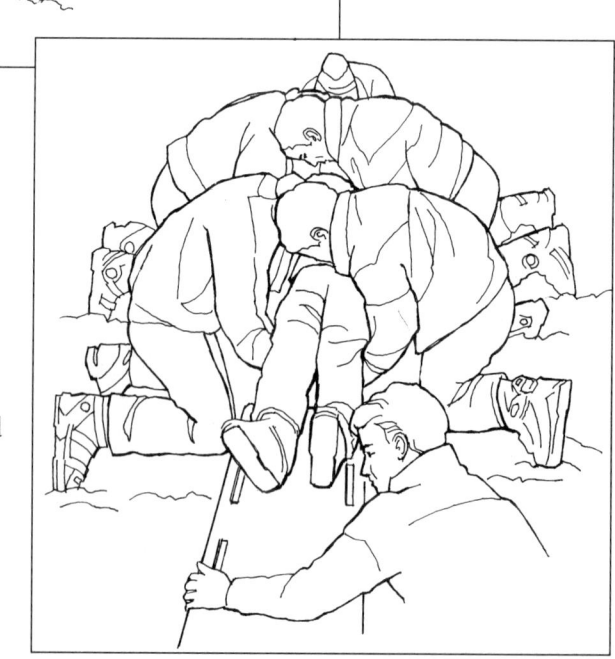

- Assures everyone's commitment and equal distribution across the bridge positions.

- Positions hands underneath the patient to lift at points of body mass (shoulders, hips).

- Lifts the patient just enough to allow a spineboard or other device to be placed underneath.

Helmet Removal

- The patient's head and neck is manually stabilized by placing a hand on each side of the helmet, fingers holding the patient's mandible.

- A second rescuer manually stabilized the patient's head and neck at the occiput and chin.

- The first rescuer spreads the sides of the helmet and eases it off the patient's head.

- The first rescuer resumes manual stabilization.

- The patient is immobilized as appropriate.

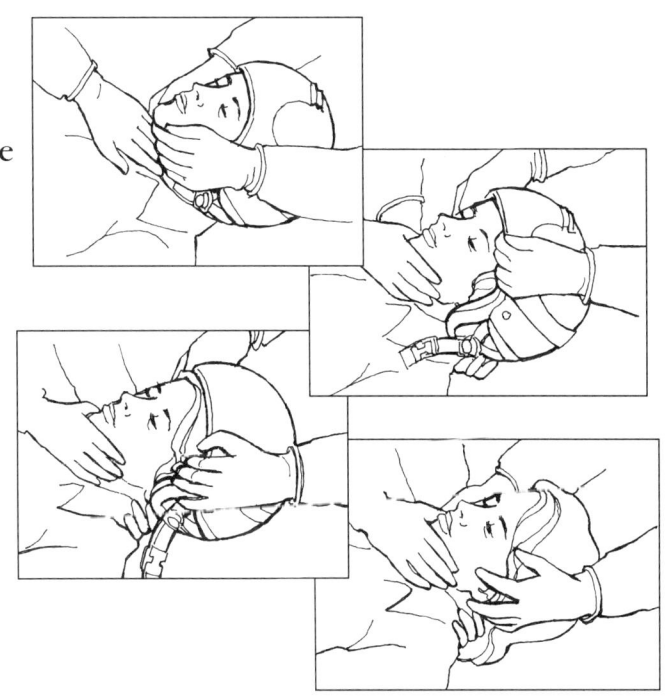

Application of a Standing Spineboard

- The first rescuer stands behind the patient and manually stabilizes the patient's head and neck

- A second rescuer inserts the board from the side between the patient and the first rescuer

- Two rescuers stand facing the patient, one on either side. Each inserts one hand under the patient's armpit and grasps the nearest handhold on the board above the armpit.

- Two rescuers grasp a handhold near the top of the board with their free hands.

- A fourth rescuer stabilizes the foot of the board.

- The board is lowered to the ground while manual stabilization of the head and neck is continually maintained

- Apply a rigid collar, center the patient by axial sliding, and strap him or her to the board using standard techniques.

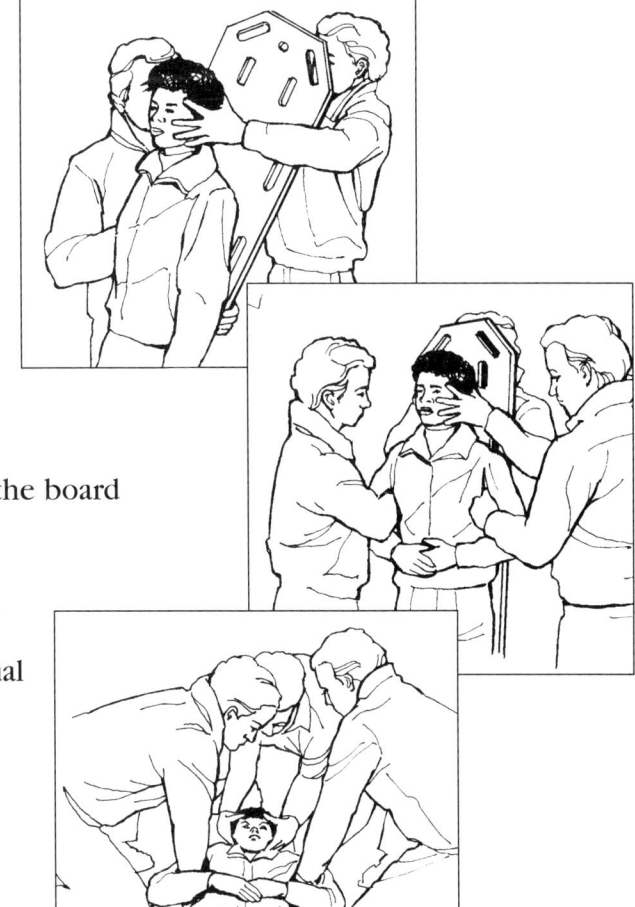

Chapter 14 Scenarios

1. An injured skier is lying in a heavily wooded area. Your first survey indicates an injury to the cervical spine. What is the first step in the process to immobilize the cervical spine? Explain your answer.

2. A 22-year-old male is skiing very aggressively on a deeply moguled expert slope when he loses his balance on an ice patch and falls forward in a "head plant." You quickly ski over to him. Although he appears stunned, he is fully responsive and exhibits no altered level of responsiveness. He tells you that he felt a sharp pain in his neck when he hit the slope. He also says that he attempted to move and sit up after the fall but laid back down when he felt a tingly sensation in his upper body. Currently, he is lying down but appears very uncomfortable and frightened. Your initial assessment reveals a pulse of 110 and respirations of 20. A second set of vital signs taken 6 minutes later yields a pulse of 88 and respirations of 16.

   Please include the answers to the following questions in your response:
   1. What problem(s) does your overall assessment indicate?
   2. What factors caused you to reach this conclusion?
   3. Are body substance isolation precautions appropriate in this circumstance?
   4. Is oxygen administration appropriate?
   5. Explain the emergency care steps you would take in the order you would take them in handling this situation.
   6. What common problems and complications might develop?
   7. Describe the transportation decisions you would make.

   _____
   _____
   _____
   _____
   _____
   _____
   _____
   _____

3. A 14-year-old male skier, while performing a double daffy jump off a mogul during a sponsored freestyle contest, is thrown backward and lands on his upper back. The patient is unresponsive initially. He regains responsiveness but has no recollection of his jump. He complains of pain in the upper thoracic spine and lower neck areas and has good movement and sensation in all extremities. Vital signs are within normal ranges.

Please include the answers to the following questions in your response:
1. What problem(s) does your overall assessment indicate?
2. What factors caused you to reach this conclusion?
3. Are body substance isolation precautions appropriate in this circumstance?
4. Is oxygen administration appropriate?
5. Explain the emergency care steps you would take in the order you would take them in handling this situation.
6. What common problems and complications might develop?
7. Describe the transportation decisions you would make.
8. What documentation is needed for this situation and why?

STUDY NOTES

LIFTING TECHNIQUES—LONG-AXIS DRAG

Objective: To demonstrate manual lifting techniques to move patients over snow or other smooth terrain.

SKILL	YES	NO	NOTATIONS

• Maintains manual stabilization of the body throughout maneuver.
  ▪ Headward drag: supports or cradles the upper torso
  ▪ Footward drag: supports or cradles the ankles and lower torso			

• Moves in a crouched position, pulling the patient slowly and smoothly about 12 inches at a time			
• Repositions, and repeats drag until reaching the desired location			
Did the trainee or patroller adequately demonstrate the performance criteria of this skill?			

COMMENTS

LIFTING TECHNIQUES—LOGROLL

Objective: To demonstrate manual techniques to move patients onto other devices

SKILL	YES	NO	NOTATIONS
• Manually stabilizes the head and neck.			
• Positions sufficient rescuers on the same side of the patient. Moves the patient as a unit while monitoring vital signs.			
• Positions hands on the far side, takes body mass into consideration.			
• Rolls the patient toward the rescuers on command from the leader (at the head), keeping the body in line. (The patient's arm may be alongside the body or elevated at local option.)			
• Places the stretcher, litter, or board alongside the patient and underneath as far as possible without excessive movement.			
• Rolls the patient onto the device on command from the leader, keeping the body in line.			
Did the trainee or patroller adequately demonstrate the performance criteria of this skill?			

COMMENTS

LIFTING TECHNIQUES—MULTIPLE-PERSON DIRECT FROM THE GROUND

Objective: To demonstrate manual techniques to move patients onto other devices

SKILL	YES	NO	NOTATIONS
• Manually stabilizes the head/neck as necessary for the injury.			
• Determines the number of lifters available and, therefore, the people pattern 5 people—3 to lift, 1 at head, 1 to move the device 6 people—4 to lift, 1 at head, 1 to move the device			
• Prepares all of the equipment needed for the lift or the device.			
• Explains the commands and procedures, and demonstrates the hand positions.			
• Executes the lift and slides the device into place, lifting the body as a unit.			
Did the trainee or patroller adequately demonstrate the performance criteria of this skill?			

COMMENTS

LIFTING TECHNIQUES—BRIDGING

Objective: To demonstrate manual lifting techniques to move patients onto other devices

SKILL	YES	NO	NOTATIONS
• Manually stabilizes the head and neck.			
• Determines the number of lifters available and, therefore, the people pattern: 5 people—3 to lift, 1 at head, 1 to move the device 6 people—4 to lift, 1 at head, 1 to move the device			
• Positions the lifters and has them form a bridge over the patient, head-to-shoulder or shoulder-to-shoulder. *(Note: All lifters must use the same configuration whether it be head-to-shoulder or shoulder-to-shoulder.)*			
• Assures everyone's commitment and equal distribution across the bridge positions.			
• Positions hands underneath the patient to lift at points of body mass (shoulders, hips).			
• Lifts the patient just enough to allow a spineboard or other device to be placed underneath.			
Did the trainee or patroller adequately demonstrate the performance criteria of this skill?			

COMMENTS

HELMET REMOVAL

Objective: To demonstrate the correct removal of a helmet from a trauma patient who may have a head or neck injury or obstructed airway.

SKILL	YES	NO	NOTATIONS
• The patient's head and neck is manually stabilized by placing a hand on each side of the helmet, fingers holding the patient's mandible.			
• A second rescuer manually stabilized the patient's head and neck at the occiput and chin			
• The first rescuer spreads the sides of the helmet and eases it off the patient's head.			
• The first rescuer resumes manual stabilization.			
• The patient is immobilized as appropriate.			
Did the trainee or patroller adequately demonstrate the performance criteria of this skill?			

COMMENTS

APPLICATION OF A STANDING SPINE BOARD

Objective: To demonstrate the application of a spineboard on a standing patient who may have a spinal injury.

SKILL	YES	NO	NOTATIONS
• The first rescuer stands behind the patient and manually stabilizes the patient's head and neck			
• A second rescuer inserts the board from the side between the patient and the first rescuer			
• Two rescuers stand facing the patient, one on either side. Each inserts one hand under the patient's armpit and grasps the nearest handhold on the board above the armpit.			
• Two rescuers grasp a handhold near the top of the board with their free hands.			
• A fourth rescuer stabilizes the foot of the board.			
• The board is lowered to the ground while manual stabilization of the head and neck is continually maintained			
• Apply a rigid collar, center the patient by axial sliding, and strap him or her to the board using standard techniques.			
Did the trainee or patroller adequately demonstrate the performance criteria of this skill?			

COMMENTS

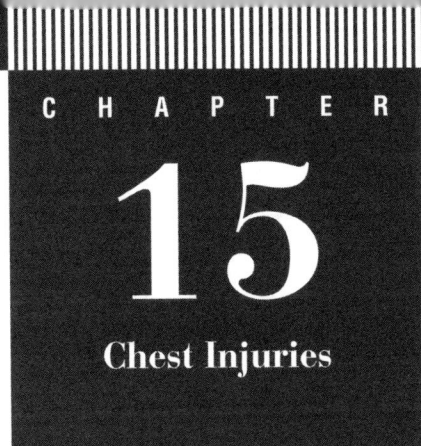

CHAPTER 15

Chest Injuries

CONCLUDING OBJECTIVES

The learner will:

Content

- List the causes and mechanisms of common types of chest injuries
- Describe signs and symptoms of common types of chest injuries

Skill Performance

- Demonstrate basic techniques for emergency care of a patient with injuries to the chest

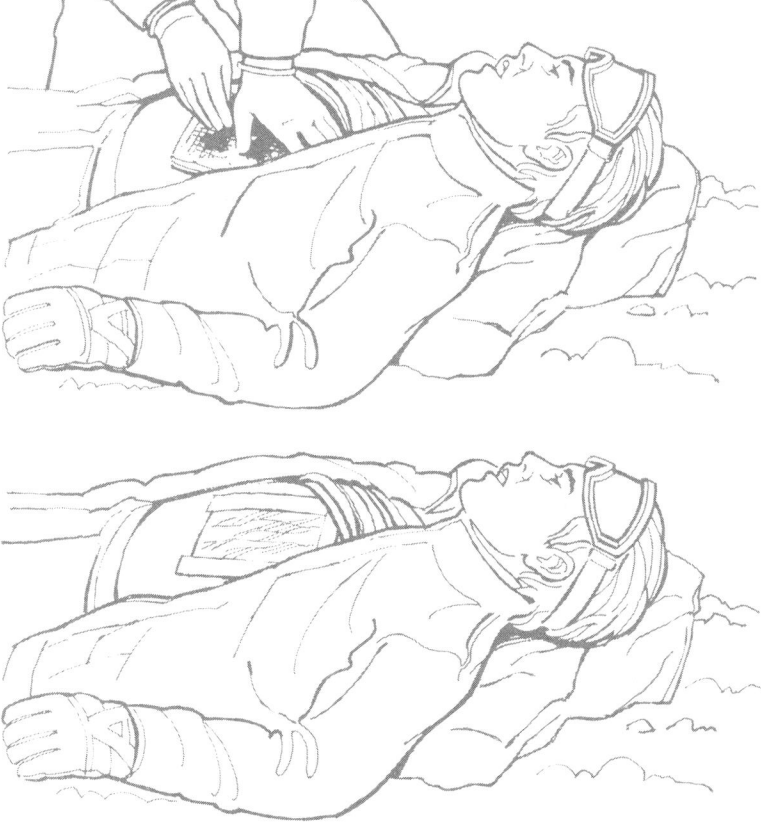

CHAPTER 15 STUDY QUESTIONS

1. Which of the following is the process in which the volume of the chest cavity increases and the lungs expand?
   A. Exhalation
   B. Compression
   C. Concussion
   D. Inhalation

2. What are the mechanisms causing common chest injuries?

Open Chest Wounds	
Closed Chest Wounds	

3. What determines the seriousness of a chest injury?
   _____
   _____

4. What are the signs and symptoms of serious chest injury?
   _____
   _____
   _____
   _____
   _____

5. When multiple rib fractures cause a portion of the chest to collapse and expand opposite to the remainder of the chest, this condition is called _____.

6. Describe the general sequence of assessment for chest injuries.
   _____
   _____
   _____
   _____
   _____
   _____

7. Identify significant factors about each of the chest wounds listed below.

Chest Wounds	Mechanisms of Injury Signs and Symptoms
Rib Fractures	
Penetrating Injuries	
Compression	
Injuries to Back of Chest	
Pneumothorax	
Tension Pneumothorax	
Hemothorax	
Subcutaneous Emphysema	
Myocardial Contusion	
Pericardial Tamponade	
Injury to the Great Vessels	

8. What is the emergency care of a patient with a chest injury?

   _____
   _____
   _____
   _____
   _____
   _____

9. An airtight dressing should be used on a sucking chest wound. For best results in applying a dressing that seals well, have the patient breathe _____ and then hold his or her breath.

10. Describe the procedure to be followed if a patient with an open chest wound suddenly gets worse.

_____
_____

11. Proper care for a patient suffering from an impaled object in the chest includes
    A. Removing the object if there is severe bleeding and backing the wound with a sterile dressing.
    B. Removing the object and sealing the wound with a sterile dressing bandaged snugly in place.
    C. Stabilizing the impaled object in place.
    D. None of the above.

12. Sometimes rib injuries may drive broken rib ends into the lung, lacerating it and producing air leakage into the chest cavity with partial collapse of the lung. This condition is called
    A. Flail chest
    B. Pneumothorax
    C. Tympanic reaction
    D. Sternal depression

13. The heart is enclosed in a sac called the
    A. Septum
    B. Foramen ovale
    C. Cuspid
    D. Pericardium

Chapter 15 Local Protocol

1. What local patrol procedures must be followed for chest injuries?

_____
_____
_____
_____
_____

2. What equipment and techniques for treatment of chest injuries are used at your area?

_____
_____
_____
_____
_____

CHAPTER 15 SKILL PERFORMANCE REQUIREMENTS

- Review *Outdoor Emergency Care* scenario 15.1

- Demonstrate basic techniques for emergency care of a patient with injuries to the chest

Skill Performance Guidelines

- Vital Signs Determination (see Chapter 3)
- Patient Assessment (see Chapter 5)
- Use of Oxygen and Airway Adjuncts (see Chapter 6)
- Control of Severe Bleeding in a Wound (see Chapter 7)

Focused Body Survey—Chest
Examines and palpates the chest for abnormality or deformity.
Questions the injured patient on the following: • Shortness of breath   • Cough   • Blood in sputum   • Pain aggravated by breathing or coughing

Chapter 15 Scenarios

1. A skier has sustained a pneumothorax from a violent accident. The patient is becoming more cyanotic and there is increased respiratory distress. The trachea is shifting to one side. What is this condition called? What is the emergency care for the patient?

   _____
   _____
   _____
   _____

2. A ski racer loses control during a race, hooks a gate, and careens from the course into the brush off an embankment. When you arrive at the scene, you find the patient responsive with abrasions on his face. He says he never lost consciousness. He details the events, but complains of severe pain the right side of the chest. Examination reveals a severe depression in the lateral right chest area. The patient's pulse is 110 and his respirations are 28. In the 5 minutes following your examination, his condition worsens noticeably.

Please include the answers to the following questions in your response:
1. What problem(s) does your overall assessment indicate?
2. What factors caused you to reach this conclusion?
3. Are body substance isolation precautions appropriate in this circumstance?
4. Is oxygen administration appropriate?
5. Explain the emergency care steps you would take in the order you would take them in handling this situation.
6. What common problems and complications might develop?
7. Describe the transportation decisions you would make.
8. What documentation is needed for this situation and why?

_____
_____
_____
_____
_____
_____
_____
_____

3. A skier who has collided with a tree is found with his chest resting against the tree. He is cyanotic and unresponsive. Upon assessment, you determined that the airway is open and that a segment of the chest bulges on exhalation.

Please include the answers to the following questions in your response:
1. What problem(s) does your overall assessment indicate?
2. What factors caused you to reach this conclusion?
3. Is oxygen administration appropriate?
4. Explain the emergency care steps you would take in the order you would take them in handling this situation.
5. What common problems and complications might develop?
6. Describe the transportation decisions you would make.

_____
_____
_____
_____
_____
_____
_____
_____

CHAPTER 16

Injuries to the Abdomen, Pelvis, and Genitalia

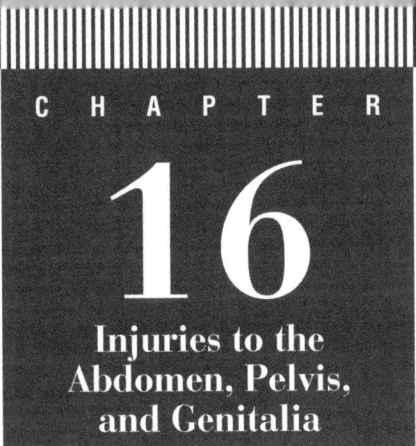

CONCLUDING OBJECTIVES

The learner will:

Content

- List the types and causes of injuries to the abdomen, pelvis, and genitalia

- Describe signs and symptoms of injuries to the abdomen, pelvis, and genitalia

Skill Performance

- Demonstrate basic techniques of emergency care for a patient with specific injuries to abdominal and pelvic areas

CHAPTER 16 STUDY QUESTIONS

1. Identify what causes open injuries in the abdomen.

2. Identify some causes of closed injuries in the abdomen.

3. List the hollow organs in the human body.

4. What happens when a hollow organ is ruptured?

5. List the solid organs in the human body.

6. What happens when a solid organ is damaged?

7. What are the signs and symptoms of peritonitis?

8. Kidney injury is usually associated with
___

9. What are the symptoms of a kidney injury?
___
___
___
___

10. What two injuries are often associated with a pelvic fracture?
___

11. How would you treat a testicle contusion?
___
___

12. How would you treat a soft-tissue injury to the external female genitalia?
___
___

13. Describe the procedures for assessing abdominal and pelvic injuries.
___
___
___
___
___
___

14. Describe an occlusive dressing.
___
___
___
___

15. Summarize the emergency care of a patient with an abdominal or pelvic injury.
___
___
___
___
___
___

16. On the ski hill, the most important emergency care for a person with severe, closed abdominal injuries is to
    A. Treat the patient for shock and rapidly transport to medical care
    B. Apply a hot pack and treat the patient for shock
    C. Apply a cold pack and treat the patient for shock
    D. Treat the patient for shock and secure the patient to a spine board

Chapter 16 Local Protocol

1. Describe local patrol procedures for the assessment, emergency care, and management of injuries to the abdomen, pelvis, and genitalia.

   _____
   _____
   _____
   _____
   _____

CHAPTER 16 SKILL PERFORMANCE REQUIREMENTS

- Review *Outdoor Emergency Care* scenario 16.1

- Demonstrate basic techniques of emergency care for a patient with specific injuries to abdominal and pelvic areas

Skill Performance Guidelines

- Vital Signs Determination (see Chapter 3)
- Patient Assessment (see Chapter 5)
- Use of Oxygen and Airway Adjuncts (see Chapter 6)
- Control of Severe Bleeding in a Wound (see Chapter 7)
- Spinal Immobililization (see Chapter 9)

Focused Body Survey
Abdomen
Examines and palpates the abdominal (all quadrants).
Questions the patient on the following: • Nausea, vomiting • Abdominal cramps • Blood in the feces or urine • Swelling of abdomen • Time of last bowel movement • Pregnancy
Pelvis
Examines and palpates the pelvic area.
Questions the patient on the following: • Trouble urinating • Blood in urine • Blood coming from urethra, vagina, or rectum • Pregnancy

Chapter 16 Scenarios

1. A teenager is sitting on the ground at the top of the mountain with her skis still on. She says she has not been feeling well for the last day or two. She was weak and tired in the morning and has a mild mid-lower abdominal pain that has slowly worsened. On the chairlift, she felt a sudden sharp, steady pain in her right lower abdomen and vomited. Now she hurts all over. She has no medical problems but is allergic to penicillin. Vital signs: initial pulse: 180, weak; respiration: 20. Based on possible mechanisms of injury, describe the potential and anticipated problems with this scenario. What problem do you suspect? What type of emergency care should you provide?

2. A 35-year-old woman skiing close to the edge of the trail on an intermediate slope loses control and falls on her left side onto the exposed runner of a moveable snow gun. Upon arrival you perform an assessment that indicates no altered level of responsiveness. The skier's initial vital signs indicate a pulse of 92 and respirations of 16. Her abdomen on the left side is tender on palpation and begins to become rigid. A second set of vitals taken 5 minutes after the first set reveals a pulse of 110 and respirations of 24.

   Please include the answers to the following questions in your response:
   1. What is your first impression of the scene telling you? What problem(s) does your overall assessment indicate?
   2. What factors caused you to reach this conclusion?
   3. What body substance isolation precautions are appropriate in this circumstance?
   4. Is oxygen administration appropriate?
   5. Explain the emergency care steps you would take in the order you would take them in handling this situation.
   6. What common problems and complications might develop?
   7. Describe the transportation decisions you would make.
   8. What documentation is needed for this situation and why?

STUDY NOTES

CHAPTER 17
Common Medical Complaints

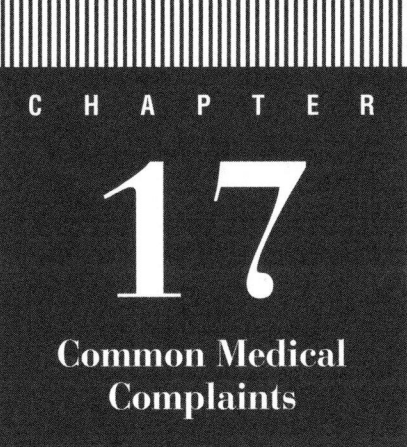

CONCLUDING OBJECTIVES

The learner will:

Content

- Describe characteristics of common medical complaints

- Describe the general principles of emergency care for patients with common medical complaints

Skill Performance

- Demonstrate assessment and management of common medical complaints

CHAPTER 17 STUDY QUESTIONS

1. How does patient assessment for a medical illness differ from that of an injury?
   _____
   _____

2. Explain the possible signs and symptoms of each respiratory complaint listed.

Complaints	Signs and Symptoms
Respiratory infections	
Pulmonary edema	
Emphysema	
Asthma	
Pulmonary embolism	
Airway obstruction	
Malignant disease	
Hyperventilation	

3. Match the medical complaints with the proper characteristics.
   ___ Pulmonary embolism
   ___ Airway obstruction
   ___ Hyperventilation
   ___ Respiratory infection

   A. Lack of air exchange, cyanosis, patient may not be able to speak or cough
   B. Runny nose, cough, green sputum
   C. Develops after trauma, surgery, blood in sputum, dyspnea, coughing
   D. Rapid breathing, tingling in fingers and toes, lack of carbon dioxide in body

4. Describe the general for emergency care of a patient with a respiratory complaint.
   _____
   _____
   _____
   _____
   _____
   _____

5. The coughing up of a bright red, frothy blood is an indication of injury to the
   A. Lung
   B. Esophagus
   C. Heart
   D. Neck

6. Too much carbon dioxide or not enough oxygen can cause
   A. Pulmonary embolism
   B. Pulmonary edema
   C. Respiratory distress
   D. Asthma

7. A condition in which the fluid part of the blood leaves the capillaries and collects in the alveoli, thus causing an interference of blood oxygen, is called
   A. Pulmonary embolism
   B. Pulmonary edema
   C. Lung cancer
   D. Asthma

8. Coughing, wheezing, and rhonchi are common in the degenerative lung disease called
   A. Emphysema
   B. Pulmonary edema
   C. Asthma
   D. Pulmonary embolism

9. Describe the assessment of patient with a respiratory complaint.

10. What is the emergency care for a patient with chest pains?

11. What chest pains should be considered serious?

12. Explain the signs and symptoms of the following chest pain complaints.

Complaint of Pain	Signs and Symptoms
Chest wall	
Due to heart disease	
Due to respiratory disease	
Due to gastrointestinal distress	
Associated with stress and anxiety	

13. Identify the anterior and posterior organs of the abdominal cavity.

Organs of the Abdominal Cavity

Organs Behind the Abdominal Cavity

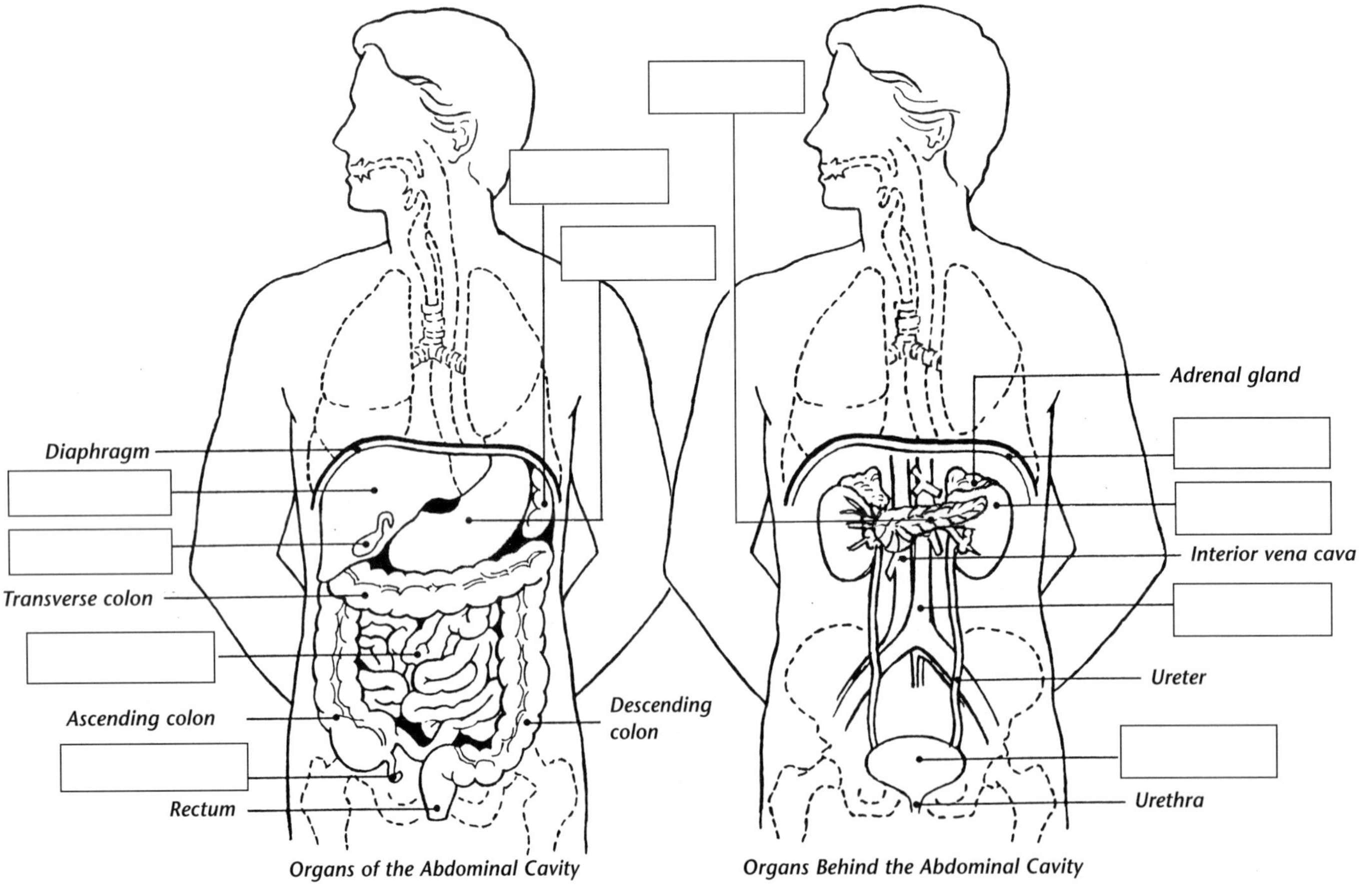

14. Shade in the most common locations of anginal pain.

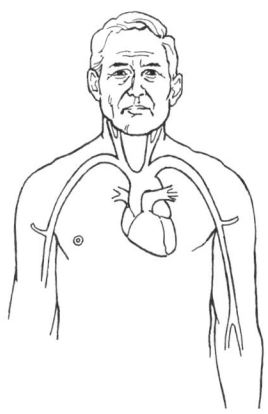

15. Explain the signs and symptoms and treatment of the following common medical complaints.

Gastrointestinal Complaint	Signs and Symptoms	Emergency Care
Indigestion		
Nausea and vomiting		
Diarrhea		
Blood in stools		
Colic		
Constipation		
Difficulty in swallowing		
Jaundice		
Acute abdomen		

Genitourinary Complaint	Signs and Symptoms	Emergency Care
Painful urination		
Blood in urine		
Incontinence		
Inability to urinate		
Abnormal menstrual flow		
Urethral/vaginal discharge		

Miscellaneous	Signs and Symptoms	Emergency Care
Vertigo, lightheadedness		
Headache		
Pain in lower back		

16. Match the following medical complaints with the proper characteristics.

    ___ Indigestion   A. Uncontrolled passage of urine and/or feces
    ___ Gastroenteritis   B. Painful or difficult urination
    ___ Jaundice   C. Yellow skin
    ___ Incontinence   D. Due to infection, overuse of alcohol, some drugs, or food poisoning
    ___ Dysuria   E. Blood in urine
    ___ Hematuria   F. Increased saliva production, heartburn, cramps, vomiting, spicy meals

17. Describe the emergency care of an acute abdomen.

    _____
    _____
    _____
    _____
    _____
    _____

18. As a patient's condition changes, a written record of observations should be kept. What are two observations this record should include?

    _____
    _____

19. During an assessment of a patient with a medical complaint, what questions should a patroller ask the patient?

    _____
    _____
    _____
    _____
    _____

20. Intermittent, severe abdominal pain due to obstruction of a hollow muscular organ may cause
    A. Colic
    B. Constipation
    C. Diarrhea
    D. Cramping

Chapter 17 Local Protocol

1. Describe local patrol procedures for handling common medical complaints.

   _____
   _____
   _____
   _____
   _____

CHAPTER 17 SKILL PERFORMANCE REQUIREMENTS

- Review *Outdoor Emergency Care* scenarios 17.1 and 17.2

- Demonstrate assessment and management of common medical complaints

    Respiratory

        Respiratory infections
    Pulmonary edema
    Emphysema
    Asthma
    Pulmonary embolism
    Airway obstruction
    Malignant disease
    Hyperventilation

    Gastrointestinal complaint

        Indigestion
    Nausea and vomiting
    Diarrhea
    Blood in stools
    Colic
    Constipation
    Difficulty in swallowing
    Jaundice
    Acute abdomen

    Genitourinary complaints

        Painful urination
    Blood in urine
    Incontinence
    Inability to urinate
    Abnormal menstrual flow
    Urethral/vaginal discharge

    Miscellaneous complaints

        Vertigo, lightheadedness
    Headache
    Pain in lower back

Skill Performance Guidelines

- Vital Signs Determination (see Chapter 3)
- Patient Assessment (see Chapter 5)
- Use of Oxygen and Airway Adjuncts (see Chapter 6)
- Control of Severe Bleeding in a Wound (see Chapter 7)
- Managing Medical and Environmental Emergencies (see Chapter 18)

Focused Body Survey—Nonspecific
Questions of the patient should include: • Tiredness or fatigue, weakness, lack of energy • Fever or chills (usually described as the sensation of being hot or cold) • Stiff neck • Loss of appetite

Chapter 17 Scenarios

1. While skiing, you come upon a skier who has fallen. He reports to you that he has twisted his knee. Your examination convinces you that he has probably sprained it. He also complains of shortness of breath, tingling in the fingers and toes, and dizziness. His respirations are above 20. He has voiced anxiety about getting off the hill and appears frightened about even being on "Suicide Slide" much less attempting to ski it.
   1) Assuming no other injuries, what is his major problem?
   2) Emergency care for this patient should include:
   3) What may happen to this patient if he continues without your care?

STUDY NOTES

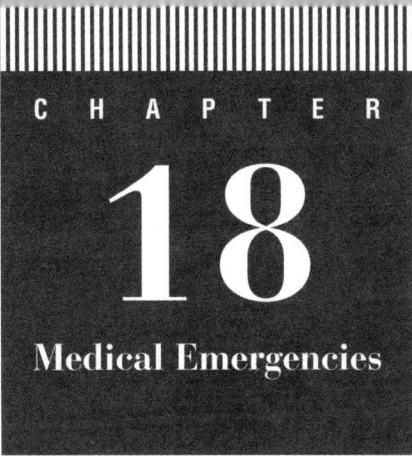

CHAPTER 18
Medical Emergencies

CONCLUDING OBJECTIVES

The learner will:

Content

- Describe the characteristics of common medical emergencies

- Describe the general principles of emergency care for patients with common medical emergencies

Skill Performance

- Demonstrate assessment and management of common medical emergencies

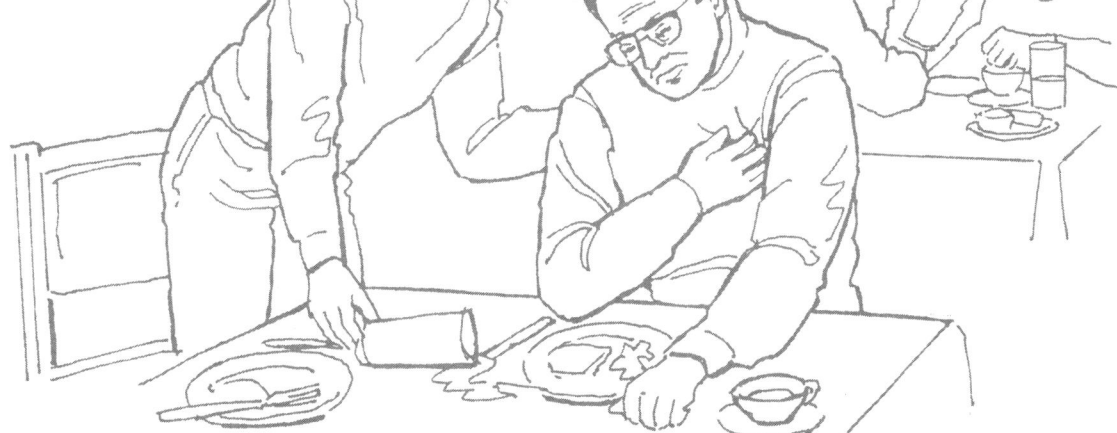

CHAPTER 18 STUDY QUESTIONS

1. Define angina pectoris.

2. Define heart attack.

3. Define myocardial infarction.

4. What condition occurs when the heart muscle is temporarily deprived of oxygen?

5. Describe the Rothberg position. Explain the benefits of placing a patient in this position.

6. List three complications of myocardial infarction.

7. Define CVA.

8. In what position should an unresponsive stroke patient be transported to a hospital?
   A. On his or her back, with the head and shoulders raised
   B. On his or her side, with the head and shoulders raised
   C. Seated with head tilted back and legs elevated
   D. Supine

9. List the signs and symptoms and emergency care for patients with heart attacks and strokes.

	Signs and Symptoms	**Emergency Care**
Heart attack		
Stroke (CVA)		

10. What is an AED and what is necessary to implement AED procedures at a resort?

_____
_____
_____
_____

11. Describe one recommended technique for administering CPR on a ski hill using a standard toboggan.

_____
_____
_____
_____
_____

12. Complete the table of comparison between diabetic hypoglycemia and ketoacidosis.

Category	Hypoglycemia	Ketoacidosis
Onset		
Mental status		
Respirations		
Pulse		
Blood pressure		
Skin		
Breath		
Weakness, fatigue		
Headache		
Hunger		
Thirst		
Seizures		
Shock		
Abdominal pain		
Blood glucose (by test strip or glucose meter)		
Treatment General care for unresponsiveness		
Sugar		
Response to treatment		

13. Define juvenile diabetes.

_____

_____

14. Define adult-onset diabetes.

_____

_____

15. Define seizure.

_____

16. Summarize the emergency care of a patient suffering a generalized seizure.

___

17. When managing a patient who is having a generalized seizure, the patroller's first responsibility is to
    A. Yell for help.
    B. Place a bite stick between the patient's teeth.
    C. Hold the patient as still as possible.
    D. Protect the patient from injury.

18. Define carbon monoxide poisoning.

___

19. The most common toxic gas associated with respiratory arrest is
    A. Carbon monoxide
    B. Nitrogen
    C. Methane
    D. Carbon dioxide

20. Define physical dependence.

___

21. Identify the common signs and symptoms, and emergency care of substance abuse patients.

Signs and Symptoms	Emergency Care

22. Match the following drug classifications with the appropriate behavior.
    ___ Alcohol   A. Disorientation
    ___ Marijuana   B. Slurred speech
    ___ Hallucinogens   C. Short-term memory impairment
    ___ Amphetamine   D. Excitement
                         E. Hallucinations

23. Constricted pupils may indicate
    A. Skull fractures
    B. Stroke
    C. Narcotics
    D. Lack of oxygen

24. Match the following medical emergencies with their signs and symptoms.
    ___ Diabetic ketoacidosis   A. Cherry-red skin
    ___ Insulin shock   B. Seizures
    ___ Carbon monoxide poisoning   C. Fruity smell
    ___ Stroke (CVA)   D. Fruity breath odor
    ___ Heart attack   E. Death of heart muscle
    ___ Myocardial infarction   F. Muscle failure on one side
    ___ Angina pectoris   G. Sudden heart malfunction
    ___ Epilepsy   H. Temporary chest pain
    ___ Diabetic coma   I. Hunger, weakness

Chapter 18 Local Protocol

1. Describe local patrol procedures for the assessment and management of common medical emergencies.

   _____
   _____
   _____
   _____
   _____

2. Describe local procedures for CPR on the hill and transporting.

   _____
   _____
   _____
   _____
   _____

CHAPTER 18 SKILL PERFORMANCE REQUIREMENTS

- Review *Outdoor Emergency Care* scenario 18.1

- Demonstrate assessment and management for common medical emergencies

  Angina Pectoris
  Heart Attack
  Stroke (CVA)
  Diabetes
      Hypoglycemia
      Diabetic Ketoacidosis
  Seizures
  Carbon Monoxide Poisoning
  Substance Abuse (management by presentation)
      Stimulants
      Depressants
      Hallucinogens

Skill Performance Guideline

- Vital Signs Determination (see Chapter 3)
- Patient Assessment (see Chapter 5)
- Use of Oxygen and Airway Adjuncts (see Chapter 6)
- Control of Severe Bleeding in a Wound (see Chapter 7)
- Managing Medical and Environmental Emergencies

Focused Body Survey—Nonspecific
Questions of the patient should include: • Tiredness or fatigue, weakness, lack of energy • Fever or chills (usually described as the sensation of being hot or cold) • Stiff neck • Loss of appetite

Managing Medical and Environmental Emergencies

- Determines level of responsiveness? (AVPU)
- Assesses ABCDE and provides priority emergency care intervention.
- Provides general care for unresponsiveness, as appropriate.
- Provides care for irrational, excited patients.
    - Does not attempt to restrain.
    - Provides care for seizures.
    - Provides care for diabetic emergencies, if indicated.
    - Does not leave patient unattended.
- Obtains a medical history (OPQRST)
    - Obtains initial vital signs.
    - If no history is available, looks for medical alert information.

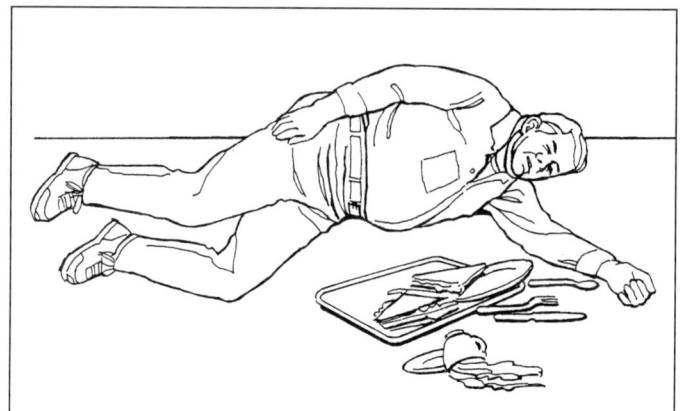

- Conducts focused body survey. Helps patient to take any medication that has been prescribed for illness if not contraindicated by patient's condition or circumstance and in accordance with local protocols.
- Stabilizes and maintains patient in a comfortable position.
- Provides protection from environment, including any necessary warming or cooling.
- Provides treatment appropriate for the medical illness, including oxygen administration.
- Arranges for transportation to a medical facility.
- Monitors vital signs at regular intervals beingalert for changes in the respiratory and circulatory systems.

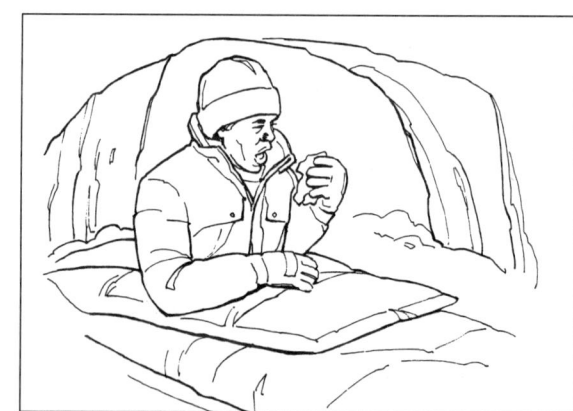

Chapter 18 Scenarios

1. A 47-year-old male complains of sudden onset of severe chest pain under his sternum that travels down his left shoulder and hand. He is short of breath, frightened, and restless. What do these symptoms indicate? What is the emergency care for the victim?

2. A 26-year-old male complains of intense thirst, headache, and vomiting. His skin is red and dry. Respirations are deep and rapid and there is a sweet or fruity smell on his breath. He is restless and merges into unresponsiveness. What condition is the victim probably suffering from? What is the emergency care for the victim?

3. A 24-year-old female complains of a sudden severe headache and collapses to the ground. She is unresponsive and her left pupil is fixed and dilated. What is the most likely cause of this condition? What is the emergency care for the victim?

4. If a patient of alcohol abuse has become unresponsive and there are no signs of trauma or distress, what actions should the rescuer take?

5. A 21-year-old advanced beginner skier falls while skiing on a steep section of an intermediate slope. He is not injured in the fall, but both of his skis release and he then slides approximately 25 feet downhill. While climbing upon to collect his skis, he begins to have difficulty breathing. He starts to wheeze and experiences tightness in his chest. Upon arrival, you find the skier diaphorectic with obvious breathing difficulty. His nostrils are flared, and he is wheezing audibly. Taking his vital signs, you note a respiratory rate of 28 and a pulse that is 120 and regular. He gives a SAMPLE history of asthma since childhood, treated with an Albuterol inhaler. He has an inhaler with him but did not think it would work because of the cold temperature.

Please include the answers to the following questions in your response:
1. What problem(s) does your overall assessment indicate?
2. What factors caused you to reach this conclusion?
3. What body substance isolation SI precautions are appropriate in this circumstance?
4. Is oxygen administration appropriate?
5. Explain the emergency care steps you would take in the order you would take them in handling this situation.
6. What common problems and complications might develop?
7. Describe the transportation decisions you would make.

_____
_____
_____
_____
_____

STUDY NOTES

MANAGING MEDICAL AND ENVIRONMENTAL EMERGENCIES

Objective: To demonstrate the skills needed to assess and manage illnesses that develop suddenly requiring emergency care intervention.

SKILL	YES	NO	NOTATIONS
• Determines level of responsiveness (AVPU).			
• Assesses ABCDE and provides with priority emergency care intervention.			
• Provides general care for unresponsiveness, as appropriate.			
• Provides care for irrational, excited patients. ▪ Does not attempt to restrain. ▪ Provides care for seizures. ▪ Provides care for diabetic emergencies, if indicated. ▪ Does not leave patient unattended.			
• Obtains a medical history (OPQRST). Obtains initial vital signs. If no history is available looks for medical alert information.			
• Conducts focused body survey. Helps patient to take any medication that has been prescribed for illness if not contraindicated by patient's condition or circumstance and in accordance with local protocols.			
• Stabilizes and maintains patient in a comfortable position.			
• Provides protection from environment, including any necessary warming or cooling.			
• Provides treatment appropriate for the medical illness, including oxygen administration.			
• Arranges for transportation to a medical facility.			
• Monitors vital signs at regular intervals being alert for changes in the respiratory and circulatory systems.			
Did the trainee or patroller adequately demonstrate the performance criteria of this skill?			

COMMENTS

CHAPTER 19

Environmental Emergencies

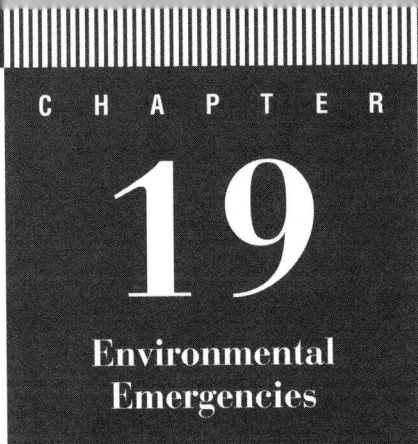

CONCLUDING OBJECTIVES

The learner will:

Content

- Describe injuries and illnesses caused by exposure to certain environmental conditions
- Describe the emergency care measures as necessary for cases of environmental emergencies

Skill Performance

- Demonstrate assessment and management of environmental emergencies

CHAPTER 19 STUDY QUESTIONS

1. Shade in the areas of the face most susceptible to frostbite and exposure.

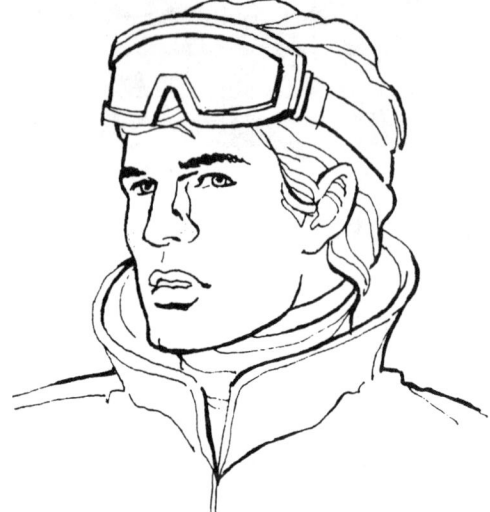

2. List each type of frostbite and its distinguishing signs and symptoms after rewarming.

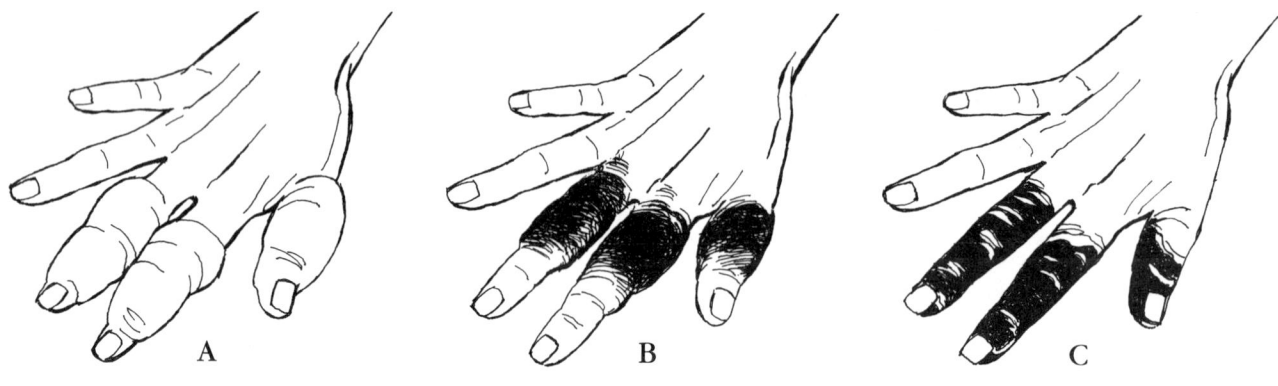

A. _____

B. _____

C. _____

3. What is the difference between superficial and deep frostbite?
   _____
   _____

4. What is the preferred emergency care for frostbite?
   _____

5. Why is refreezing the worst thing for a frostbitten part?
   _____

6. Hypothermia can be divided into categories by duration of exposure. Match each category to its description.

   ___ Acute   A. Exposure occurs in several hours to a day.
   ___ Chronic   B. Exposure occurs in several minutes to an hour.
   ___ Subacute   C. Exposure occurs in more than a day.

7. What body temperature differentiates between mild and severe hypothermia?
   _____
   _____

8. When can hypothermia occur?
   Immersion
   _____
   _____

   Field
   _____
   _____

   Urban
   _____
   _____

   Submersion
   _____
   _____

9. List the emergency care of a hypothermic patient.
   1) General Measures
   _____

   2) Mild Hypothermia
   _____

   3) Severe Hypothermia
   _____

10. List the signs and symptoms and emergency care for heat stroke and heat exhaustion.

	Signs and Symptoms	Emergency Care
Heat Stroke		
Heat Exhaustion		

11. List at least five signs and symptoms of altitude sickness.

_____

_____

_____

_____

_____

12. Complete the table on acute mountain sickness.

	Early Symptoms	Late Symptoms	Emergency Care
HACE			
HAPE			

13. What is the cornerstone of emergency care for the acute mountain sickness (AMS) patient?

_____

14. If unable to walk, the acute mountain sickness patient should be carried in which of the following positions?
    A. Sitting
    B. Prone
    C. Semiprone
    D. Supine

15. What is the emergency care for a patient with high-altitude illness at ski areas and other resorts?

16. Describe the characteristics of physical and chemical sunscreen preparations.

17. What is the best way to prevent sunburn?

18. Snowblindness is
    A. The result of frostbitten eyelids
    B. Caused by moisture building up on the eyelashes, which leads to the eyes freezing shut
    C. Sunburn of the conjunctiva
    D. A momentary condition which manifests itself only minutes after being exposed to the bright reflection of the sun off the snow.

19. Describe windburn and how to treat it.

20. What is the assessment and emergency care for an electrical/lightning injury?

21. If a person have been found alive following an avalanche incident, what possible environmental or medical problems may exist?

22. If an avalanche victim is found alive, what emergency care procedures may be required?

Chapter 19 Local Protocol

1. Describe the general local procedures for handling environmental emergencies.

   Frostbite

   Hypothermia

   Heat Illness

   Acute Mountain Sickness and Altitude Sickness

Sunburn

Windburn

Snowblindness

Lightning and Electrical Injury

Avalanche Injuries

CHAPTER 19 SKILL PERFORMANCE REQUIREMENTS

- Review *Outdoor Emergency Care* scenario 19.1

- Demonstrate assessment and management of environmental emergencies

    Frostbite
    Hypothermia
    Heat Illness
        Heat Stroke
        Heat Exhaustion
    Acute Mountain Sickness
        HAPE
        HACE
    Sunburn
    Windburn
    Snowblindness
    Lightning and Electrical Injury
    Avalanche Injuries

Skill Performance Guidelines

- Vital Signs Determination (see Chapter 3)
- Patient Assessment (see Chapter 5)
- Use of Oxygen and Airway Adjuncts (see Chapter 6)
- Control of Severe Bleeding in a Wound (see Chapter 7)
- Managing Medical and Environmental Emergencies

Chapter 19 Scenarios

1. A frantic woman approaches you as you come in from sweep. Her friend, who was skiing on an intermediate nordic trail, is missing. A search and rescue is organized, and you have two sectors to cover with another patroller. You are given a pack containing two blankets, splints, matches, and a radio. Two hours into the search you find the missing skier, semi-responsive. You radio for a snowmobile, which will take 30 minutes to arrive.

   The patient is lying semi-prone, left side down. Her left arm is straight out from the body and will not bend. She is responsive only to painful stimulus secondary to hypothermia. Her hands and feet are frostbitten, and she has a fractured left humerus. Vital signs sequence: 1) initial: pulse 58, respirations 10; 2) five minutes: pulse 54, respirations 12; 3) 10 minutes: pulse 52, respirations 12.

Based on possible mechanisms of injury, describe the potential and anticipated problems of this scenario. What equipment would be needed? What type of emergency care should you provide?

_____

_____

_____

_____

_____

2. You are skiing in a light, misty rain on a windy day. The temperature is 34 F. Halfway down a run, you see an overweight woman who looks to be about 45 years old. She is not wearing a hat and is sitting on the snow. Upon approaching her, you see that the woman is shivering and having difficulty zipping her jacket. When you ski up to her, she excitedly tells you that this is her first day on skis and despite frequent falls she has been at it for about four hours. At the moment, she is having a hard time getting her ski boot back into her binding. Upon taking a SAMPLE history you find that the woman is an adult-onset diabetic and although she recalls taking her oral diabetic medication that morning, further questioning reveals a poor memory of other events of the day.

   Please include the answers to the following questions in your response:
   1. What problem(s) does your overall assessment indicate?
   2. What factors caused you to reach this conclusion?
   3. Is oxygen administration appropriate?
   4. Explain the emergency care steps you would take in the order you would take them in handling this situation.
   5. What common problems and complications might develop?
   6. Describe the transportation decisions you would make.

   _____

   _____

   _____

   _____

   _____

3. A teenage girl is skiing without a hat. The outside temperature is 36 degrees F and a light rain is falling intermittently. The skier traveled almost all night to reach the ski area, slept very little, and skipped breakfast before skiing. She caught an edge and took a minimal fall. You find her sitting on the beginner's trail close to the bottom of the area, her right ski off. Somewhat confused and shivering, she is unable to reattach her ski. There is no evidence of other injury. Her vital signs indicate a pulse of 100, respirations of 18, and a core temperature in the patrol room of 95 degrees F.

Please include the answers to the following questions in your response:
1. What problem(s) does your overall assessment indicate?
2. What factors caused you to reach this conclusion?
3. Is oxygen administration appropriate?
4. Explain the emergency care steps you would take in the order you would take them in handling this situation.
5. What common problems and complications might develop?
6. Describe the transportation decisions you would make.

___

4. A middle-aged skier who lives in the southeastern United States was skiing for the first time in Colorado and at an elevation of 10,000 feet. He stops at an aid station complaining of shortness of breath, severe fatigue after only four runs, headache, and nausea. The skier says he had "worked out at home" before the ski trip and thought he was in good shape.

Please include the answers to the following questions in your response:
1. What problem(s) does your overall assessment indicate?
2. What factors caused you to reach this conclusion?
3. Is oxygen administration appropriate?
4. Explain the emergency care steps you would take in the order you would take them in handling this situation.
5. What common problems and complications might develop?
6. Describe the transportation decisions you would make.

___

STUDY NOTES

MANAGING MEDICAL AND ENVIRONMENTAL EMERGENCIES

Objective: To demonstrate the skills needed to assess and manage illnesses that develop suddenly requiring emergency care intervention.

SKILL	YES	NO	NOTATIONS
Determines level of responsiveness. (AVPU)			
• Assesses ABCDE and provides with priority emergency care intervention.			
• Provides general care for unresponsiveness, as appropriate.			
• Provides care for irrational, excited patients. ▪ Does not attempt to restrain. ▪ Provides care for seizures. ▪ Provides care for diabetic emergencies, if indicated. ▪ Does not leave patient unattended.			
• Obtains a medical history (OPQRST). Obtains initial vital signs. If no history is available looks for medical alert information.			
Conducts focused body survey. Helps patient to take any medication that has been prescribed for illness if not contraindicated by patient's condition or circumstance and in accordance with local protocols.			
• Stabilizes and maintains patient in a comfortable position.			
• Provides protection from environment, including any necessary warming or cooling.			
• Provides treatment appropriate for the medical illness, including oxygen administration.			
• Arranges for transportation to a medical facility.			
• Monitors vital signs at regular intervals being alert for changes in the respiratory and circulatory systems.			
Did the trainee or patroller adequately demonstrate the performance criteria of this skill?			

COMMENTS

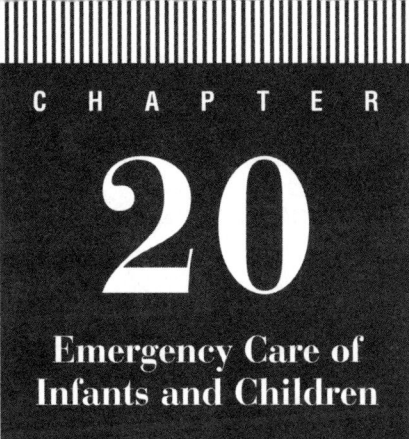

CHAPTER 20

Emergency Care of Infants and Children

CONCLUDING OBJECTIVES

The learner will:

Content

- Describe the causes of and emergency care for illnesses and injuries to infants and children

- Identify anatomical differences between pediatric and adult patients

- Describe special aspects of pediatric emergency care

Skill Performance

- Explain and demonstrate assessment of the pediatric patient

- Explain and demonstrate the emergency care for illnesses and injuries of infants and children

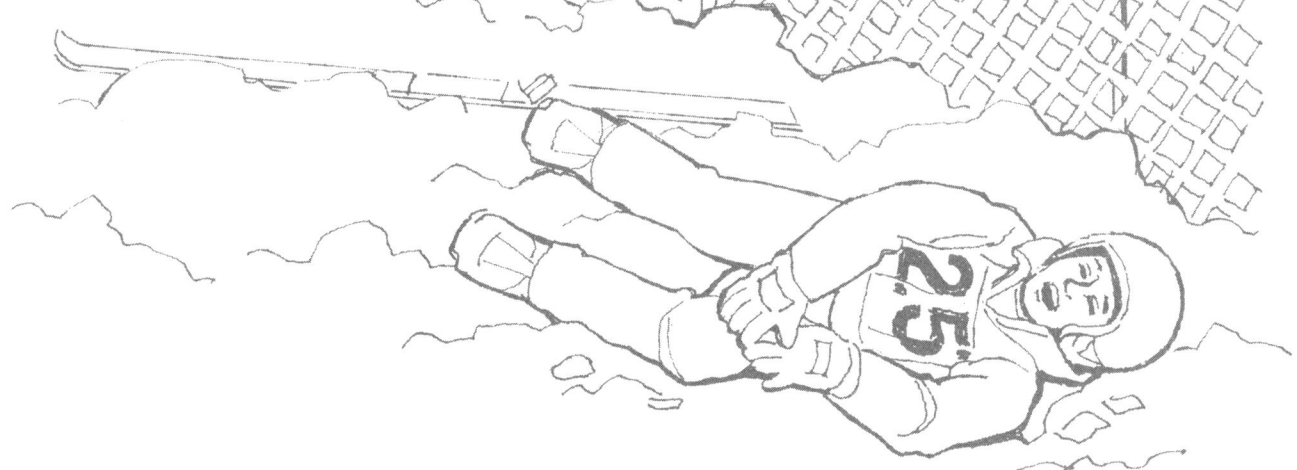

CHAPTER 20 STUDY QUESTIONS

1. What are the ages that define each of the following?
   Neonate _____
   Infant _____
   Toddler _____
   Preschooler _____

2. Identify the anatomical and physiologic differences between pediatric and adult patients.
   _____
   _____
   _____
   _____
   _____
   _____
   _____
   _____

3. What pulse should be assessed on children under the age of one year?
   _____

4. What are the major causes of cardiac arrest in children?
   _____

5. Describe some modifications that may be used when giving oxygen to a responsive child whom refuses a mask.
   _____
   _____
   _____

6. Give two reasons why pediatric patients are more susceptible to respiratory distress.
   _____
   _____

7. Explain when capillary refill is considered abnormal in a pediatric patient.
   _____
   _____

8. Describe how to assess responsiveness in young children.

9. Why are pediatric patients more susceptible to hypothermia and hyperthermia?

10. When performing assessments on a pediatric patient, what considerations should be taken?

11. Describe how retractions occur during respiratory distress.

12. What emergency care should be given to all patients with stridor?

13. In its early stages, shock is harder to diagnose in children than in adults.
    ☐ True   ☐ False

14. What is the emergency care of a pediatric patient with shock?

15. Because of the physiological distinctions among infants and young children, describe some differences in the patterns of injury.

16. What modifications must be made in placing a child younger than eight years of age on a spineboard?

_____
_____
_____
_____

17. Describe emergency care of the injured pediatric patient.

SPECIFIC INJURY/ILLNESS	EMERGENCY CARE
Burns	
Poisoning	
Drowning	
Seizures	
Hyperthermia	
Hypothermia	
Severe Infection (Sepsis)	
Dehydration	
Child Abuse	

Chapter 20 Local Protocol

1. Describe the special equipment your patrol has for dealing with pediatric patients.

_____
_____
_____
_____

2. Explain your patrol's local procedures for giving emergency care to a pediatric patient.

_____
_____
_____
_____

3. Explain what forms and procedures are required at your area for gaining parental consent to treat a pediatric patient.

___
___
___
___
___

CHAPTER 20 SKILL PERFORMANCE REQUIREMENTS

- Review *Outdoor Emergency Care* scenarios 20.1 and 20.2

- Explain and demonstrate the emergency care for illnesses and injuries of infants and children

- Explain and demonstrate assessment of the pediatric patient

Skill Performance Guidelines

- Vital Signs Determination (see Chapter 3)
- Patient Assessment (see Chapter 5)
- Use of Oxygen and Airway Adjuncts (see Chapter 6)
- Control of Severe Bleeding in a Wound (see Chapter 7)

Pediatric Assessment
First impression • Note if the child is injured or ill, active or quiet.
Approach the patient at eye level
Access level of responsiveness
Perform ABCs • Maintain airway in sniffing position • Use brachial artery for neonates and infants; use radial or carotid in older patients
Rescue breathing is given at a rate of 20 breaths per minute (one breath every three seconds) if necessary
Obtain a SAMPLE history from parents
Perform an rapid body survey or whole body survey. Start with uninjured areas.

Chapter 20 Scenario

1. A 10-year-old was skiing powder in an out-of-bounds (non-patrolled) area with his father when he lost control on a steep pitch and hit a small stand of trees. He is lying between two small trees with little room. He is crying and complaining of pain in his right mid-thigh. There is a significant lump mid-shaft. He also has abrasions on his forehead and face, and is missing two teeth. His pulse is 120 and strong, respirations are 26, and his capillary refill is 1.5 seconds. He complains loudly if his leg is moved. The father is very concerned, attempting to help the administration of care, and does not want any movement that causes pain to his child. The child is shivering slightly and complaining of being cold. It is a 30-minute hike with a toboggan back to the area with no open terrain nearby. What do you suspect? What is the emergency care you provide? Explain your answers.

2. You are called to the scene of a tubing accident involving two children ages 7 and 10. The children were sliding down the hill at the same time when the older child slid headfirst into the younger child, striking him in the chest area. The older child is complaining of a sore shoulder. The younger child is crying and blaming the other child for the accident. Your survey of the younger child's chest and breathing does not reveal any significant injury but the child insists is hurts. The older child is surveyed and is found to have pain and tenderness in the shoulder and neck. Given this information, describe the possible injuries to each patient and explain the emergency care (including transportation decisions) you would give to both.

STUDY NOTES

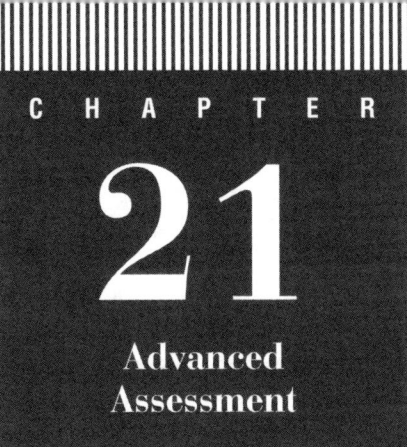

CHAPTER 21
Advanced Assessment

CONCLUDING OBJECTIVES

The learner will:

Content

- Further develop assessment techniques as initially learned in Chapters 4 and 5

Skill Performance

- Fully assess a situation, name and describe probable injuries or illnesses, and report emergency care

- Obtain a relevant medical history from a responsive patient

- Properly prioritize treatment of multiple injuries and/or multiple patient situations

CHAPTER 21 STUDY QUESTIONS

1. Review the basic protocol for assessing a responsive patient.

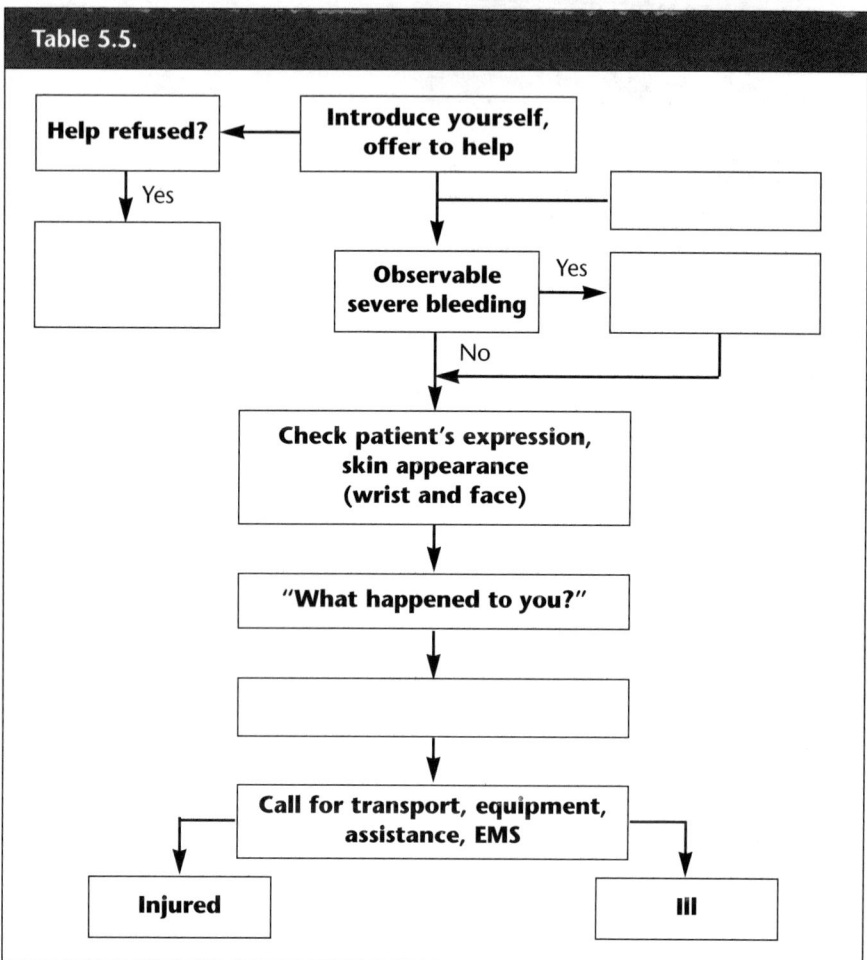

2. What major decision must a rescuer make before performing assessment and providing care of a responsive patient?

_____

3. Review the basic protocol for assessing an unresponsive patient.

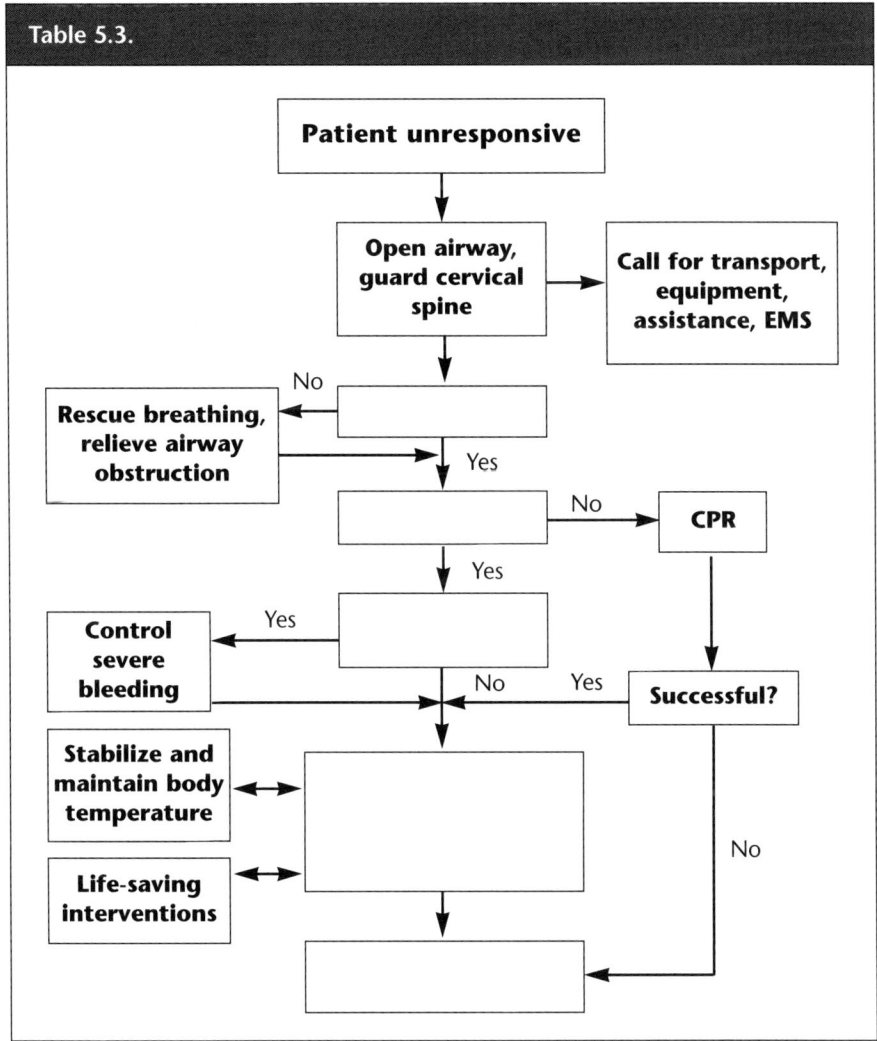

4. What is the major branching point for both assessment and care of an unresponsive patient?
   _____

5. List illnesses and injuries that could be an immediate or potential threat to life.
   _____
   _____
   _____
   _____
   _____
   _____
   _____

6. List illnesses or injuries that could represent a serious disability.

   _____

   _____

   _____

   _____

7. What situation indicates the need to assess the pupils and response to pain during the urgent survey and why?

   _____

   _____

8. Identify the advantages and disadvantages of taking a pulse in three different locations. What is the approximate single blood pressure value by this pulse?

Location of Pulse	Advantages/Disadvantages	Single Blood Pressure Value
Carotid		
Radial		
Femoral		

9. What does capillary refill indicate?

   _____

10. What might asymmetry of the face in a trauma patient indicate?

    _____

11. What do you do and ask the patient to do in order to test the major nerves of the lower extremity?

    _____

    _____

    _____

    _____

12. List the early signs of death.

13. Assessing a patient requires applying your total knowledge of illness to make an accurate assessment. Although first impressions, location, weather, and mechanism of injury may be significant factors, your thorough understanding of potential problems is crucial. Describe what it might mean if you find...

    ...an ill patient complaining of pain

    ...an ill patient with a fever or an acute infection

    ...an unresponsive patient with strong pulse at normal rate

    ...an unresponsive patient with weak, fast pulse

    ...a patient with slow pulse

    ...a responsive patient with rapid pulse with normal skin color, moisture, temperature

    ...a patient with rapid pulse with red, hot skin, elevated temperature

    ...a patient with high blood pressure

    ...a patient with normal blood pressure

    ...a patient with low blood pressure

    ...a patient with increased respiratory rate

    ...a patient with decreased respiratory rate

14. The whole body survey consists of exposing each area in turn and looking, feeling, listening, and smelling. Describe what to include in each:

Look	Feel	Listen	Smell

15. Describe the body substance isolation procedures that you initiate before each survey.

___

Chapter 21 Local Protocol

1. What procedures does your ski area follow in the event of a difficult multi-injury/ multi-patient emergency care?

___

2. What procedures must be followed at your area in the event of a death on the hill?

3. What are local procedures for interviewing witnesses and/or family members? Are there any special forms or reports that must be completed?

CHAPTER 21 SKILL PERFORMANCE REQUIREMENTS

- Review *Outdoor Emergency Care* scenarios 21.1 and 21.2

- Fully assess a situation, name and describe probable injuries or illnesses, and report emergency care

- Obtain a relevant medical history from a responsive patient

- Properly prioritize treatment of multiple injuries and/or multiple patient situations

Skill Performance Guidelines

- Vital Signs Determination (see Chapter 3)
- Patient Assessment (see Chapter 5)
- Use of Oxygen and Airway Adjuncts (see Chapter 6)
- Control of Severe Bleeding in a Wound (see Chapter 7)
- Traction Splinting (see Chapter 9)
- Spinal Immobililization (see Chapter 9)
- General Management of Long Bone Fractures (see Chapter 11)
- General Management of a Fracture or Dislocation At or Near a Joint (see Chapter 11)
- Alignment of Angulated or Displaced Fracture (see Chapter 11)
- General Management of an Open Fracture (see Chapter 12)
- Ski Boot Removal (see Chapter 14)
- Lifting Techniques (see Chapter 14)
- Helmet Removal (see Chapter 14)
- Application of a Standing Spineboard (see Chapter 14)
- Managing Medical and Environmental Emergencies (see Chapter 18)

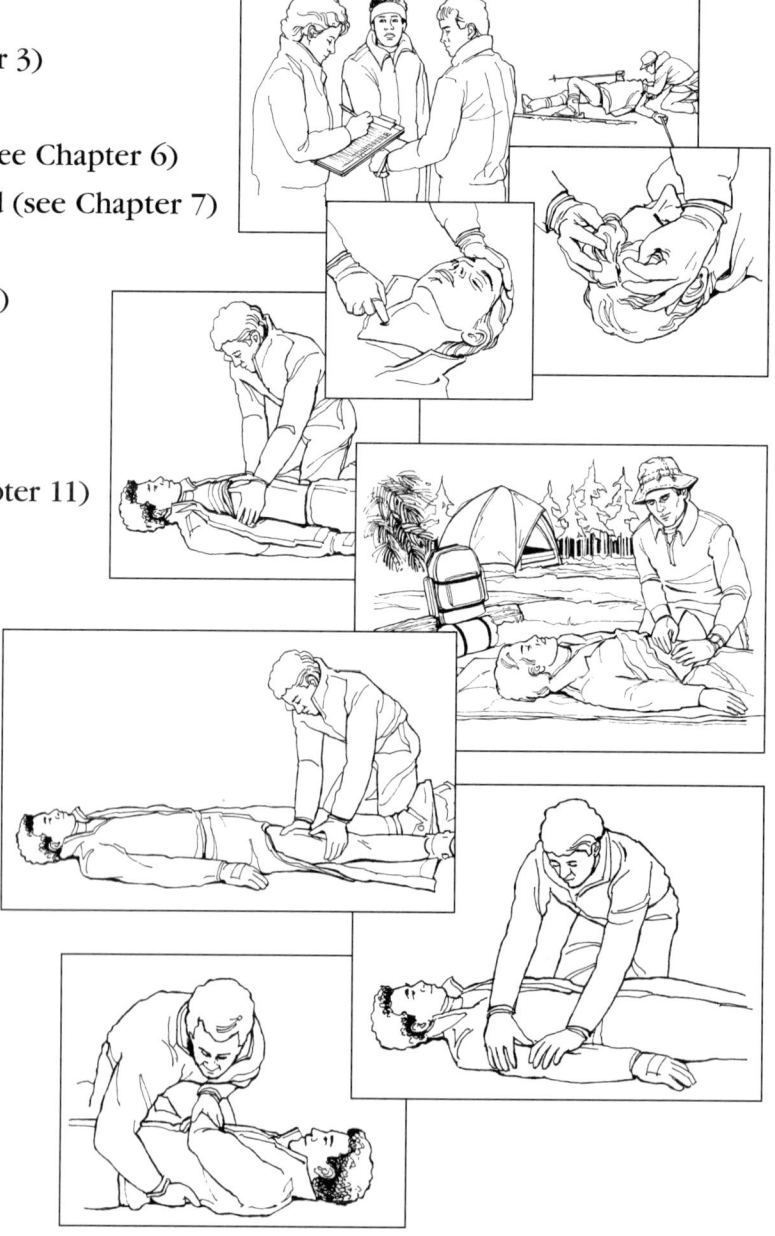

Chapter 21 Scenarios

1. Patient came off "more difficult" slope at high speed and struck pop fence that tripped him, causing him to fall forward. Patient is conscious of pain in his jaw and has the feeling that his teeth aren't meshing properly. Patient also has low level of responsiveness (LOR) and cannot recall the accident. He is a minor (16 years old), and parents are not present, but scout leader has consent form. Based on possible mechanisms of injury, describe advanced assessment procedures, identify the potential and anticipated problems with this scenario. What emergency care procedures should you provide?

2. There has been a flash fire by an area equipment shed, cause is unknown at the time of the problem. The employee who was in the shed at the time has first-degree burns to the face, and first and small areas of second-degree burns to the backs of his hands. He stumbled out of the shed and fell into a fellow employee, striking him in the face, breaking his glasses and knocking him down. Based on possible mechanisms of injury, describe advanced assessment procedures, identify the potential and anticipated problems with this scenario. What emergency care procedures should you provide?

3. It is late in the afternoon, and a beginner skier has decided to give the "bowl" one try before going home. The slope is hard packed and icy, so he does not go far before losing control. He goes over a mogul and is thrown backwards, hitting his head sharply on the ice. His skis release, but one hits him in the head. He then slides at an accelerated speed into the snow fence along the woods. He hooks his leg on a post, which brings him to an abrupt stop. Based on possible mechanisms of injury, describe advanced assessment procedures, identify the potential and anticipated problems with this scenario. What emergency care procedures should you provide?

STUDY NOTES

CHAPTER 22
Rescue Techniques

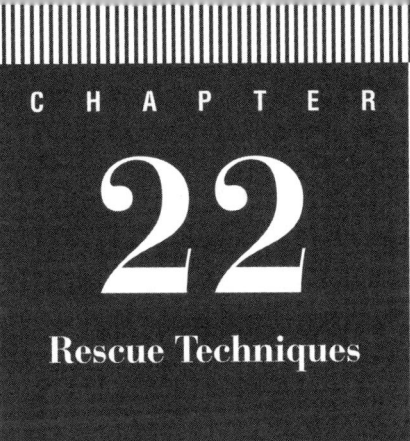

CONCLUDING OBJECTIVES

The learner will:

Content

- Describe techniques for obtaining access to, extricating, transferring, packaging, and transporting patients who may be found in remote areas, unstable positions, and/or awkward positions

Skill Performance

- Align an injured person into a supine neutral position

- Perform emergency and non-emergency patient moves, lifts, and carries

- Demonstrate extricating or moving an injured person from a difficult or confining location

CHAPTER 22 STUDY QUESTIONS

1. What is extrication?
   _____
   _____

2. Describe two ways in which a rescuer might represent a potential source of danger to the patient.
   _____
   _____

3. If the terrain is unique, steep, or technically challenging, search and rescue should be conducted only by _____.

4. Describe the six basic anatomical positions in which a patient may be found.
   _____
   _____
   _____
   _____
   _____
   _____
   _____
   _____
   _____
   _____
   _____
   _____

5. The ultimate goal of extrication is to have an injured patient in position _____ on the ground or on a long spineboard.

6. What are the three important reference points for "neutral position?"
   _____
   _____
   _____

7. During multi-rescuer lifts and carries, one rescuer should be designated as the leader. Where is this person usually located, and what is he or she doing?

___

8. Never move a patient's body _____.

9. When lifting a patient, the lifting should be done by the rescuer with the
   A. Hips and back rather than the legs
   B. Back and arms only
   C. Hips and legs rather than the back
   D. Hips, back and arms with arms slightly flexed.

10. Explain the difference between an emergency and non-emergency move.
    Emergency Move

    ___

    Non-emergency Move

    ___

11. What are three reasons why a rescuer might use an emergency lift or carry?

    ___

12. Explain the appropriate situations in which to use these carries.

    Fireman's Drag

    ___

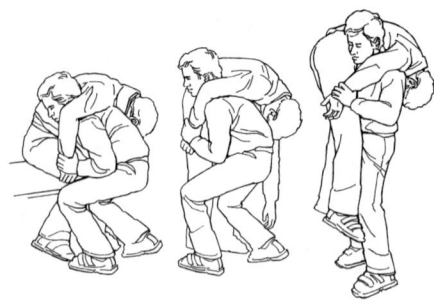

Fireman's Carry

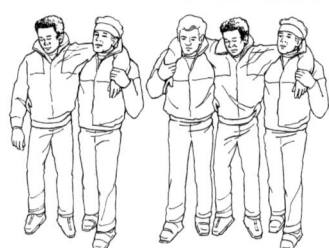

Human crutch

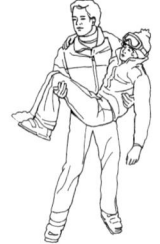

Front cradle

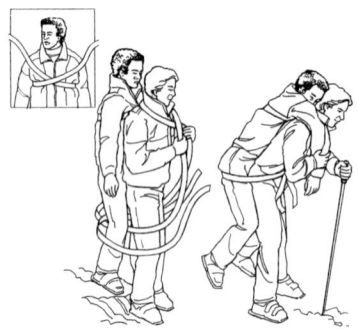

Back Carry

13. Describe the technique of a bridge lift for a patient with a spinal injury.

   _____
   _____
   _____
   _____
   _____
   _____
   _____
   _____

14. Describe the techniques of a direct ground lift and when you should use this lift.

   _____
   _____
   _____
   _____
   _____
   _____
   _____
   _____
   _____

Chapter 22 Local Protocol

1. Describe your resort's overall rescue process within area boundaries.

   _____
   _____
   _____
   _____
   _____

   Outside area boundaries

   _____
   _____
   _____
   _____
   _____

2. Explain local patrol procedures for:
   Emergency one-rescuer moves with possible spine injury

   _____
   _____
   _____

   Emergency two-rescuer moves with no spine injury

   _____
   _____
   _____

   Nonemergency direct ground lift and carry with no spine injury

   _____
   _____
   _____

   Extremity lift, fractures splinted—two or more rescuers

   _____
   _____
   _____

3. Describe local patrol procedures for removing an injured patient from:
   a tree well

   _____
   _____
   _____

   machinery (snow making equipment, lifts)

   _____
   _____
   _____

   a vehicle (snowcat, snowmobile, car)

   _____
   _____
   _____

4. Review the extraction equipment available at your local area and its uses.

CHAPTER 22 SKILL PERFORMANCE REQUIREMENTS

- Review *Outdoor Emergency Care* scenarios 22.1, 22.2, and 22.3

- Align an injured person into a supine neutral position

- Perform emergency and non-emergency patient moves, lifts, and carries.

    Emergency, One-Rescuer Techniques—Spine Injury Unlikely
        Fireman's Drag
        Fireman's Carry
        Human Crutch
        Front Cradle
        Back Carries

    Emergency One-Rescuer Moves—Possible Spine Injury
        Long Axis Drag

    Emergency Two-Rescuer Moves—No Spine Injury
        Seated Carries
        fore-and-aft Carry

    Nonemergency Moves—One or Multiple Rescuers
        Direct Ground Lift and Carry—No Spine Injury
        Direct Ground Lift and Carry—Possible Spine Injury
        Extremity Lift, Fractures Splinted—Two or More Rescuers
        Canvas Stretcher or Blanket Lift and Carry—No Spine Injury
        Bridge Lift—Possible Spine Injury

- Demonstrate extricating or moving an injured person from a difficult or confining location

Skill Performance Guidelines

- Lifting Techniques

    Long-axis Drag (see Chapter 14)

    Logroll (see Chapter 14)

    Multi-person Direct from the Ground (see Chapter 14)

    Bridge Lift (see Chapter 14)

    Lift into a Toboggan (see Chapter 23)

Chapter 22 Scenario

1. An employee was moving a portable snow gun into place when it rolled over on him. Hoses are wound around his torso and pelvis and the snow gun is resting across his lower legs, pinning him to the ground. He tells you that the snow gun rolled on him. He is complaining of pain in his lower abdomen. His respirations are shallow and somewhat rapid, his pulse slightly elevated, but strong. What emergency care procedures should you provide?

_____
_____
_____
_____
_____

STUDY NOTES

LIFTING TECHNIQUES—LONG-AXIS DRAG

Objective: To demonstrate manual lifting techniques to move patients over snow or other smooth terrain.

SKILL	YES	NO	NOTATIONS
• Maintains manual stabilization of the head and neck throughout maneuver. ▪ Headward drag: supports or cradles the upper torso ▪ Footward drag: supports or cradles the ankles and lower torso			
• Moves in a crouched position, pulling the patient slowly and smoothly about 12 inches at a time			
• Repositions, and repeats drag until reaching the desired location			
Did the trainee or patroller adequately demonstrate the performance criteria of this skill?			

COMMENTS

LIFTING TECHNIQUES—MULTIPLE-PERSON DIRECT FROM THE GROUND

Objective: To demonstrate manual techniques to move patients onto other devices

SKILL	YES	NO	NOTATIONS
• Manually stabilizes the head/neck as necessary for the injury.			
• Determines the number of lifters available and, therefore, the people pattern 5 people—3 to lift, 1 at head, 1 to move the device. 6 people—4 to lift, 1 at head, 1 to move the device.			
• Prepares all of the equipment needed for the lift or the device.			
• Explains the commands and procedures, and demonstrates the hand positions.			
• Executes the lift and slides the device into place, lifting the body as a unit.			
Did the trainee or patroller adequately demonstrate the performance criteria of this skill?			

COMMENTS

LIFTING TECHNIQUES—LOGROLL

Objective: To demonstrate manual techniques to move patients onto other devices

SKILL	YES	NO	NOTATIONS
• Manually stabilizes the head and neck.			
• Positions sufficient rescuers on the same side of the patient. Moves the patient as a unit while monitoring vital signs.			
• Positions hands on the far side, takes body mass into consideration.			
• Rolls the patient toward the rescuers on command from the leader (at the head), keeping the body in line. (The patient's arm may be alongside the body or elevated at local option.)			
• Places the stretcher, litter, or board alongside the patient and underneath as far as possible without excessive movement.			
• Rolls the patient onto the device on command from the leader, keeping the body in line.			
Did the trainee or patroller adequately demonstrate the performance criteria of this skill?			

COMMENTS

LIFTING TECHNIQUES—BRIDGING

Objective: To demonstrate manual lifting techniques to move patients onto other devices

SKILL	YES	NO	NOTATIONS
• Manually stabilizes the head and neck.			
• Determines the number of lifters available and, therefore, the people pattern: 5 people—3 to lift, 1 at head, 1 to move the device. 6 people—4 to lift, 1 at head, 1 to move the device.			
• Positions the lifters and has them form a bridge over the patient, head-to-shoulder or shoulder-to-shoulder. *(Note: All lifters must use the same configuration whether it be head-to-shoulder or shoulder-to-shoulder.)*			
• Assures everyone's commitment and equal distribution across the bridge positions.			
• Positions hands underneath the patient to lift at points of body mass (shoulders, hips).			
• Lifts the patient just enough to allow a spineboard or other device to be placed underneath.			
Did the trainee or patroller adequately demonstrate the performance criteria of this skill?			

COMMENTS

CHAPTER 23
Snowsport and Mountain Bike Injuries

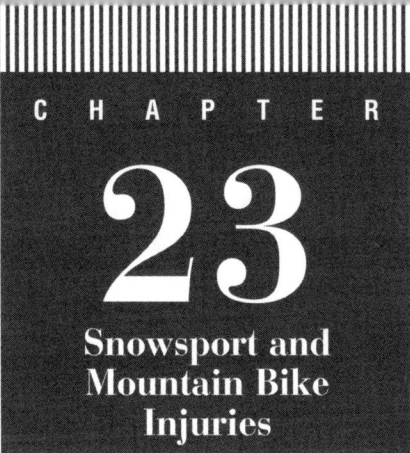

CONCLUDING OBJECTIVES

The learner will:

Content

- Describe basic types of skiing (alpine, nordic) and snowboarding accidents and common injuries resulting from each accident type

- Describe the safety aspects of modern alpine and nordic ski equipment, and of snowboards

- Describe methods of preventing accidents

- Describe the correct approach to an accident scene with a rescue toboggan

- Define positioning of patients in the toboggan

- Describe common off-road bicycling injuries

Skill Performance

- Demonstrate loading an injured skier into a toboggan and securing the patient

- Demonstrate the principles of boot removal

CHAPTER 23 STUDY QUESTIONS

1. Identify some of the most common injuries with each snowsport.

Alpine Skiing	Nordic Skiing	Snowboarding	Monoskiing	Tubing

2. What is the most frequent upper-body injury? How does it occur?

   _____

   _____

   _____

3. What are the two basic types of ski accidents?

   _____

4. What is the difference between a rotational and nonrotational fall.
   Rotational _____

   _____

   Nonrotational _____

   _____

5. List ski injuries that may result from a rotational fall.

   _____

   _____

   _____

6. List the ski injuries that may result from a nonrotational fall.

7. What are contributing factors in determining the likelihood of a ski injury?

8. Describe recommendations to prevent ACL injuries.

9. List the six rules of the Skier's Responsibility Code.

10. Why is the general rule to position the injury uphill on a toboggan?

11. Describe general positioning guidelines for a patient in the toboggan.

    Head downhill _____

    _____

    _____

    Head uphill _____

    _____

    _____

    On injured side _____

    _____

    _____

    Semiprone or recovery position _____

    _____

    _____

12. What condition takes preference in toboggan positioning, if patient has multiple serious injuries?

    _____

    _____

13. List common snowmobiling injuries.

    _____

    _____

    _____

14. List common off-road bicycling injuries.

    _____

    _____

    _____

    _____

15. List characteristics of backcountry toboggans.

Commercial	Improvised

Chapter 23 Local Protocol

1. Describe ways that your patrol works at increasing skiability and preventing accidents.

2. Describe local patrol procedures for approaching an accident site with a toboggan.

3. Describe local patrol procedures for removing a boot and when you would remove the boot.

CHAPTER 23 SKILL PERFORMANCE REQUIREMENTS

- Review Outdoor Emergency Care Scenarios 23.1 and 23.2
- Demonstrate loading an injured skier into a toboggan and securing the patient
- Demonstrate the principles of boot removal

Skill Performance Guidelines

- Lift into a Toboggan
- Ski Boot Removal

Lift Into A Toboggan

Assesses the factors:
- position of the patient in the toboggan.
- nature and extent of the injury.
- patient responsive/unresponsive.
- patient mobility—ability to assist.
- number of people able to assist.
- terrain (steep or flat).
- conditions (icy/hard; poor footing; soft, deep powder)
- type of toboggan (with/without baskets—height of edges).

Positions the toboggan and all of the other equipment.

Ensures all lifters are in appropriate position.

Ensures that the patient clears the side of the sled.

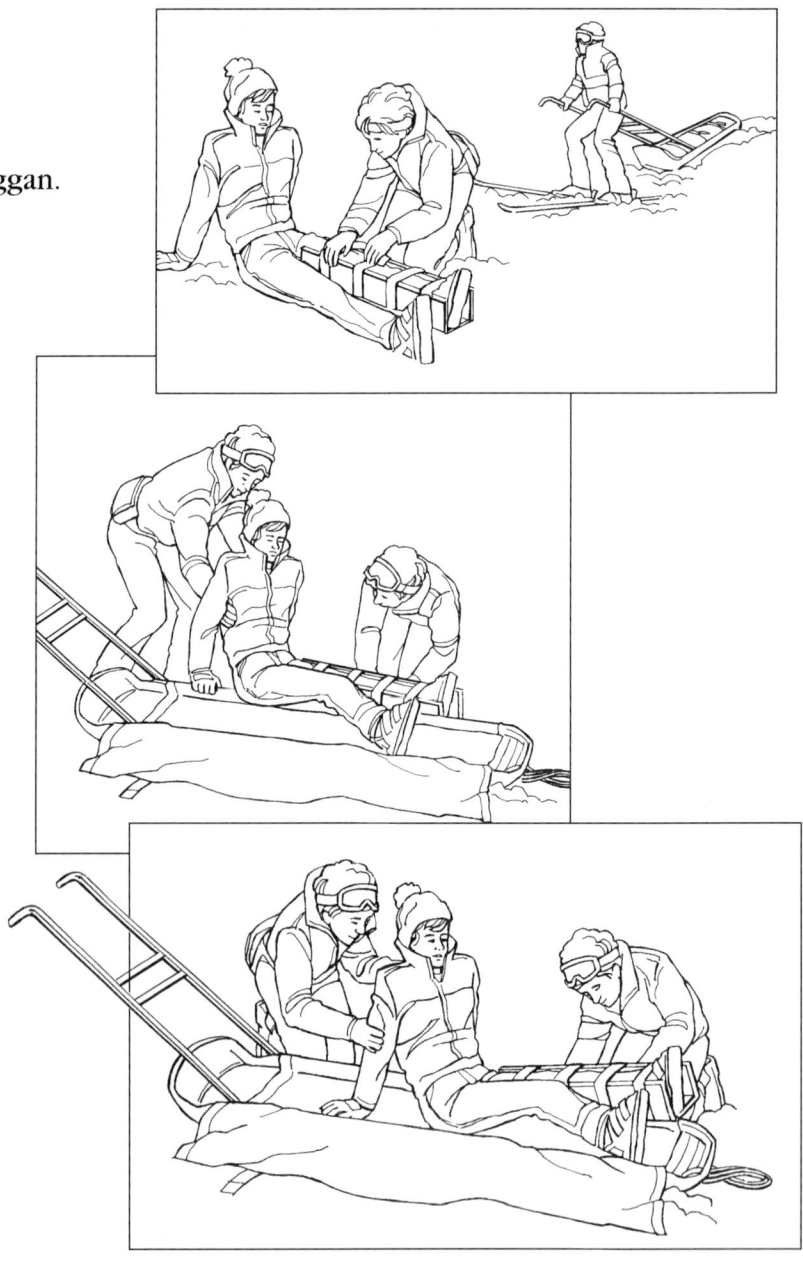

Ski Boot Removal

Note: The decision to remove a ski boot from an injured leg is based on local protocols.

- Stabilize and manually immobilize the lower leg and the ski boot.

- While maintaining manual immobilization, spread boot shell, pulling tongue out or opening rear entry boot, as wide as possible. Loosen all devices and provide instructions to assisting patroller.

- With the boot shell held open and the leg immobilized, apply tension to the boot. Firmly and smoothly pull and rotate boot off the foot.

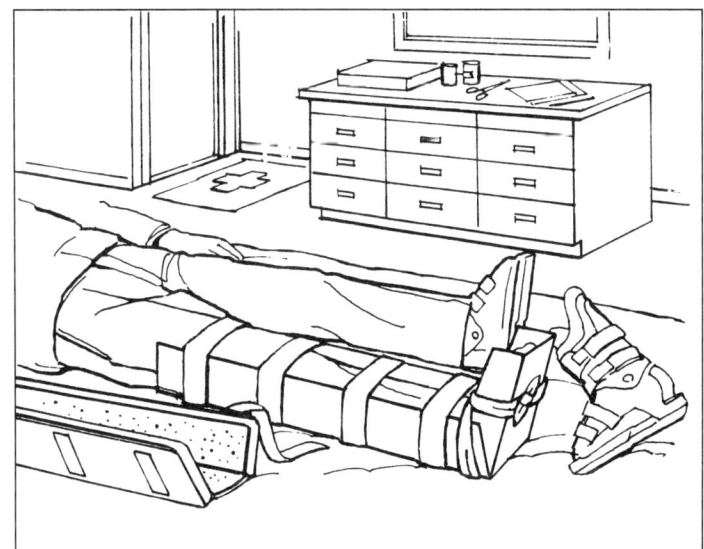

- Monitor patient for indications of excessive pain or resistance. Stop or modify procedure as appropriate.

- Assess distal circulation and neurological function, swelling, displacement, bruising, etc. (remove clothing).

- Prepare to splint the lower extremity.

Chapter 23 Scenarios

1. A 34-year-old female beginner skier decided to go to the top of the mountain after lunch. She said she caught the inside edge of her downhill ski. She said her foot rotated in and her knee popped. She cannot put weight on the knee. What injury do you suspect and why? How would you transport her in the toboggan?

   _____
   _____
   _____
   _____

2. A 24-year-old male mountain biker was attempting to bunny-hop a log. The back wheel of the bike failed to clear the log causing the rider to be thrown over the handlebars and hit the ground on his right shoulder. When you arrive, he is alert and sitting on the ground cradling his right arm against his chest. Upon inspection, you find he has tenderness and there is a deformity on the anterior portion of his shoulder. Describe the steps you would take in assessing the patient (include the questions you would ask him). What injuries do you suspect he has? Given the description of the accident, what injuries would you want to rule out before making a transport decision? Assuming his only injury is to the shoulder area, what emergency care would you give?

   _____
   _____
   _____
   _____
   _____

LIFTING TECHNIQUES—LIFT INTO A TOBOGGAN

Objective: To demonstrate loading an injured person into a toboggan and securing the patient.

SKILL	YES	NO	NOTATIONS

• Assesses the factors:
  • position of the patient in the toboggan.
  • nature and extent of the injury.
  • patient responsive/unresponsive.
  • patient mobility—ability to assist.
  • number of people able to assist.
  • errain (steep or flat).
  • conditions (icy/hard; poor footing; soft, deep powder).
  • type of toboggan (with/without basket—height of edges).			

• Positions the toboggan and all of the other equipment.			
• Ensures all lifters are in appropriate position.			
• Performs the lift smoothly without compromising the injury.			
• Ensures that the patient clears the side of the sled.			
Did the trainee or patroller adequately demonstrate the performance criteria of this skill?			

COMMENTS

SKI BOOT REMOVAL

Objective: To demonstrate the removal of a typical ski boot without compromising an injured leg.

SKILL	YES	NO	NOTATIONS
• Stabilizes and manually immobilizes the lower leg and the ski boot.			
• While maintaining manual immobilization, spreads boot shell, pulling tongue out or opening rear entry boot, as wide as possible. Loosens all devices and provides instructions to assisting patroller.			
• With the boot shell held open and the leg immobilized, applies tension to the boot. Firmly and smoothly pulls and rotates boot off the foot.			
• Monitors patient for indications of excessive pain or resistance. Stops or modifies procedure as appropriate.			
• Assesses distal circulation and neurological function, swelling, displacement, bruising, etc. (removes patirnt's clothing).			
• Prepares to splint the lower extremity.			
Did the trainee or patroller adequately demonstrate the performance criteria of this skill?			

COMMENTS

CHAPTER 24
Triage

CONCLUDING OBJECTIVES

The learner will:

Content

- Explain the purpose and use of the triage process

Skill Performance

- Apply the four color-coded categories to a multiple-casualty incident
- Apply the sequence of emergency care for a single patient with multiple injuries

CHAPTER 24 STUDY QUESTIONS

1. Define a multiple casualty incident.

   _____

   _____

   _____

2. In the outdoors triage situation, what patients are provided care?

   _____

3. Classify these patients in triage priority 1 through 4:

   ___ A middle-aged woman who is screaming hysterically. She has a large lump on her forehead and a fractured wrist. Her respirations and capillary refill are normal; she tells you that she hurt her head and wrist when the gondola fell.

   ___ A middle-aged man who is lying in the gondola wreckage, unresponsive, breathing normally, frowning, and spontaneously moving all four extremities. His capillary refill time is one second.

   ___ An elderly man with an obvious crushed chest. He has no detectable pulse and is not breathing.

   ___ A young woman who is lying quietly. Her ski is pale, cold and clammy, her pulse if fast, her respirations are rapid and shallow, and her capillary refill time is delayed. She complains weakly of abdominal pain.

   ___ An obnoxious, middle-aged man who is yelling, cursing, and threatening to sue the ski area. He does not appear to be hurt.

   ___ A young man who is lying quietly on his side, complaining of pain in the back between the should blades. He says that he cannot move his legs. His breathing and capillary refill time seem normal.

   ___ An elderly woman who appears basically healthy and vigorous for her age. She is in respiratory distress and is complaining of chest pain. A brief inspection of the site of pain discloses a flail segment of chest wall.

   ___ A middle-aged woman who seems calm and does not appear to be injured.

4. Fill in the blanks on the following table summarizing the triage categories.

Priority	Handling	Color Code	Description	Examples
1		Red	1. Hypoxia or shock is present or pending. 2. Survival is likely with rapid care and transport. 3. Care is not time-consuming.	
2	Delayed			Severe burns without respiratory distress, back or spinal cord injuries, multiple or major fractures, stable abdominal injuries, eye injuries, severe head or chest injuries
3		Green	1. Injuries are not life-threatening. 2. Patient may be ambulatory. 3. A minimum of emergency care is needed. 4. Patient is able to wait several hours before transport.	
4		Black		

5. Explain the steps and decisions used in the START triage plan.

_____
_____
_____
_____
_____
_____

6. Fill in the blanks on the following table comparing triage assessment with standard assessment.

Standard Assessment	Triage Assessment (Survival Scan)
1. A—Open the airway and guard the cervical spine. Ask, "Are you okay?"	
2. B—	2. Assess breathing. Do not give rescue breathing. Have a green-priority patient keep the airway open if needed.
3. C—Assess circulation and bleeding. Assess the carotid or radial pulse. Control bleeding if required. Give CPR if necessary.	
4.	4.
5. Conduct a nonurgent survey.	5.

7. Describe the "golden hour."

   _____
   _____
   _____

8. Life-threatening injuries usually involve _____, _____, and _____ systems.

Chapter 24 Local Protocol

1. Outline your patrol's procedures for a multiple casualty incident.

   _____
   _____
   _____
   _____
   _____

CHAPTER 24 SKILL PERFORMANCE REQUIREMENTS

- Review *Outdoor Emergency Care* scenarios 24.1 and 24.2

- Apply the four color-coded categories to a multiple-casualty incident

- Apply the proper sequence of emergency care for a single patient with multiple injuries

- Triage skills require scenario application using all the skill performance guidelines as applicable

Skill Performance Guidelines

- Vital Signs Determination (see Chapter 3)
- Patient Assessment (see Chapter 5)
- Use of Oxygen and Airway Adjuncts see Chapter 6)
- Control of Severe Bleeding in a Wound (see Chapter 7)
- Traction Splinting (see Chapter 9)
- Spinal Immobililization (see Chapter 9)
- General Management of Long Bone Fractures (see Chapter 11)
- General Management of a Fracture or Dislocation At or Near a Joint (see Chapter 11)
- Alignment of Angulated or Displaced Fracture (see Chapter 11)
- General Management of an Open Fracture (see Chapter 12)
- Ski Boot Removal (see Chapter 22)
- Lifting Techniques (see Chapters 14 and 22)
- Helmet Removal (see Chapter 14)
- Application of a Standing Spineboard (see Chapter 14)
- Managing Medical and Environmental Emergencies see Chapter 18)

Chapter 24 Scenarios

1. There is a small avalanche in which skiers are found alive and breathing.
   #1 is unresponsive and has a crushed chest.
   #2 is responsive and has a dislocated hip and a scalp laceration.
   #3 is unresponsive with a bruise on his head.
   #4 is responsive, has a broken jaw, facial abrasions, and a broken clavicle.
   #5 is responsive and has a broken wrist.

   Three patrollers and two toboggans are available. How should they proceed with the injured skiers and in what order?

   _____
   _____
   _____
   _____
   _____

2. In the late afternoon on a warm spring day, a deck attached to the base lodge collapses. Twenty guests fall 15 feet to the ground. Your initial triage reveals that one person is pulseless and apneic; 10 people are "walking wounded," six have serious injuries, and three have life-threatening injuries. Five minutes after the incident, two other patrollers join you at the site.

   Please include the answers to the following questions in your response:
   1. What BSI precautions are appropriate in this circumstance?
   2. Is oxygen administration appropriate?
   3. Explain the emergency care steps you would take in the order you would take them in handling this situation.
   4. What common problems and complications might develop?
   5. Describe the transportation decisions you would make.
   6. What documentation is needed for this situation and why?

   _____
   _____
   _____
   _____
   _____

STUDY NOTES

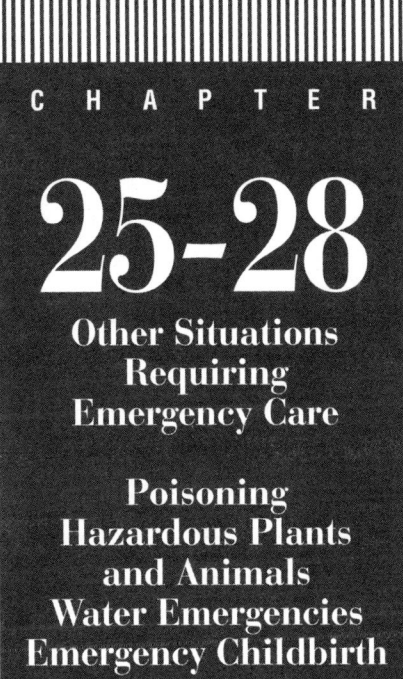

CHAPTER 25-28

Other Situations Requiring Emergency Care

Poisoning
Hazardous Plants and Animals
Water Emergencies
Emergency Childbirth

CONCLUDING OBJECTIVES

The learner will:

Content

- Describe the causes of and the general emergency care for illness and injuries from poisoning through ingestion, inhalation, injection, or absorption

- Describe the causes of and general emergency care for illness and injuries from contact with hazardous plants and animals

- Describe the dangers of and typical injuries associated with water sport recreation activities and the emergency care for submersion injuries

- Describe the handling and treatment for newborn and mother prior to, during, and following a normal out-of-hospital childbirth delivery

Skill Performance

- Explain and demonstrate the local procedures for handling illness and injuries that are not typical of the winter environment

CHAPTERS 25, 26, 27, and 28 STUDY QUESTIONS

1. Identify four ways that poisonous substances can enter the body.

2. List signs and symptoms of poisoning.

3. What are the important aspects of assessment and emergency care when poisoning is suspected?

4. Insect, spider, and snakebites follow emergency procedures for injected poisons. Those general procedures are:

5. List the common groups of signs and symptoms that can occur with injuries associated with hazardous plants.

6. What types of diseases can be carried and transmitted to humans by ticks?

7. In addition to general emergency protocols, what specific procedures are necessary with bites with envenomation?

8. Describe the general care of patients with warm-blooded animal bites.

9. What steps should be taken when encountering an animal that is believed to have rabies?

10. What will the emergency department physician need to know about a submersion patient?

11. What is the emergency care of a submersed-injury patient?

12. Labor is divided into three stages. Describe the key points of each stage.

    First stage _____

    Second stage _____

    Third stage _____

13. List the signs that determine when a pregnant woman should be taken to a hospital for delivery.

14. What criteria determine out-of-hospital emergency childbirth delivery?

15. Describe the general care required for some possible complications that may be encountered in emergency childbirth.

Complications of Childbirth	
Nonbreathing baby	
Abnormal presentation or prolapsed cord	
Abnormal bleeding	
Prolonged delivery	

16. Which bone(s) can be easily fractured as the result of diving into shallow water?
    A. Clavicle
    B. Cervical vertebrae
    C. Humerus
    D. Scapulae

17. To allow the victim to reach the shore, or a rescuer to safely reach a victim who has broken through an ice-covered body of water, the rescue should
    A. Be undertaken immediately with as many rescuers as possible
    B. Be undertaken only if the rescuer is wearing a wet suit of full-exposure suit
    C. Be performed so that weight is widely distributed over the ice surface
    D. Always involve helicopter assistance

Chapters 25-28 Local Protocol

1. Identify potential poisons that could be at your resort during any season and where they are located.

   Ingested poisons _____
   _____

   Inhaled poisons _____
   _____

   Injected poisons _____
   _____

   Contact poisons _____
   _____

2. What are the local procedures for handling poison incidents? Do the procedures vary during off-season?

   _____
   _____
   _____
   _____
   _____

3. Identify any poisonous plants, insects, arachnids, and snakes found in your local area.

Plants	Insects	Arachnids	Snakes

4. Are there any environmental features at your area that could potentially create a water emergency? If so, what are the local procedures?

　

5. Identify local protocols, if any, to handle an emergency childbirth.

CHAPTER 25-28 SKILL PERFORMANCE REQUIREMENTS

- Review *Outdoor Emergency Care* scenarios 26.1 and 27.1

- Explain and demonstrate the local procedures for handling illness and injuries that are not typical of the winter environment

    Poisoning through ingestion, inhalation, injection, or absorption

    Contact with hazardous plants and animals

    Water and submersion injuries

    Out-of-hospital childbirth delivery

Skill Performance Guidelines

- Vital Signs Determination (see Chapter 3)
- Patient Assessment (see Chapter 5)
- Use of Oxygen and Airway Adjuncts (see Chapter 6)
- Control of Severe Bleeding in a Wound (see Chapter 7)
- Traction Splinting (see Chapter 9)
- Spinal Immobililization (see Chapter 9)
- General Management of Long Bone Fractures (see Chapter 11)
- General Management of a Fracture or Dislocation At or Near a Joint (see Chapter 11)
- Alignment of Angulated or Displaced Fracture (see Chapter 11)
- General Management of an Open Fracture (see Chapter 12)
- Lifting Techniques (see Chapters 14 and 22)
- Helmet Removal (see Chapter 14)
- Application of a Standing Spineboard (see Chapter 14)
- Managing Medical and Environmental Emergencies (see Chapter 18)

STUDY NOTES

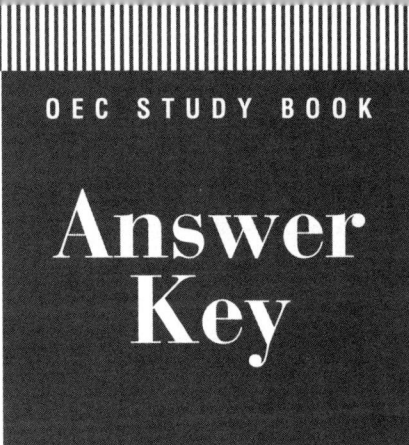

OEC STUDY BOOK

Answer Key

CHAPTER 1 STUDY QUESTIONS

1. 1) Oxygen
   2) Maintenance of body temperature
   3) Water
   4) Food
   5) Physical integrity
   6) Confidence, the will to survive

2. In the alveoli

3. **Insufficient oxygen in the outside air**
   1) High altitude
   2) Burial in a snow or dirt avalanche
   3) Poorly ventilated snow cave or other confined space
   4) Malfunction of underwater breathing apparatus
   5) Near drowning
   6) Smoke or other substance in air replaces oxygen

   Obstruction of the upper airway
   1) Relaxation of the tongue or pharyngeal tissue in an unresponsive person
   2) Aspirated food, vomitus, dentures, or other foreign material
   3) Injury to the face or neck

   Obstruction of the lower airway
   1) Inhaled foreign body
   2) Inability to cough up blood, pus, or mucus

   Interference with lung function
   Acute
   1) Filling of the alveoli with pus, blood, or fluid, as in pneumonia, lung hemorrhage, or pulmonary edema
   2) Partial or total collapse of the lung because of blood, fluid, or air pressing on the outside of the lung
   3) Spasm and thickening of bronchial walls and plugging of small bronchi with mucus, as in an attack of asthma

   Chronic
   1) Thickening of the alveoli walls, as in pulmonary fibrosis
   2) Loss of some alveoli, enlargement of others, and narrowing of the bronchi, as in emphysema
   3) Replacement of lung tissue by tumor (benign or malignant)

   Interference with chest integrity or function
   1) Paralysis of the nerve supply to the diaphragm and/or chest muscles, as in spinal cord injury
   2) Crushing injury to the chest, as in flail chest caused by multiple rib fractures
   3) Open chest wounds

Interference with the brain's control of breathing
1) Head injury
2) Meningitis
3) Stroke
4) Poisoning overdose of depressants

Abnormal function of the circulatory system
Illness
1) Heart attack
2) Chronic heart failure
3) Fluid in the sac around the heart
4) Blood clot in the lung blocking blood flow through its vessels (pulmonary embolus)

Injury
1) Shock
2) Direct injury to the heart or blood vessels

Interference with the blood's oxygen-carrying capacity
1) Anemia
2) Carbon monoxide poisoning

4.
1) Rate and depth of breathing increases
2) Blood absorbs oxygen more efficiently
3) Blood carries oxygen more efficiently
4) Heart and skeletal muscle action become more efficient

5. A. Hypoxia

6. **Involuntary**
   1) Shivering
   2) Foot stamping and other semiresponsive activity
   3) Non-shivering thermogenesis

   Voluntary
   1) Muscular activity
   2) Eating—heat from hot food and drink
   3) Food—energy
   4) Stove, fire, sun

7.
1) The direct transfer of heat from a warm body to a cooler object
2) The transfer of heat when air that is cooler than body temperature moves across the body's surface
3) The loss of heat when water or another volatile liquid on the body's surface is converted into vapor
4) Heat loss from the body through infrared waves
5) Body heat that is lost through respiration as inhaled air is warmed to body temperature before being exhaled

8. **Involuntary**
   1) Decrease sweating
   2) Shunt blood away from the shell
   3) Decrease body surface area

   Voluntary
   1) Add clothing
   2) Seek shelter

9. The relationship between actual temperature, wind velocity, and "effective" temperature at the skin surface. As the wind velocity rises, the "effective" temperature drops.

10. 1) Attain and maintain a high state of physical fitness. Allow time for acclimatization.
    2) Maximize body heat loss by exposing as much skin to the air as possible, wearing loose, light colored, cotton clothing; maintaining hydration to promote sweating; and acclimatize
    3) Minimize heat gain from the environment by wearing protective clothing, seek shade during the heat of the day, avoid touching hot objects, and do not lie directly on the ground
    4) Minimize body heat production by decreasing muscular activity

11. B. Are warm even when wet

12. It is important to wear garments that trap a layer of still, warm air around the body and maintain a microclimate despite extremes of wind, wet, and cold temperatures. Layering allows flexibility because one or more layers may be added or subtracted as necessary.

13. To prevent overheating or chilling by adding/subtracting layers of clothing

14. To reduce heat loss from radiation and convection, wear a hat. Up to 70 percent of the heat produced by the body can be lost from an uncovered head.

15. 60 percent

16. 1) Light in weight
    2) High in energy
    3) Not require cooking or complicated preparation
    4) Resistant to spoilage

17. **Carbohydrates**
    1) Vegetables
    2) Cereals
    3) Fruits
    4) Sugar

    Proteins
    1) Eggs
    2) Dairy products
    3) Meat
    4) Poultry
    5) Cereals
    6) Fish
    7) Peas
    8) Beans
    9) Nuts

    Fat
    1) Butter
    2) Lard
    3) Cooking oil
    4) Mayonnaise
    5) Ice cream
    6) Cereals
    7) Fried foods
    8) Dairy products
    9) Meat
    10) Eggs
    11) Nuts
    12) Vegetables
    13) Chocolate

Minerals
1) Calcium
2) Phosphorus
3) Magnesium
4) Iron
5) Sodium
6) Potassium
7) Chlorine
8) Sulfur
9) Chromium
10) Cobalt
11) Copper
12) Fluorine
13) Iodine
14) Manganese
15) Molybdenum
16) Nickel
17) Selenium
18) Silicon
19) Tin
20) Vanadium
21) Zinc

Vitamins
1) B_1, B_2, B_6, B_{12}
2) Niacin
3) Pantothenic acid
4) Biotin
5) Choline
6) Folic acid
7) C, A, D, E, K

Water
1) 2,500 milliliters (2.7 quarts) daily

18. Four to five

19. Upper and lower extremities

20. 1) A warm-up period
    2) Selected calisthenics
    3) A period of rhythmical, non-stop training
    4) A cooling-down period

21. 1) Cardiovascular or aerobic (oxygen-requiring) fitness: Develops the heart and circulatory system to meet the body's changing needs for blood
    2) Motor fitness: Develops and enhances strength, power, endurance, balance, agility, and flexibility

Chapter 1 Scenario

1. Since winds will be high and it may rain/snow/sleet, prepare to layer clothing. By layering you can stay the warmest and driest. Start with polypropylene long underwear. Outerwear should include wind or rain pants. Definitely have a hat, gloves, and waterproof boots with good traction in case trails get slick. Equipment should include shelter such as a tent and a ground cloth for extra insulation.

CHAPTER 2 STUDY QUESTIONS

1.

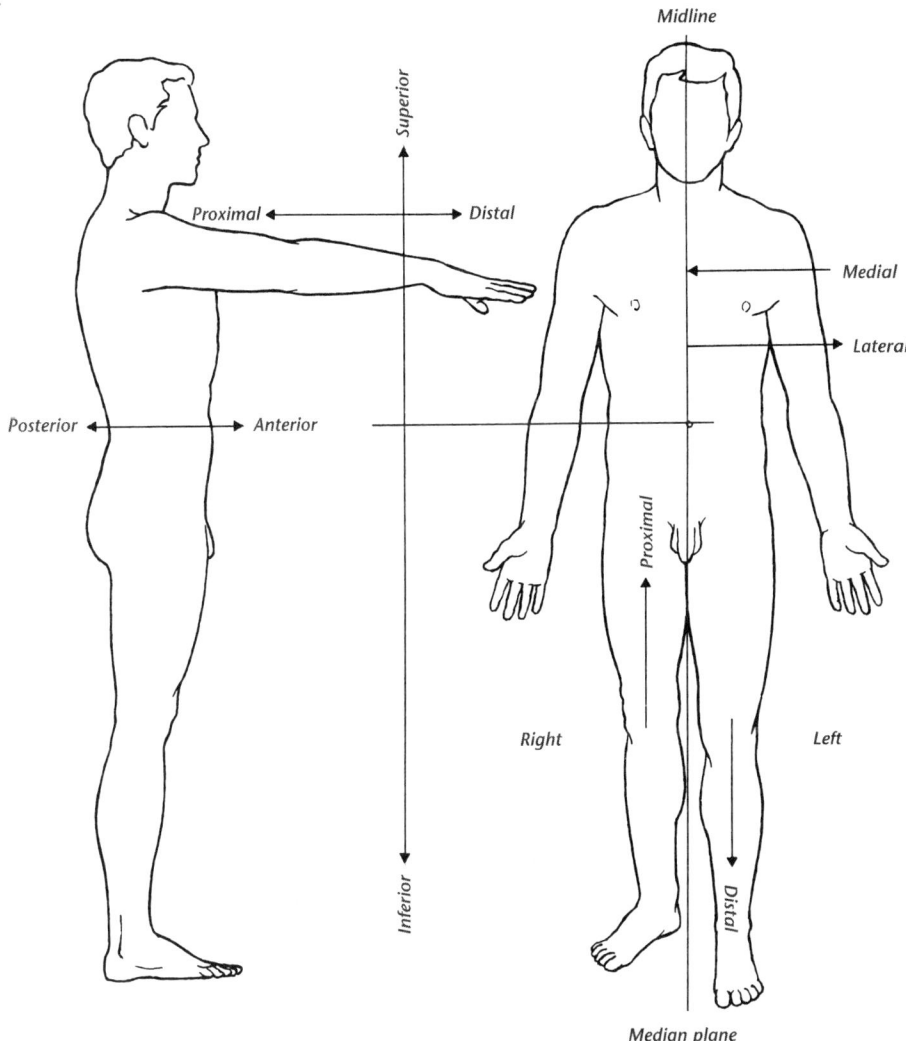

2. G
   C
   D
   H
   F
   E
   A
   B
   I
   J

3. D
   A
   F
   E
   B
   G
   C
   H

4. The ability of muscle cells to function without immediate oxygen supply and make it up later

5. Blood from the body returns to the heart through the right atrium, then to right ventricle that pumps it into the pulmonary arteries to the lungs to be oxygenated in the alveoli. Then blood returns through left atrium via pulmonary veins to left ventricle through aorta to systemic system to vena cava.

6. C. Aorta

7.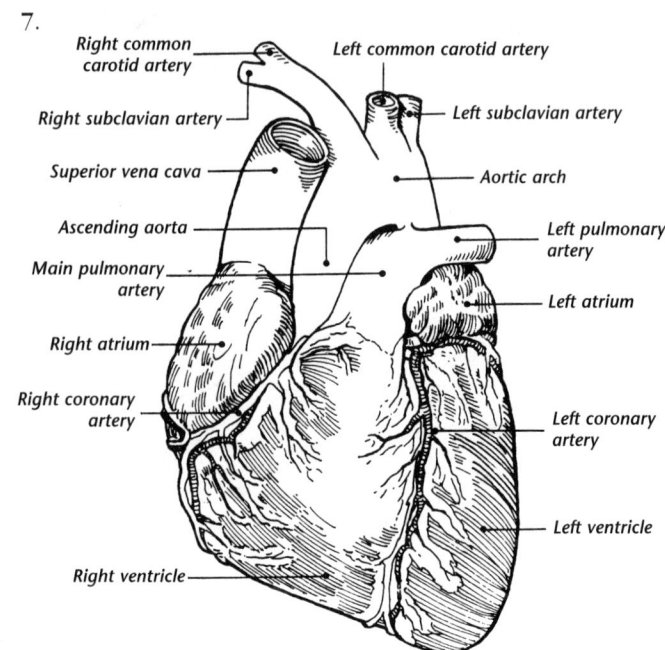

8.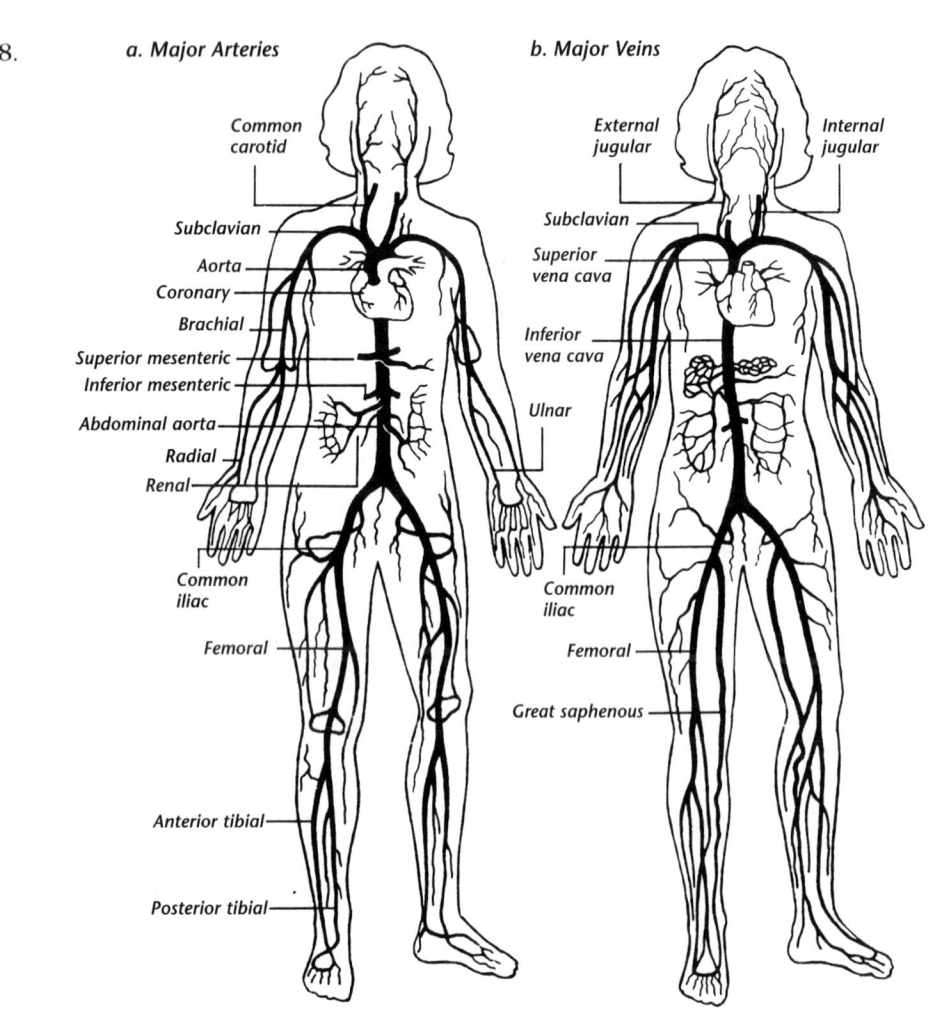

9. **Platelets** Aid blood clotting
   White Fight infection
   Red Carry oxygen

10.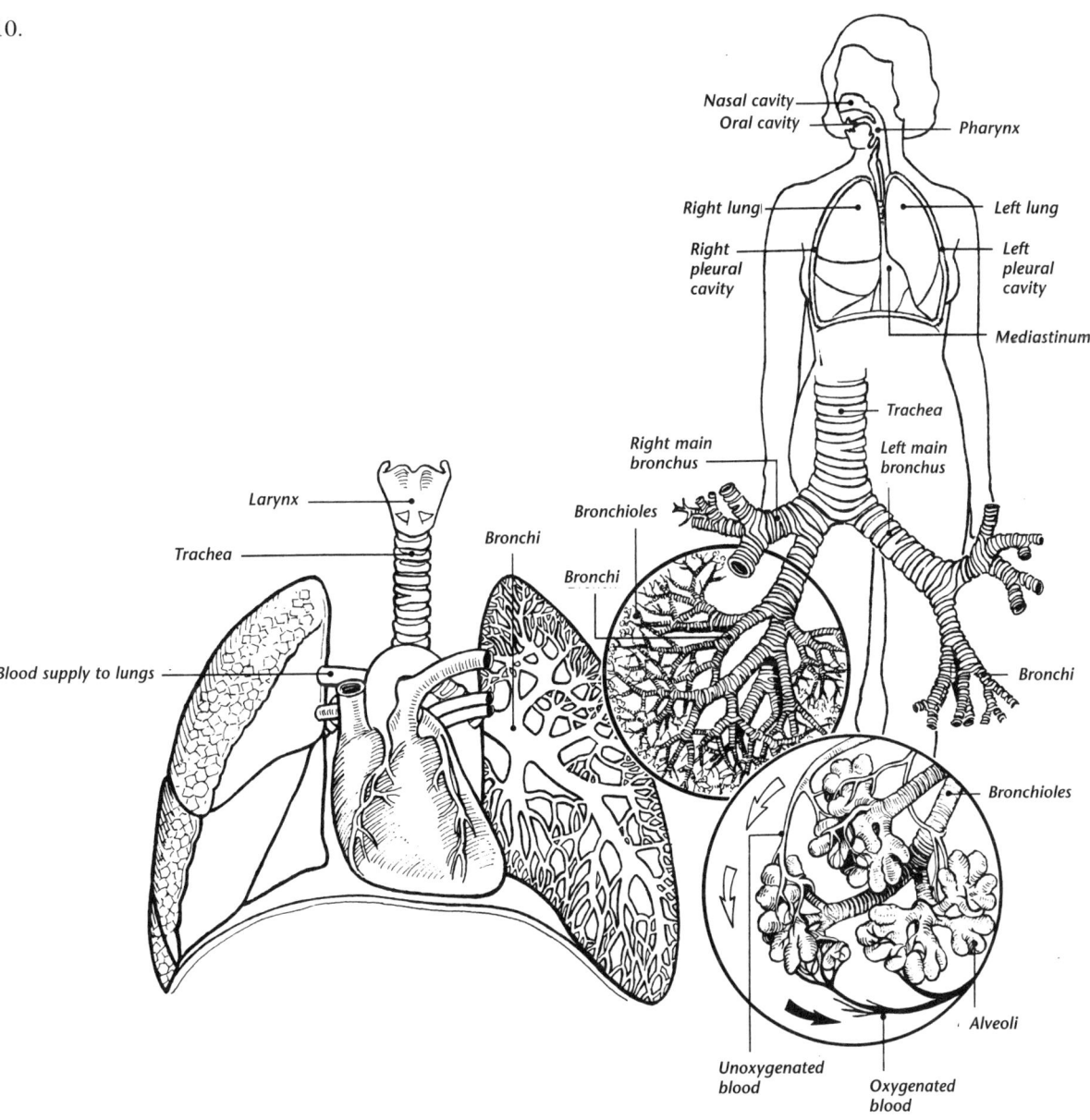

11. C. Larynx

12. The air enlarges the chest cage, and the inside pressure becomes lower than the outside pressure. Air flows in to equalize the pressure, and the lungs are pushed out by the air. The air is forced out by chest pressure, and the chest cage returns to its previous size.

13. D. B and C.

14.

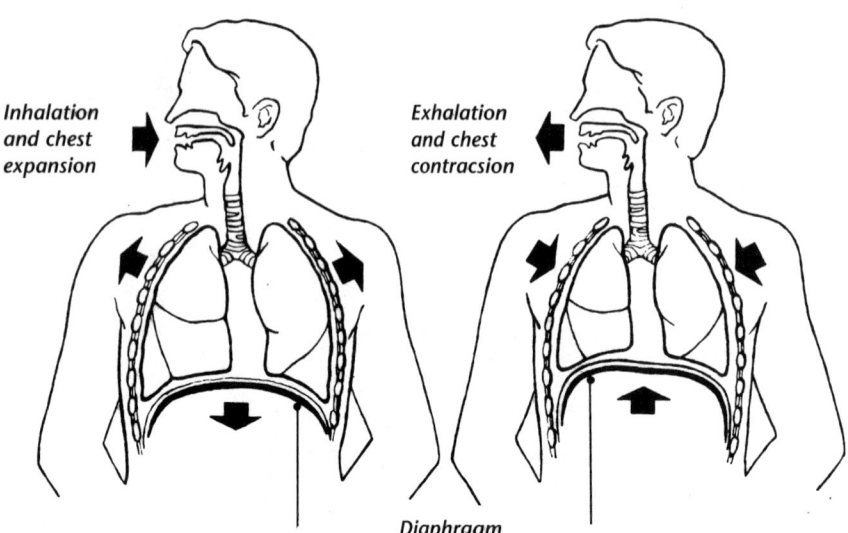

15. 1) The central nervous system
    2) The peripheral nervous system

16. Central nervous system

17. Somatic—Controls voluntary activities such as eating, walking, and talking
    Autonomic—Controls bodily activities not under responsive control

18. C
    E
    D
    A
    B

19. C
    D
    A
    B

20. The autonomic nervous system

21. At the base of the brain

22. The head

23. To the muscles

24. To the brain

25. The radial nerve

26. Flex

27.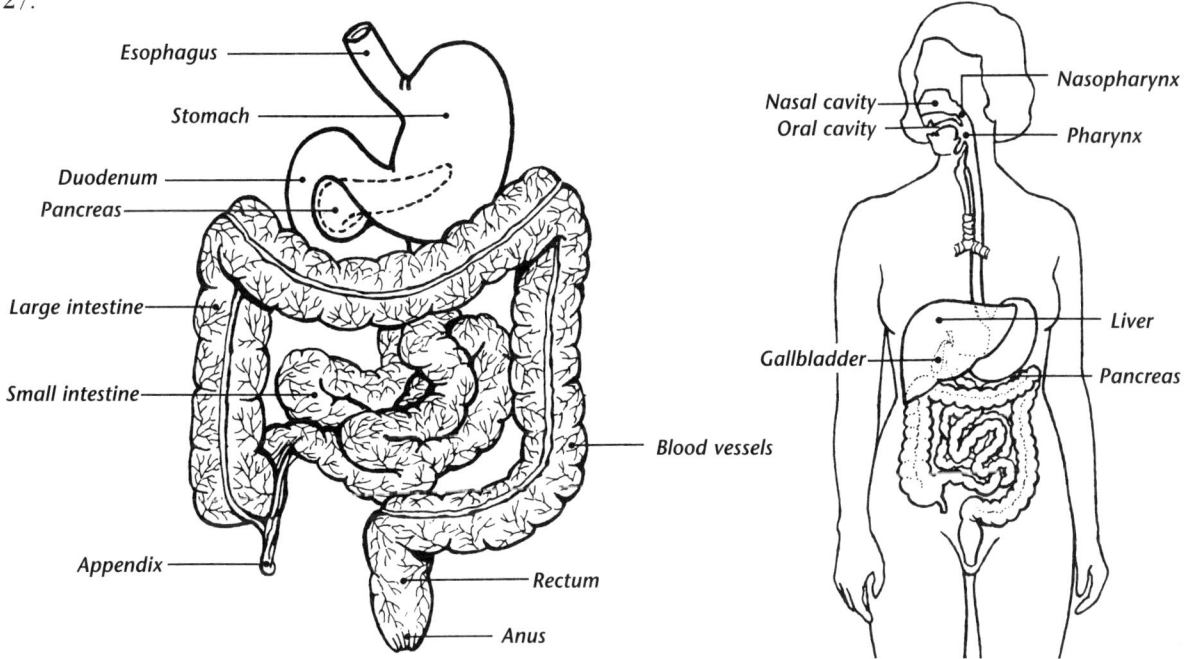

28. Food enters the mouth, where it is chewed into small pieces by the teeth and mixed with saliva. Saliva moistens the food and starts the digestive process with an enzyme that breaks down starch. The tongue helps move the food and contains taste buds. The chewed and moistened food then passes through the oropharynx and esophagus into the stomach, where it is mixed with gastric juice. The partly digested food enters the first part of the small intestine, where it is mixed with bile and pancreatic juice. Most of the digested food is absorbed in the small intestine. The undigested residue enters the large intestine, which concentrates the residue by removing most of the water. The resulting fecal matter is stored in the lower part of the large intestine until it can be expelled.

29. 1) Kidneys
    2) Uterus
    3) Bladder
    4) Urethra

30. C. Blood

31.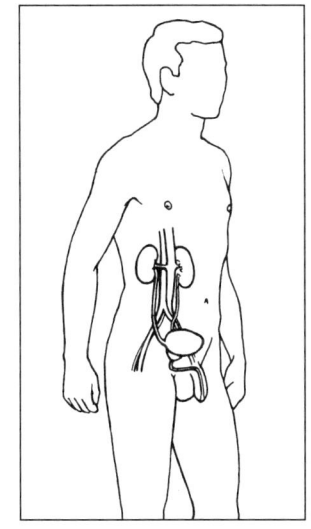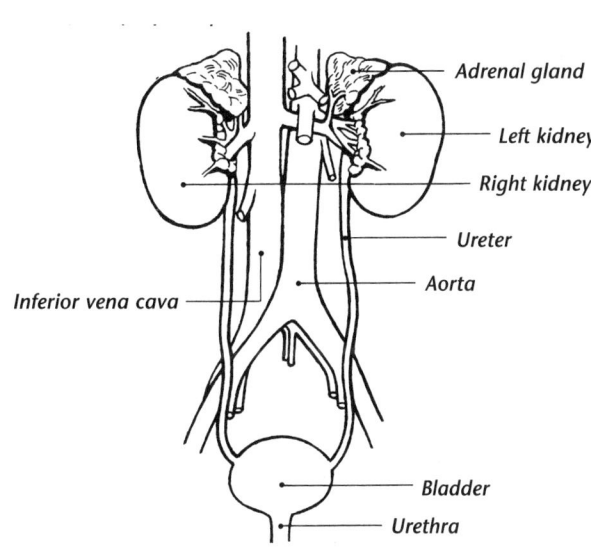

32.

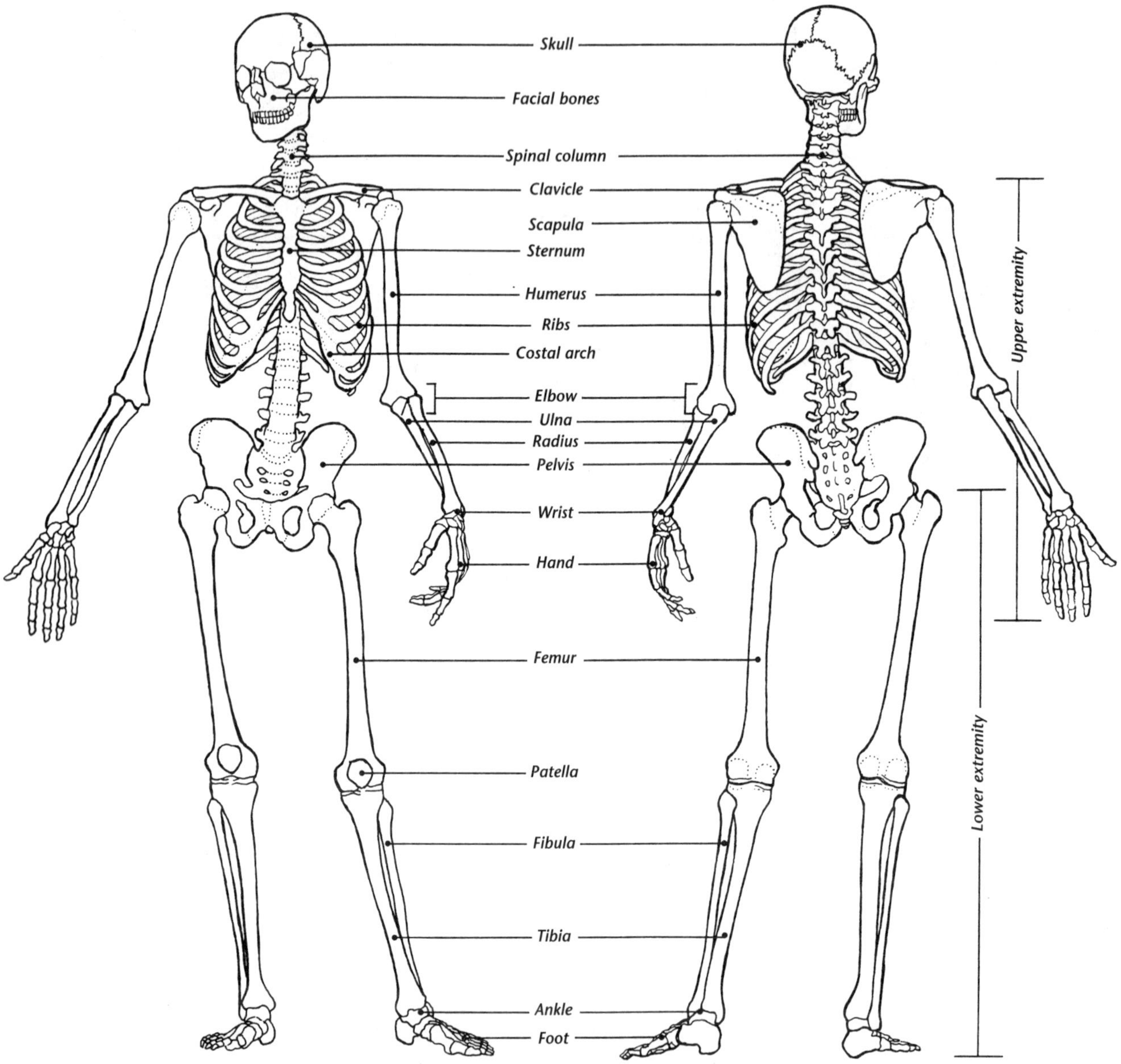
Skull
Facial bones
Spinal column
Clavicle
Scapula
Sternum
Humerus
Ribs
Costal arch
Elbow
Ulna
Radius
Pelvis
Wrist
Hand
Femur
Patella
Fibula
Tibia
Ankle
Foot
Upper extremity
Lower extremity

33.

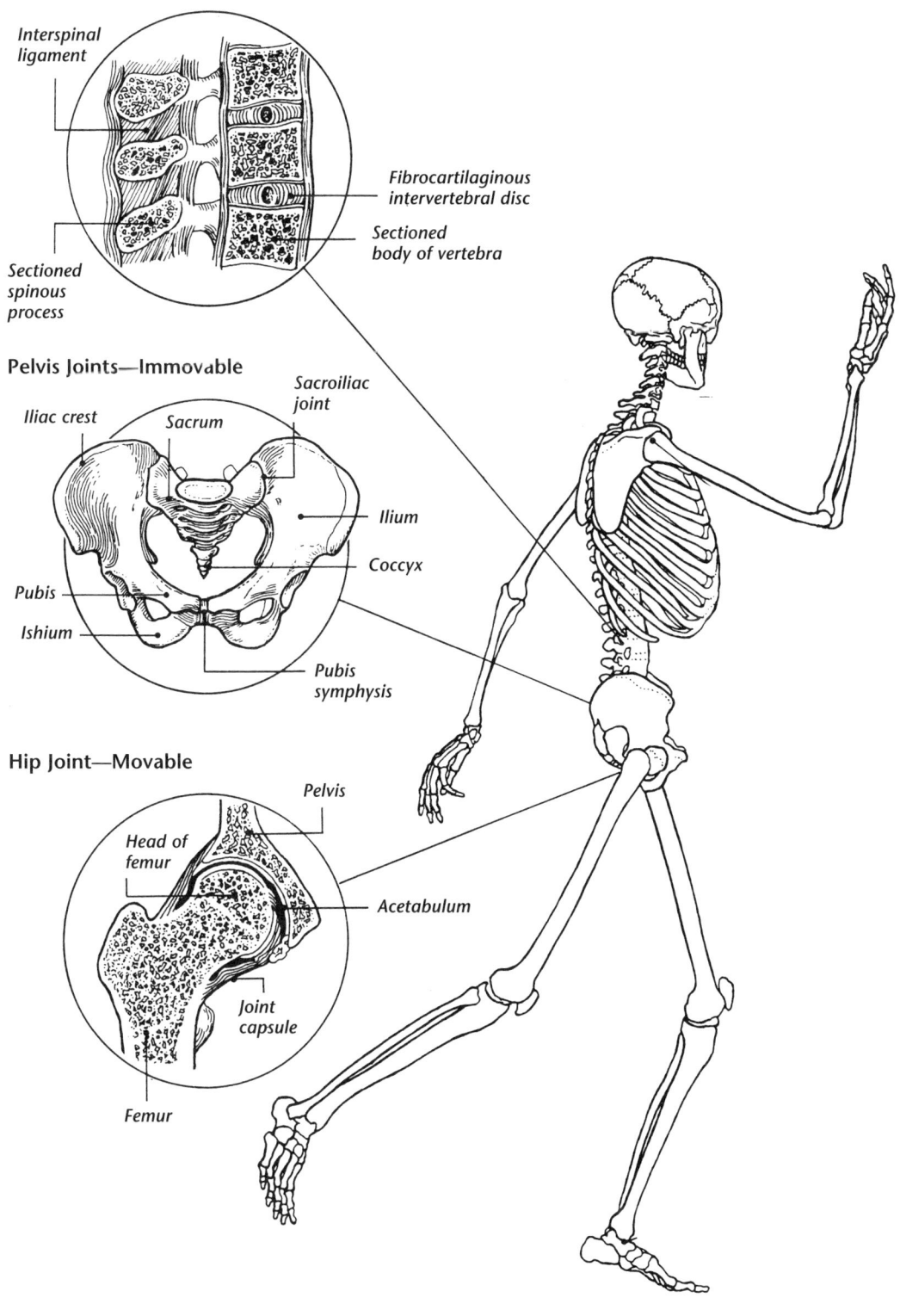

34.

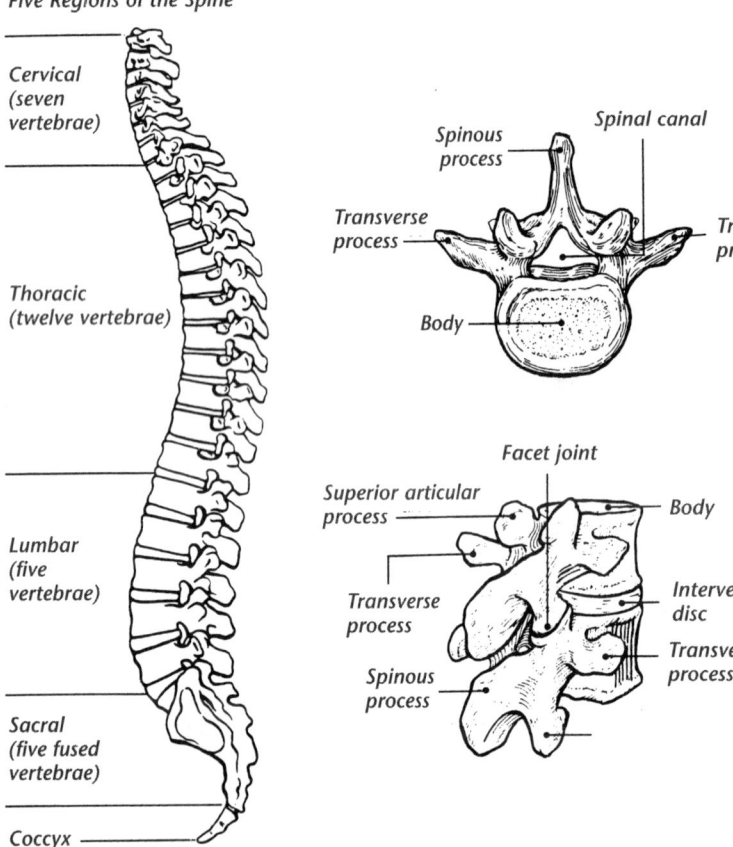

35.

Five Regions of the Spine

Cervical (seven vertebrae)

Thoracic (twelve vertebrae)

Lumbar (five vertebrae)

Sacral (five fused vertebrae)

Coccyx

36.

37.

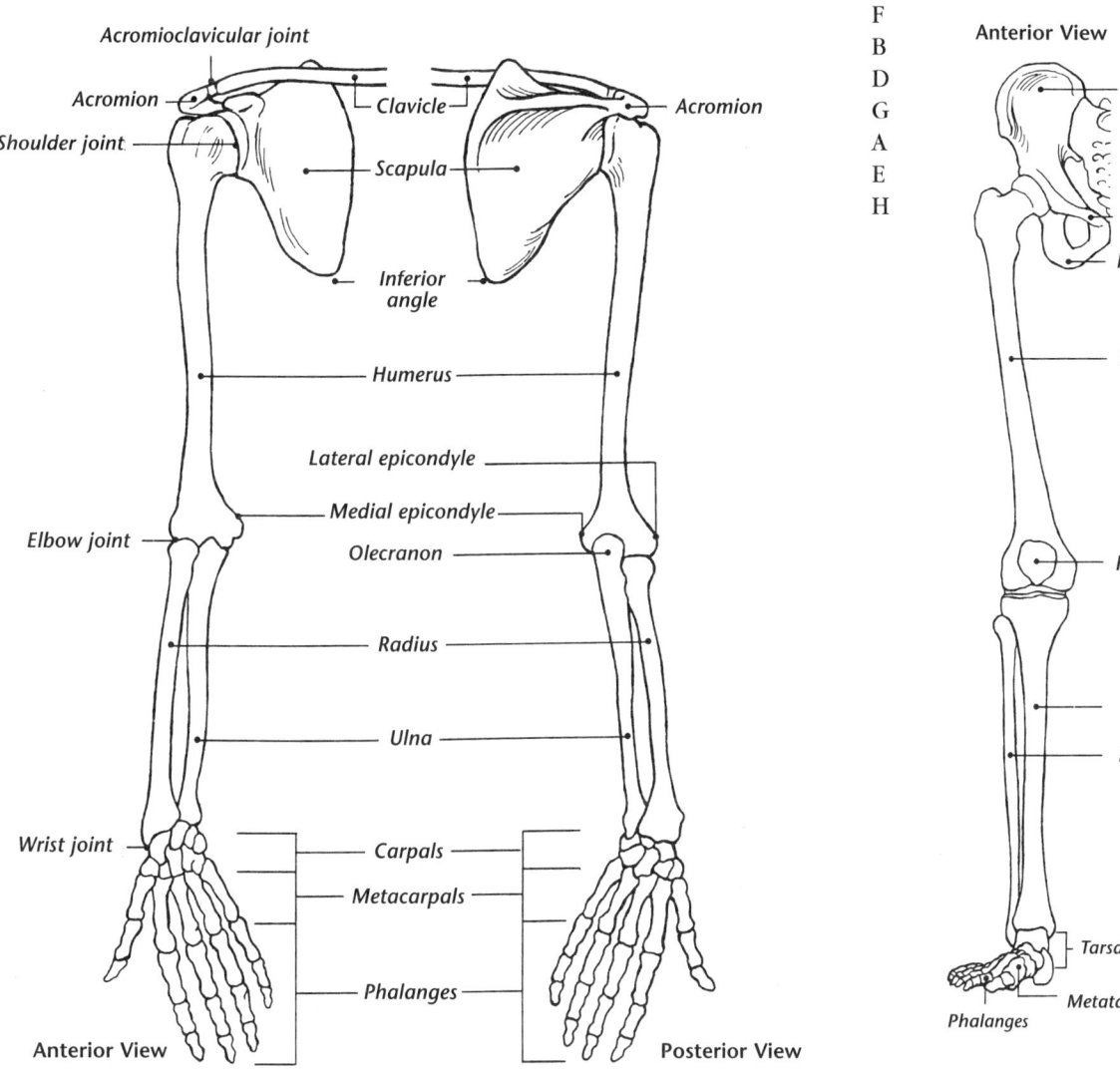

38. C
F
B
D
G
A
E
H

40. B. Lumbar

41.

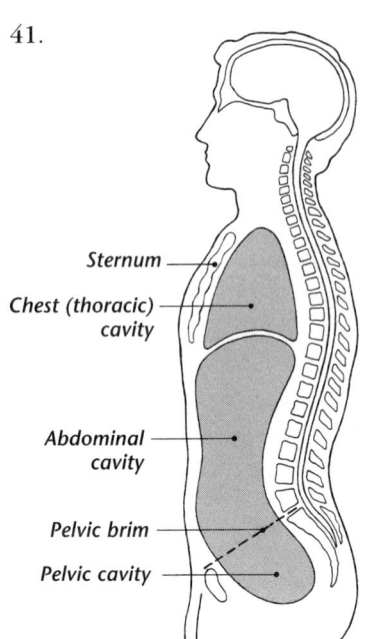

42.

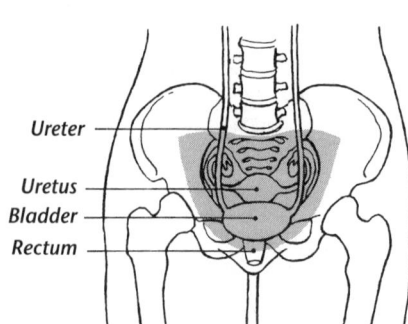

43.

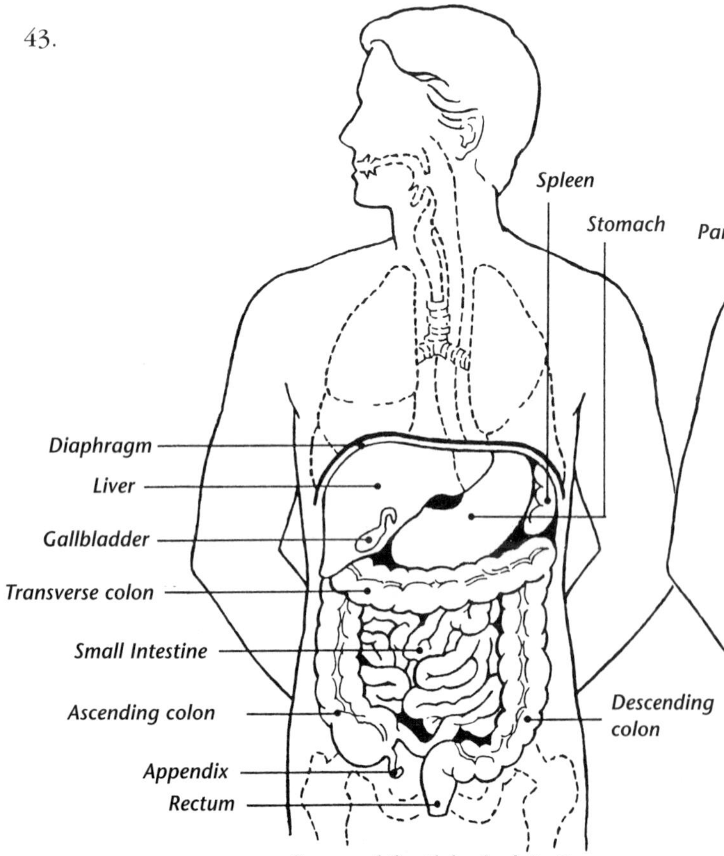

Organs of the Abdominal Cavity

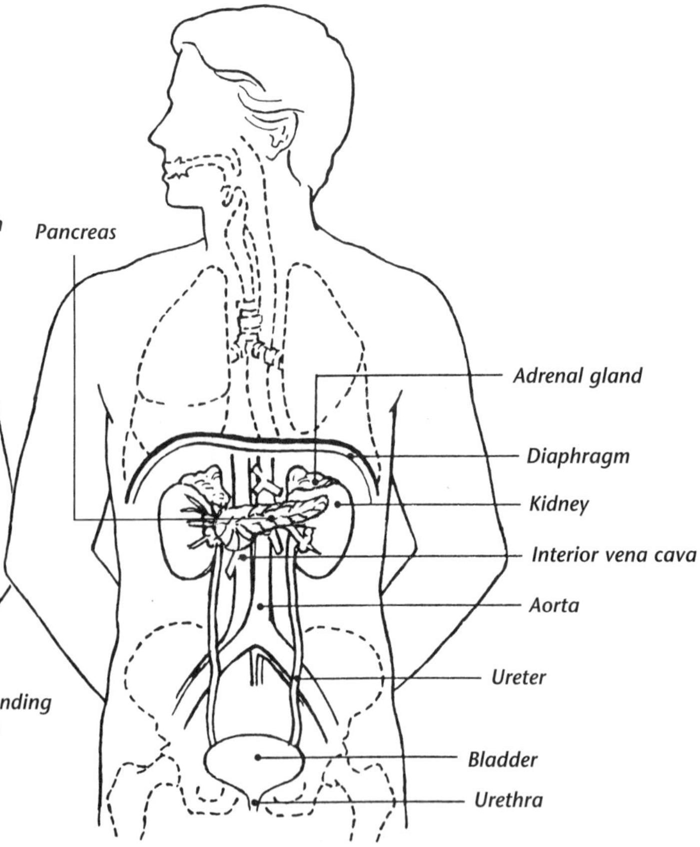

Organs Behind the Abdominal Cavity

44. **Smooth Muscle Tissue** Forms in sheets rather than fibers and is under automatic control. Found in hollow organs of respiratory, circulatory, digestive, urinary, and reproductive systems. Helps carry out much of the body's automatic internal work.

Cardiac Muscle Tissue Striated muscle under automatic control. Never stops working. Requires constant supply of oxygen and glucose furnished by uninterrupted blood flow.

Skeletal Muscle Tissue Voluntary muscles allowing body movement. Extend joints and attach at points proximal and distal to joints.

45. I
    H
    G
    E
    C
    D
    F
    B
    A
    J

46. Epidermis
    Dermis

47. B.   Dermis

48.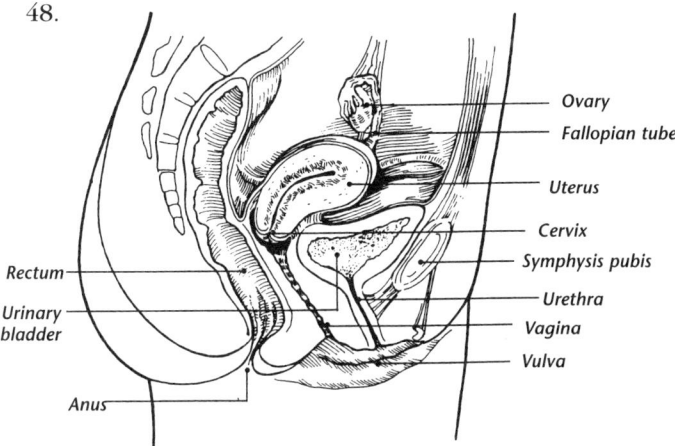

49.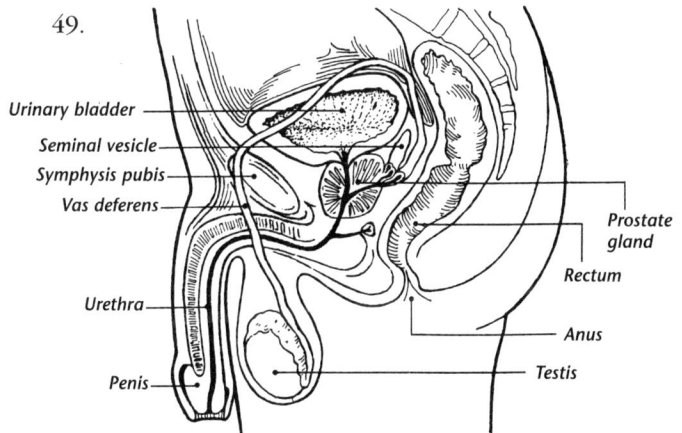

50. The pituitary gland

51. A. Adrenal
    B. Pituitary
    C. Thyroid
    D. Pancreas (islet cells)
    E. Ovaries
    F. Testicles

CHAPTER 3 STUDY QUESTIONS

1.

2. B
   D
   A
   C
   E
   F

3.

4.

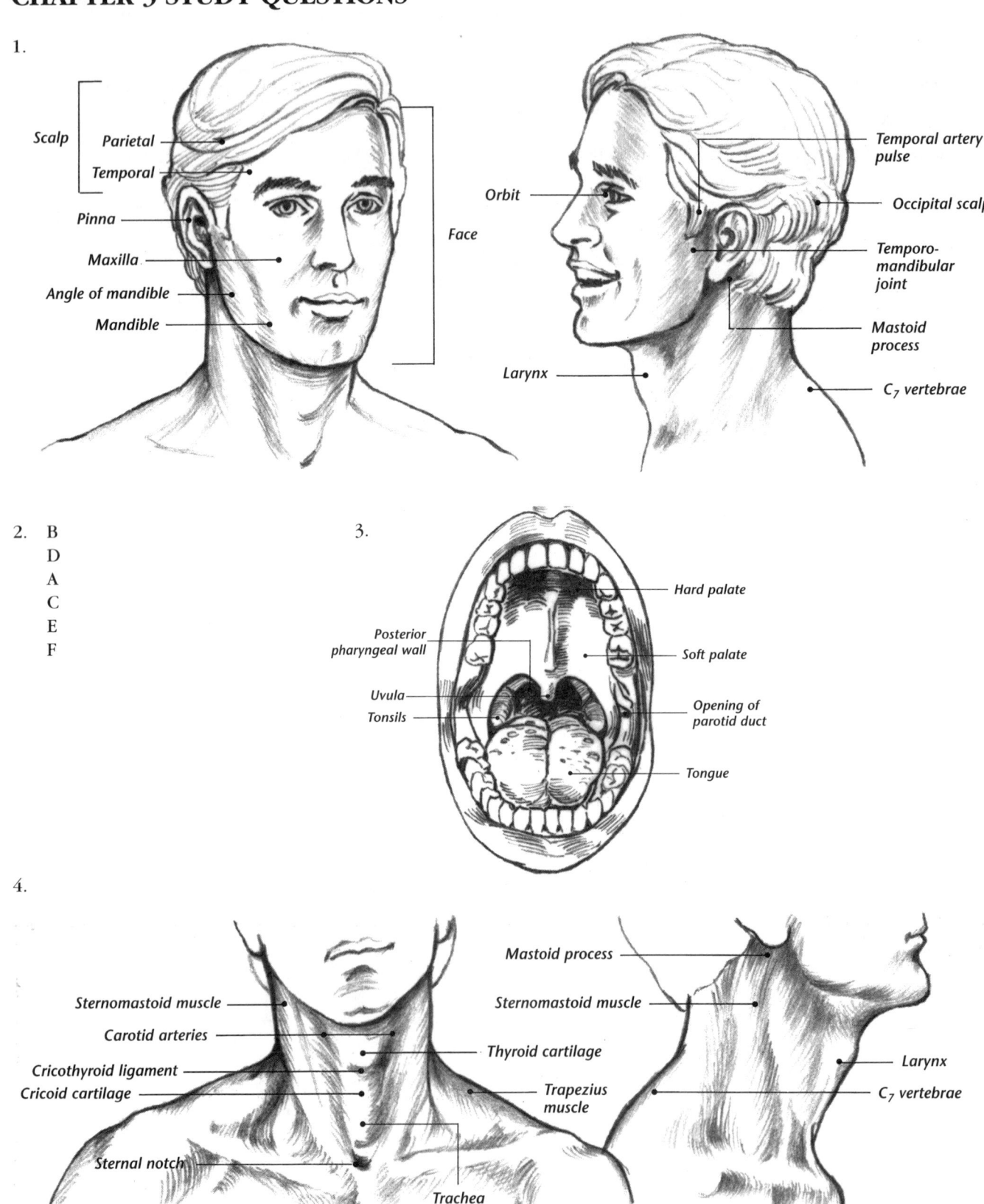

5. Seven

6.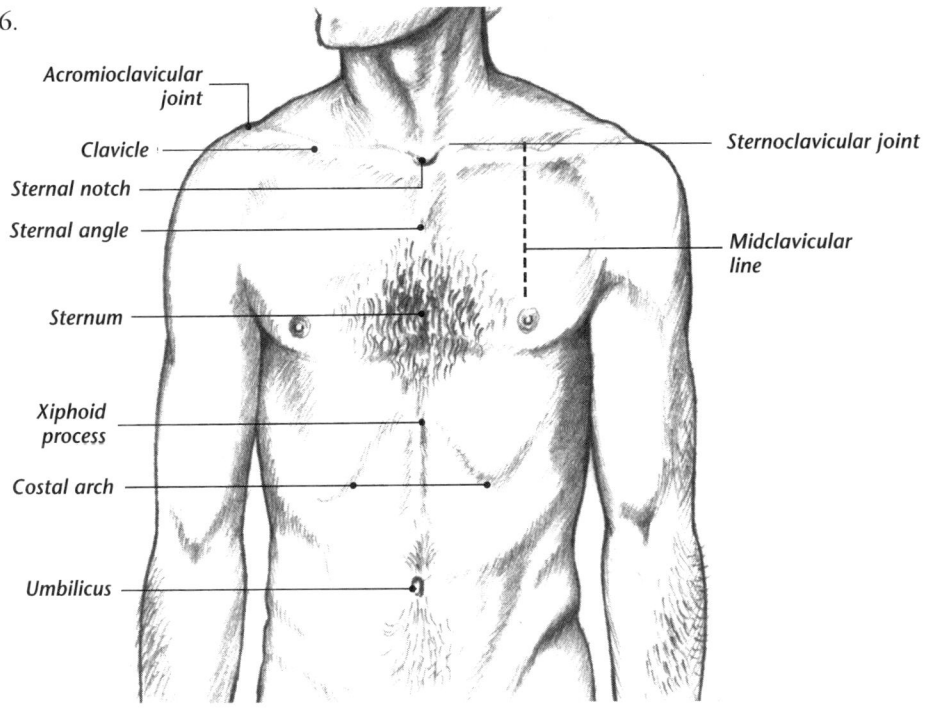

7.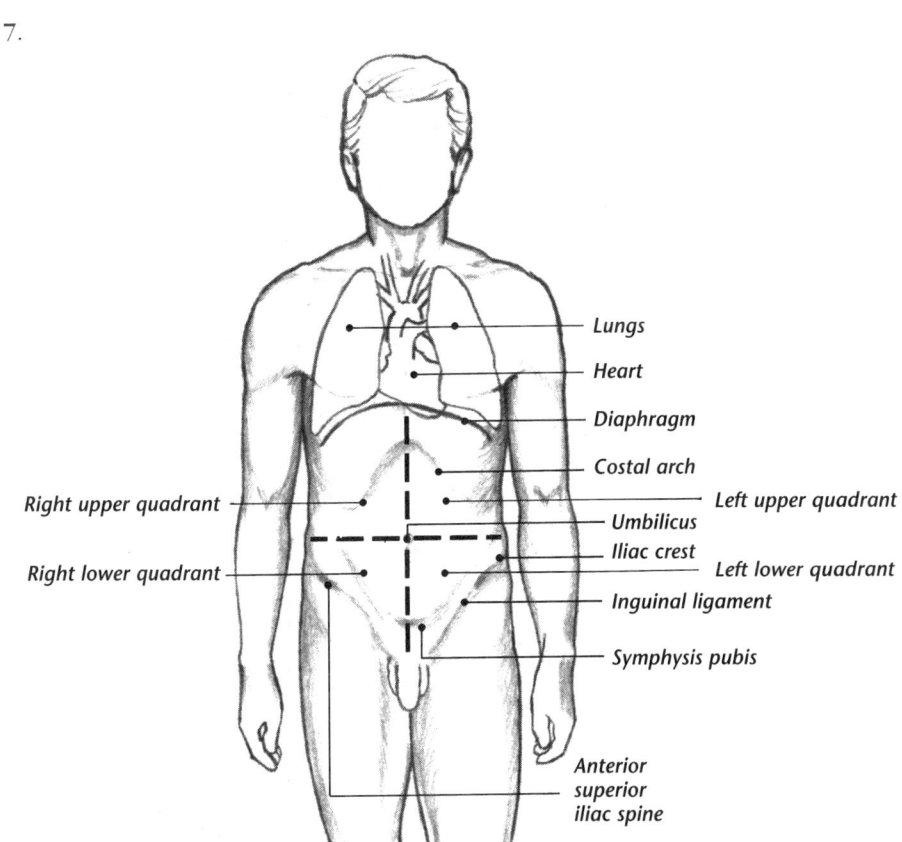

8.

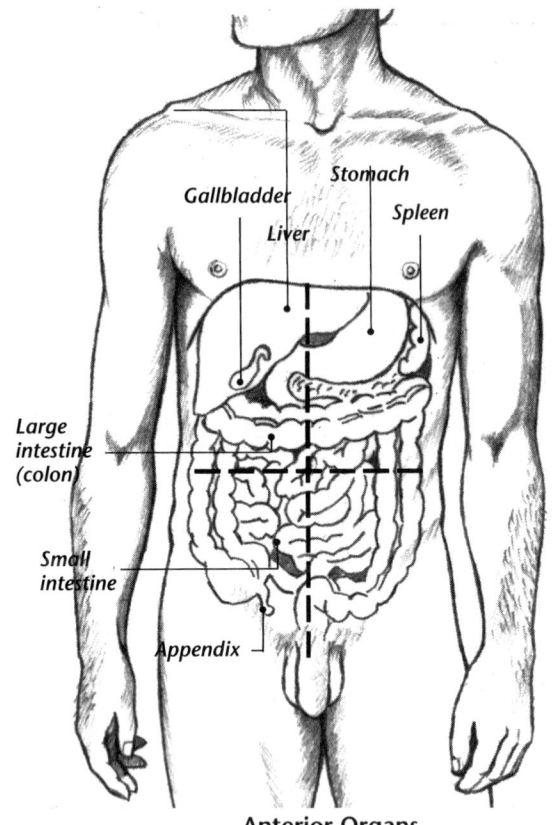
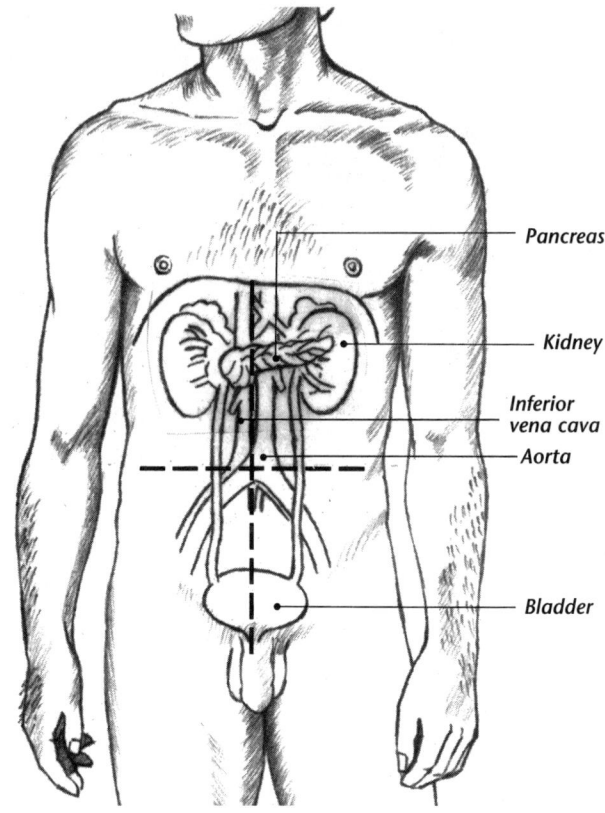

Anterior Organs   Posterior Organs

9.

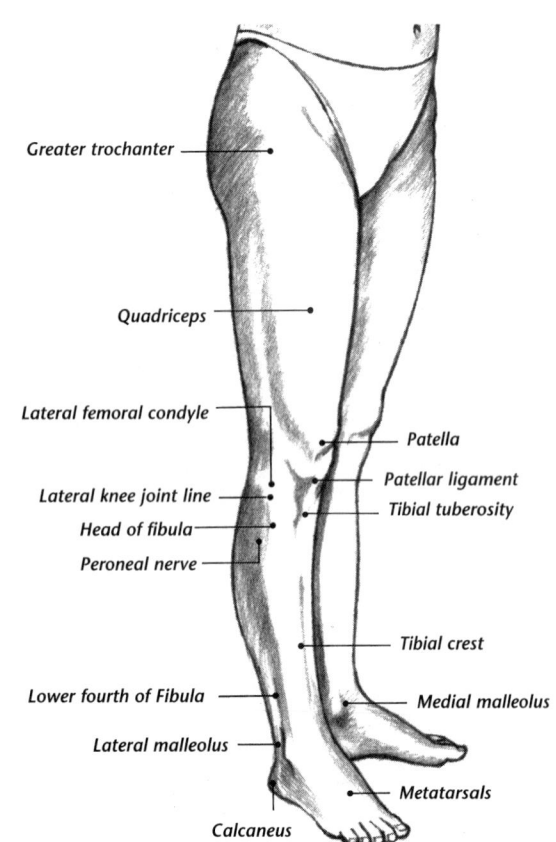

10.

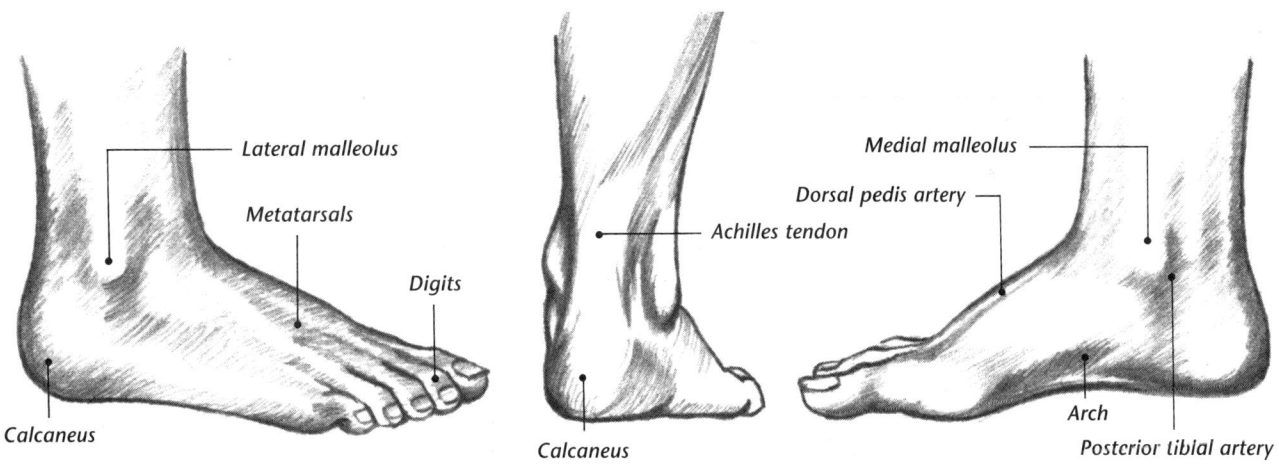

11.

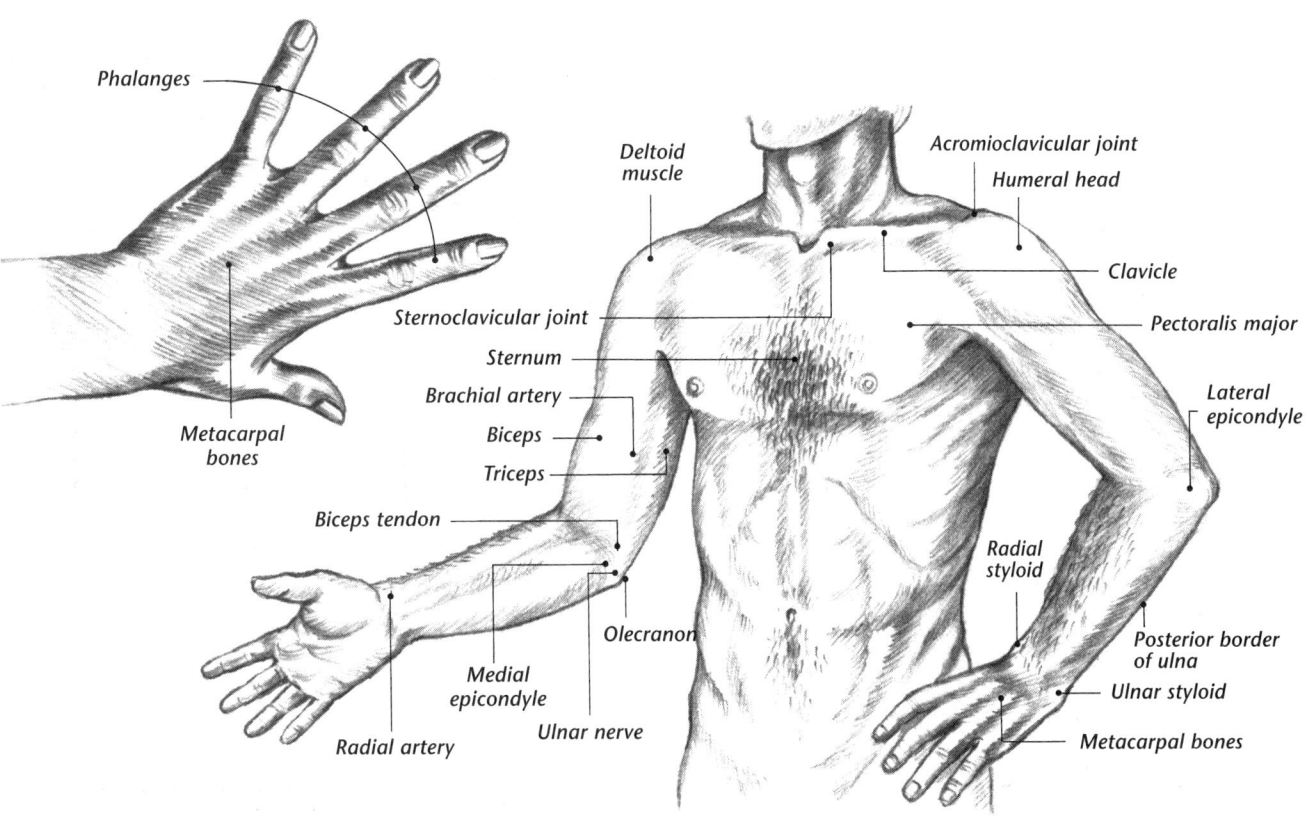

12.

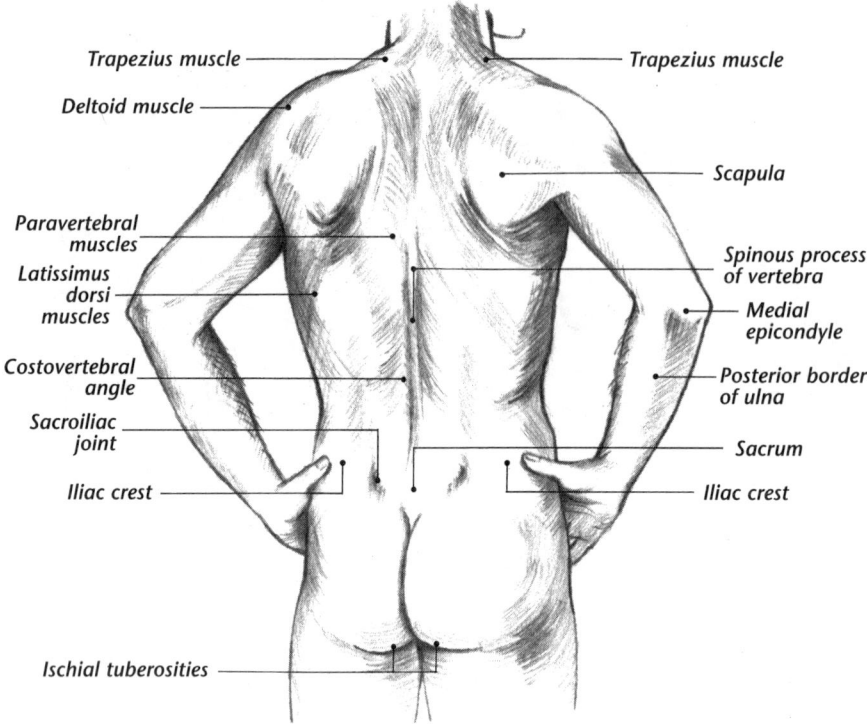

13. 1) Pulse
    2) Respiration
    3) Temperature
    4) Blood pressure
    5) Level of responsiveness

14. **Sign** An important characteristic of illness or injury that the observer notes by looking, feeling, listening, or smelling

    Symptom An important characteristic that the patient notes and discusses with the observer

15. **Normal level of responsiveness:** patient responds fully to your questions and appears alert.
    Other than completely responsive state: altered mental status determined by the AVPU scale

16. **Alert:** The patient appears normal, talks coherently to the examiner, knows his or her own identity, location, address, telephone number, day, and date.

    Responds to Verbal Stimuli: The patient is not alert, the eyes do not open spontaneously, but the patient responds in some way when spoken to.

    Responds to Pain: The patient does not respond to verbal stimuli, but moves or cries out in response to pain, i.e. a firm pinch. This response is not valid if the extremity is numb or paralyzed.

    Unresponsive: The patient responds neither to verbal stimuli nor to pain.

17. The pressure wave in the arteries each time the heart beats

18. The patient's arterial channel is open and the heart is beating strongly enough to be felt

19. 1) The heart is not beating
    2) The arterial channel is blocked
    3) The examiner's fingers are in the wrong place

20. 1) Rate
    2) Rhythm
    3) Strength

21. 50 to 90 times a minute

22. Weak and fast

23. 1) The carotid artery
    2) The femoral artery

24. Because thumbs have a pulse that may be confused with the pulse of the patient

25.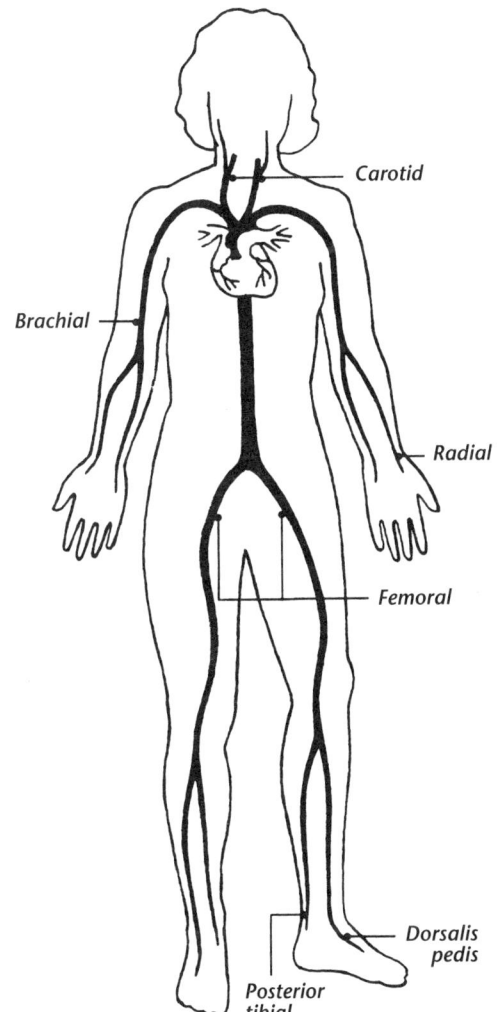

26. 12 and 20

27. Labored breathing

28. C. Because the blood is not properly oxygenated

29. 1) Orally   98.6 F
    2) Armpit   97.6 F
    3) Rectally 99.6 F

30. **Normal (normothermic)**—patients with acute injuries or non-infectious illnesses

    Low (hypothermic)—patients with fall in body temperature due to shock or failure of heat mechanism

    High (hyperthermic)—patients with elevated temperature due to infection or breakdown of the normal body-heat regulating mechanisms

31. 1) Pulse rate
    2) Cardiac output
    3) Amount of blood in the vessels
    4) Tone of the blood vessel walls

32. Systolic pressure and diastolic pressure

33. 1) Skin temperature, moisture, and color
    2) Pupils of eyes
    3) Capillary refill
    4) Ability or inability to move on command
    5) Reaction to touch and pain

34. **Level of Responsiveness** An individual with a *normal* level of responsiveness is alert, oriented, talks coherently to the examiner, and can easily answer questions about identity, location, day, date, and time of day.

Pulse Normal resting pulse is 50 to 90 beats per minute in an adult and 90 to 110 beats per minute in a child. Important features are its rate, rhythm, and strength.

Respiration Normal respiratory rate is 12 to 20 breaths per minute for adults and somewhat higher for children and infants.

Temperature Normal body temperature is about 98.6 degrees.

Blood Pressure The blood pressure of a healthy young adult is usually about 120/80; pressures from 85/50 to 140/90 are within the normal range.

Skin Temperature, Moisture and Color Skin temperature varies according to the difference between the temperature of the environment and the temperature of the blood; skin wetness depends on the activity of the sweat glands; skin color depends on the state of the surface blood vessels and the blood within them.

Capillary Refill Normal capillary refill means that the small vessels refill after the blood has been squeezed out of them.

Reaction of the Pupils Pupils normally constrict in response to bright light—inability to do so may indicate cardiac arrest. Pupils normally are the same size—unequalness may indicate serious head injury. Abnormal dilation may indicate drug use, fear, or unresponsiveness.

Reaction to Pain Test for normal feeling by pinching the skin or scratching with a fingernail. An inability to feel pain usually means damage to the nerve pathways running from that body part to the brain.

Ability to Move Test for impaired movement by asking the patient to move or wiggle fingers and toes and to squeeze your hands. A responsive patient who is unable to comply is said to be paralyzed.

CHAPTER 4 STUDY QUESTIONS

1. 1) Detect life-threatening conditions rapidly and care for them immediately
    2) Determine whether you need to attend to any other problems
    3) Transport the patient rapidly to further definitive medical care when indicated
    4) Miss nothing significant
    5) Do nothing that would make the patient worse
    6) Arrange for timely interface with the EMS system

2. A lack of thorough or systematic assessment; a lack of knowledge

3. Interventions

4. Supporting breathing by opening a blocked airway
    Supporting circulation by controlling bleeding or caring for shock
    In an unresponsive patient, inserting an airway
    In a patient with suspected neck injury, stabilizing the neck
    Giving care for serious injuries such as splinting

5. First impression, urgent survey, nonurgent survey, ongoing survey

6. A: open airway
   B: assess breathing
   C: assess circulation

7. Your initial reaction to the patient and the patient's initial reaction to the rescuer

8. Document the patient's refusal according to local protocol and get a witness

9. Stay with the patient until you are satisfied that everything is under control.

10. Position yourself at eye level with the child
    Make eye contact
    Move slowly
    Explain procedures, especially painful ones, before they are carried out
    Use simple terms

11. 1) Psychological reactions such as sadness, guilt, lack of enthusiasm, inability to concentrate, irritability, lack of motivation, a desire to quit emergency care activities, and a lack of interest in family and friends. Difficulty going to sleep or awakening during the night and not being able to get back to sleep is common.
    2) Physical sensations such as headache, backache, fatigue, indigestion, decreased appetite, changes in bowel habits, and weight loss
    3) Persistent thoughts about death, suffering, or pain
    4) Unintentional recalls ("flashbacks") of the stressful experience
    5) Feelings such as "if only I had done something differently"

12. A program developed to aid caregivers in dealing with these serious injuries so that the process of normal grieving is facilitated and significant psychological problems are prevented

13. HIV (human immunodeficiency virus)

14. By blood, semen, or vaginal secretions

15. Human blood; body fluids such as semen, amniotic fluid, and cerebrospinal fluid; any body fluid contaminated with blood; any unknown body fluid; clothing or bedding soiled with blood or body fluids

16. 1) Use rubber gloves
    2) Wash hands after touching a patient
    3) Wash unbroken skin with soap and water
    4) If you receive a splash onto a mucous membrane, flush the area
    5) Use protective clothing such as surgical masks, face shields, and gowns
    6) Handle soiled patient care equipment with care
    7) Use mouth shield or pocket face mask when performing CPR
    8) Handle contaminated bed linen and laundry properly
    9) Consider hepatitis B vaccine

17. Getting an infected patient's blood or other high risk substances on non-intact skin or splashed into an eye, mouth, or nose; or from accidentally cutting yourself while working on an infected patient.

18. Avoid contact with all body fluids.

19. Rubber (latex) gloves, ski goggles, facemask or shield, water-resistant parka and pants. A pocket mask or mouth shield should be in every aid belt.

20. Wear rubber utility gloves while cleaning. Disinfect reusable equipment with a substance that will effectively inactivate HIV and hepatitis viruses: 0.3% hydrogen peroxide, 25% ethyl alcohol, 35% isopropyl alcohol, 0.5% Lysol, 0.25% povidone-iodine, 1:10 to 1:100 dilution of sodium hypochlorite (household bleach). Blood can be removed from clothing with hydrogen peroxide and the clothing cleaned in an automatic washer (hot water cycle) or dry cleaned.

21. Propane, cleaning chemicals, gasoline, solvents

22. Call 911 and inform the dispatcher that there has been a hazmat incident so that specially trained personnel can respond.

23. Care provided in an emergency outside a physician's office or hospital by persons who are not licensed to practice medicine.

24. Care performed as any other reasonable, prudent person with similar training would perform under the same circumstances

25. The patient can be turned over to qualified personnel who can continue the care

26. Laws to help out voluntarily in emergencies

Chapter 4 Scenarios

1. Since both hands are bleeding profusely, BSI includes rubber/vinyl gloves at a minimum. If the blood is actually spurting, consider goggles, faceshield, and a gown. Pull out all supplies to be used before you actually come in contact with any blood. Make sure to clean up all blood from the snow and place it in a labeled bag.

2. Since the patient refuses help, have him sign an emergency care refusal form. Make sure you explain what he is signing and obtain a witness signature. Also, stay with the patient until he leaves.

CHAPTER 5 STUDY QUESTIONS

1. First impression, urgent survey, nonurgent survey, ongoing survey

2. How many patients are there?
   Will triage be required?
   Is there danger?
   What extrication will be required?
   What help will be required?
   What occurred? What is the mechanism of injury?
   Is the patient responsive or unresponsive?
   Is there bleeding

3. Initiate body substance isolation (BSI) procedures

4. Prone: patient lying face down
   Semi-prone: patient lying face down on one side
   Supine: patient lying face up

5. Determine the patient's level of responsiveness

6. If the patient is less than fully alert

7. Breathing normal, no neck/back injury: turn to the supine position by single rescuer turning
   Breathing normal, possible neck/back injury: if there is time, wait for help
   Breathing not normal: open airway, turn patient supine using single rescuer turning

8. Shout for help, call 911, or radio for rapid transportation. Assess breathing and, if breathing is abnormal, open the airway

9. The possibility of aggravating a neck or back injury

10. Kneel by the patient's shoulder, far enough away so the patient can be rolled toward you. Cross the patient's far ankle over the nearer one and move both of the patient's arms to the sides to help splint the spine. With one hand, grasp the patient's neck just below the back of the head. Place your other hand under the patient's far armpit so that your hand is against the anterior part of the patient's shoulder. Gently roll the patient toward you with the least possible bending or twisting of the neck or back.

11. The tongue, because the muscles of the upper airway may relax allowing the tongue to fall back and close the airway

12. Head tilt/chin lift

13. Jaw thrust

14. Assessing breathing by observing whether the chest rises and falls, listening for escape of air, and feeling for the flow of air

15. A reflex that causes the patient to attempt to vomit when the back of the tongue or back of the throat is touched with a foreign object such as a tongue blade

16. Insert an oral or nasal airway

17. Vomiting

18. Rescue breathing

19. Take a deep breath, seal your lips or mouthpiece of the device around the patient's lips and blow into the patient's mouth. Give the patient two breaths.

20. To protect yourself from diseases such as AIDS, hepatitis, tuberculosis, and other contagious diseases

21. Assess circulation by feeling the carotid artery for 5 to 10 seconds

22. Then begin CPR

23. Spinal injury

24. To identify as much critical information about the patient's well being as you can.

25. Control the bleeding as rapidly and efficiently as possible with direct pressure

26. Obtain a SAMPLE history from witnesses and family; do a rapid body survey

27. S   signs and symptoms
    A   allergies
    M   medications
    P   pertinent past history
    L   last meal
    E   events

28. Rapid body survey, whole body survey

29. Hands-on/clothes-on survey performed as quickly as possible

30. By systematically looking, feeling, listening, and smelling from head to toe in a comfortable environment

31. **D**eformities
    Contusions
    Abrasions
    Punctures, **P**enetrations
    Burns, **B**leeding
    Tenderness
    Lacerations
    Swellings

32. Circulation: assessed by checking extremity pulses
Motion: assessed by watching movement in response to pain (in unresponsive patient) or ability to move (in responsive patient)
Sensation: assessed by observing whether the patient responds to a pinch in extremities

33. **Head**   Reassess the level of responsiveness and reexamine eyes and pupils. Inspect scalp and face for open wounds, bleeding, bruises, swellings, and depressions. Gently feel scalp for bumps and depressions. Inspect ears and nose for a clear or bloody discharge. Check mouth for dentures, foreign objects, wounds, and bleeding. Note whether lower jaw is properly aligned under upper jaw. Smell breath for unusual odors.
    Neck   Inspect for open and closed wounds, bleeding, swellings, bruises, asymmetry, engorged neck veins, and unusual positions. Feel back of the neck for tender areas, lumps and deformities, swellings and impression of "Rice Krispies" produced by air under the skin. Check sternal notch to make sure trachea is in the midline. Feel for masses and swellings.
    Chest   Open clothing for adequate assessment. Inspect for open and closed wounds, bleeding, bruises, lumps, swelling, asymmetry, and deformities. Note effort required for breathing. Feel thoracic cage to detect swellings, tenderness, and subcutaneous emphysema. Place one hand on either side of anterior chest to see whether both sides are expanding equally with inhalation; listen for audible wheezes and other noises.
    Abdomen and Pelvis   Open clothing to assess abdomen and pelvis. Inspect abdominal skin for open and closed wounds, bleeding, bruises, and distention. Palpate abdominal wall to check for tenderness, rigidity, swellings, masses, and tightening of abdominal muscles. Note audible gurgling noises.
    Lower Extremities   Inspect thighs, legs, and feet for open and closed wounds, bleeding, bruises, deformities, abnormal shortening, and unusual positions. Compare injured extremity with opposite normal extremity. Locate and palpate pulses. Feel skin for tender areas, swellings, and depressions. Ask if patient feels numbness or tingling in legs or feet. Check sensation. Ask patient to move toes and ankles.
    Upper Extremities   Inspect skin of each arm, forearm, and hand for open and closed wounds, bleeding, bruises, deformities, swellings, abnormal shortening, and unusual positions. Compare injured extremity with opposite normal extremity. Feel radial pulse. Check skin of each extremity for abnormal swellings, tender areas, and depressions. Ask patient if there is numbness or tingling. Check for sensation. Test strength.
    Back   For other than suspected spinal cord injury, logroll patient onto one side. Inspect skin of back and buttocks for open and closed wounds, bleeding, bruises, swelling, deformities, or unusual positions.

34. Hard contact lenses: with a special suction cup made for this purpose, or can be slid from the clear part of the eye onto the white of the eye.
    Soft contact lenses: lift them off by pinching them gently between your thumb and index finger

35. If the patient has sustained a direct injury to the eye

36. "Rice Krispies" crackle of air under the skin

37. Circulation, Motion, Sensation (CMS)

38. So you can test the patient's strength and compare the grip of one hand with the other

39. Immediate emergency care measures designed to halt or manage life-threatening or serious conditions discovered during the urgent survey. These are urgent measures performed on the hill to treat or stabilize a patient immediately, and are usually directed toward reestablishing proper function of the respiratory and circulatory systems.

40. The patient is placed on his or her side which will help protect the airway

41. The first hour after the injury

42. 30 minutes

43. Offer to assist. Assess ABCs. Control patient for severe bleeding. Observe patient expression and skin condition. Determine the chief complaint. Call for transport, equipment, assistance, and/or EMS as needed. Obtain trauma/medical history and confirm MOI. Conducts focused body survey. Stabilize and maintain body temperature, Determine pulse and respiration rates. If patient has abnormal ABCs, significant MOI, or has poor general impression, perform rapid body survey, SAMPLE history, interventions, and rapid transport. Provide care for chief complaint. Transport off the hill.

44. What happened, how it happened, when it happened, why it happened, where is the damage, how bad does it hurt

45. Did you hit your head, neck, or back?
    Does your neck or back hurt?

46. **General:** weakness, light-headedness, or excessive fatigue; any bleeding
    Head injury: headache; dizziness; loss of responsiveness, even momentary; double vision or inability to see normally
    Neck or back injury: numbness, tingling, weakness, inability to move; difficulty breathing
    Chest injury: shortness of breath; cough; blood in sputum; pain aggravated by breathing or coughing
    Abdominal injury: nausea, vomiting; abdominal cramps; blood in the feces or urine; swelling of the abdomen; time of last bowel movement; possibility of pregnancy
    Pelvic injury: trouble urinating; blood in urine; blood coming from urethra, vagina, or rectum; possibility of pregnancy
    Extremity injury: pain on motion; inability to move or use extremity; numbness or tingling; inability to bear weight on lower extremity

47. Focused body survey

48. Assess each site in questions, looking for bleeding wounds. Give appropriate care.

49. Rapid body survey

50. Fever, pain, variations from normal functions

51. **Non-specific:** tiredness, weakness, lack of energy; fever or chills; stiff neck; loss of appetite; depression or other alteration of the emotional state
    Respiratory system: sore throat; runny or stuffy nose; postnasal discharge; earache; cough; chest pain; chest pain aggravated by cough or deep breath; shortness of breath, wheezing; pus in the sputum or nasal secretions; hoarseness
    Circulatory system: palpitations; chest pain; shortness of breath; leg swelling
    Digestive system: pain or difficulty on swallowing; heartburn; sour stomach; nausea; vomiting; vomiting blood; diarrhea, constipation, or other changes in bowel habits; blood in bowel movements; abdominal pain or cramps
    Genitourinary
    Musculoskeletal/Neurologic: soreness, aching, pain on motion of a body part; weakness, clumsiness, or paralysis of a body part; numbness or tingling of a body part; double vision, blurring or blindness of one or both eyes; difficulty with balance; headache; backache; stiffness, pain or swelling of joints
    Cutaneous: itching, rash; localized swelling or lump; swollen lymph nodes

52. Ask the patient to describe the details of the pain or specific symptom. Determine the chief complaint. Obtain a SAMPLE history.

53. O: Onset
    P: Pain
    Q: Quality
    R: Radiation
    S: Severity
    T: Time

54. Head   assess pupils, check the patient's throat
    Neck   feel both sides of the jaw, listen for hoarseness
    Chest   note wheezes and rattles, inspect any material coughed up
    Abdomen   check for distention, tenderness, and rigidity
    Skin   look for redness, swelling, and tenderness
    Extremities compare strength with the good side
    Back   assess for tenderness

55. Rapid body survey, if the patient has abnormal ABCs or poor general impression

56. Once you have the patient in the aid room

57. Assesses and records LOR and vital signs, including pulse, respirations, and blood pressure. Updates SAMPLE history. Performs whole body survey. Cared for all problems found. Arranges or provides for transportation.

58. If injuries are minor and the patient can clearly indicate there are no additional problems

59. To reassess the patient to catch possible changes

60. Stable: every 15 minutes
    Unstable: every 5 minutes

61. Reassessing mental status, airway, breathing, pulse, blood pressure, and skin temperature. Requestioning the patient regarding changes and rechecking interventions.

62. 4
    3
    5
    6
    7
    1
    2

Chapter 5 Scenarios

1. Initiate BSI. The first impression includes noting single patient, making sure the scene is safe, note the bleeding, and the fact that the patient appears unresponsive. The urgent survey includes shouting for help and calling 911. Determine the level of responsiveness with AVPU. Open the airway, determine the patient is breathing by using the jaw-thrust. Check the carotid pulse to determine there is a pulse. Next, control the bleeding. Insert an oral airway and provide high flow oxygen when it arrives. Stabilize the cervical spine and obtain a history from witnesses or friends. Do a rapid body head-to-toe survey to determine injuries. Transport the patient and perform the nonurgent survey once inside. The nonurgent survey includes reassessing responsiveness, recording vitals and performing a whole body head-to-toe survey. The ongoing survey includes monitoring the patient until advanced transportation arrives.

2. Initiate BSI. The first impression includes noting single patient and the scene is safe. Note the patient is responsive. The urgent survey includes introducing yourself and asking his name and if you can help. Then, determine the chief complaint. Once you determine what happened is not trauma related, perform the medical history and focused body survey. Obtain a SAMPLE history and assess the body depending on his symptoms. Transport the patient and perform the nonurgent survey. The nonurgent survey includes reassessing responsiveness, recording vitals and performing a whole body head-to-toe survey. The ongoing survey includes monitoring the patient until advanced transportation arrives.

3. Initiate BSI. The first impression includes noting single patient and the scene is safe. Note the patient is responsive and his location in the snowboard park. The urgent survey includes introducing yourself and asking his name and if you can help. Then determine the chief complaint. Once you determine what happened is trauma related, perform the trauma history and focused body survey. Make sure he did not hit his head or neck. Assess the shoulder and care for it. While waiting to transport, obtain a SAMPLE history and a rapid body survey. Perform the nonurgent survey. The nonurgent survey includes reassessing responsiveness, recording vitals and performing a whole body head-to-toe survey. The ongoing survey includes monitoring the patient until advanced transportation arrives.

CHAPTER 6 STUDY QUESTIONS

1. 21 percent

2. 25 percent
   16 percent oxygen

3. Pounds per square inch

4. **D cylinder**   360 liters of oxygen, time: 36 minutes
   E cylinder   625 liters of oxygen, time: 62? minutes
   M cylinder   3,000 liters of oxygen, time: 300 minutes

5. If the pressure guage reads 1,000 psi, the cylinder is about half full. When the guage reads less than 200 psi, the cylinder should be replaced by a full cylinder.

6. 1) Those who are breathing and need supplemental oxygen
   2) Those who are not breathing

7. **Give oxygen to any patient who has one or more of the following:**
   1) Shortness of breath
   2) Cyanosis (bluish skin and mucus membranes)
   3) Chest injuries other than the most trivial
   4) Serious injury, particularly with head or spinal cord injuries; femur, hip, or pelvic fractures; multiple injuries; or severe burns, especially those of the respiratory tract
   5) Serious illness, such as cardiac arrest, heart attack, and stroke
   6) Altered mental status, shock, or anticipated shock
   7) High-altitude illness
   8) Injuries or illnesses that are more than trivial at altitudes above 8,000 feet (2,438 meters)
   9) Significant bleeding, external or internal
   10) Probability of benefiting from supplemental oxygen, in the opinion of the experienced rescuer

8. **Non-rebreather mask** Transparent mask fitted with a plastic reservoir bag and a one-way valve. Patient can inhale oxygen from the bag, but cannot exhale into the bag. Mask can provide greater than 90 percent oxygen at flow rates of 10 to 15 liters per minutes.

   Pocket mask with oxygen inlet Use for mouth to mask ventilation. Has soft bladder to make a good seal. Keep fitted with one-way valve to protect rescuer. Oxygen inlet nipple on the mask allows the patient to be ventilated with air from the rescuer's lungs enriched by oxygen added from a tank.

   Mouth shield Inexpensive, compact, disposable device designed for CPR only. The mouthpiece has a one-way valve.

   Nasal cannula Delivers low concentrations of oxygen at lower flow rates. Provides 25-40 percent oxygen at flow rates of 2 to 6 liters per minute.

   Bag-valve-mask Mask attached to a self-inflating bag that is squeezed rhythmically by the rescuer. Provides 90 percent oxygen.

9. Here are the steps for providing supplemental oxygen
   1) Place the cylinder upright and position yourself to the side. Using the wrench, open the tank valve for a second to clean any debris from the outlet. This process is called "cracking" the tank.
   2) Close the regulator flow valve and attach the regulator to the tank. With a yoke-style regulator, make sure the "O" ring gasket is in place and that the key prongs and oxygen outlet are lined up correctly. Tighten it securely by hand.
   3) Open the tank valve slowly to one-half turn beyond the point where the regulator becomes pressurized. Note the tank pressure registered on the pressure gauge of the regulator (in pounds per square inch, or psi). If the psi is less than 200, go to steps 8, 9, and 10 (except that since you have not yet connected the mask or cannula tubing, you will not have to remove it), replace the tank with a full one, and start again with step 1.
   4) Attach the tubing of the mask or cannula to the regulator output nipple.
   5) Open the regulator flow valve until the desired flow rate in liters per minute (lpm) registers on the flow gauge, or turn the dial to the desired rate on the fixed-orifice flowmeter. The valve may turn in a direction opposite from what you expect. The flow rate for a non-rebreather mask should not be *less* than 6 lpm and the flow rate for a nasal cannula should not be *more* than 6 lpm.
   6) Explain to the patient why he or she needs oxygen and what you are going to do. If using a cannula, test the output on yourself by feeling it on the back of your hand. If using a non-rebreather mask, set it at 10 lpm and cover the hole between the reservoir bag and the mask with your finger until the bag is partially inflated. Then, adjust the liter flow to the desired rate, position the mask on the patient's face, and adjust the elastic strap to keep the mask in place.
   7) When you have finished administering oxygen, remove the mask or cannula from the patient and turn the regulator flow valve until the rate on the flow gauge registers zero.

8) Shut off the main tank valve and remove the delivery tubing from the regulator output nipple.
9) Bleed the valves and gauges by opening the regulator flow valve again until the flow rate stays at zero.
10) Close the regulator flow valve. Be sure the valve wrench is secured to the tank or regulator in such a way that it cannot be lost. Discard a used cannula or mask, since these are *not* designed for reuse.

10. Cracking procedure. Open and close the tank valve slowly with a wrench to clean debris.

11. Remember that the contents of an oxygen tank are under very high pressure, and therefore this device can be as lethal as a missile if mishandled. Here are some general safety precautions for handling oxygen equipment.
    1) Do *not* position any part of your body or the patient's body directly over the tank valve—a loose-fitting regulator can be blown off the top of the cylinder with enough force to maim or kill. Do *not* expose oxygen tanks to excessive heat, and always secure them so there is no danger that a tank can topple over and knock off the valve. *Never* drop a tank.
    2) *Never* use an oxygen tank without a properly fitting regulator. *Never* use tape and other "foreign" material on oxygen equipment.
    3) Close all valves when a tank is not in use, even if it is empty.
    4) Oxygen will not explode when exposed to fire but *will* cause a burning object such as a cigarette to flare up, which presents the danger of setting other combustibles on fire. Smoking and other sources of open flame are prohibited where oxygen is being used. Flammable materials such as oil or grease should not come in contact with oxygen equipment.
    5) *Never* move an oxygen cylinder by rolling it on its side or its bottom.
    6) Inspect valve seat inserts and gaskets regularly. Do *not* lose your "O" rings, and always have extra "O" rings on hand.
    7) Store oxygen cylinders in a cool, ventilated area. Avoid exposing cylinders to temperatures below freezing and above 125°F (52°C).
    8) Have oxygen cylinders hydrostatically tested at regular intervals. The dates of previous tests are stamped on the top of the cylinder near the valve stem.

12. Use a protective mask with a one-way valve

13. It should extend from the corner of the mouth to the angle of the jaw

14. 1) Determine proper size
    2) Open the mouth using the crossed-finger technique
    3) Insert the airway with the tip up
    4) Rotate the airway

15. Anytime the upper airway is in danger of being blocked by sputum, edema fluid, blood, vomitus, or foreign material such as snow. Snoring, noisy rattling, or crowing sounds coming from the upper respiratory tract.

16. A stable side position for all responsive or semi-responsive patients without neck or back injuries to allow vomitus to flow out and avoid the possibility of having to aspirate.

Chapter 6 Scenarios

1. 1) The cannula is preferred with patients of chronic obstructive pulmonary disease because they do not need a high concentration of oxygen.

   2) A flow rate of no more than 2 liters per minute is recommended in order not to stop the breathing that is being driven by hypoxia

2. Consider the cylinder empty. Follow local patrol procedures to indicate empty and get refilled.

3. 1) First choice: Pocket mask with high flow of oxygen input, because with a single rescuer the pocket mask is easier to maintain a seal.

    Second choice: The bag-valve-mask with two rescuers, because it delivers oxygen at a higher concentration than a pocket mask or nasal cannula.

    2) Oxygen flow is set at 15 lpm for either device and ventilations are delivered at a rate of 12 per minute or one ventilation every 5 seconds.

CHAPTER 7 STUDY QUESTIONS

1. A. Direct pressure

2. **Direct pressure** Apply pressure locally with sterile dressing, directly over the wound. Elevate and immobilize the wound if on an extremity.

    Pressure points Pressure over a major artery supplying the area of injury. Use several fingers or the palm of the hand to press the artery against the underlying bone.

    Pneumatic counterpressure devices Provide direct pressure to an entire extremity. Especially effective for extensive skin and soft-tissue extremity injuries with widespread bleeding.

    Tourniquet Use only when bleeding cannot be controlled in any other way. The wound is so severe risking the loss of limb must be part of the decision to apply a tourniquet.

3. 1) A suitable mechanism of injury such as a blunt or penetrating injury to the head, neck, chest, abdomen, pelvis, thigh, or multiple sites
   2) Signs and symptoms of shock following trauma when there is no external bleeding or other obvious cause of shock, or when the severity of shock is not explained by the extent of obvious injuries
   3) A history of indigestion or abdominal pain, accompanied by abdominal tenderness and associated with signs and symptoms of shock
   4) Progressive pain, tenderness, nausea, vomiting, rigidity, and enlargement of the abdomen following abdominal trauma
   5) Progressive respiratory distress following chest trauma
   6) Progressive enlargement, pain, tenderness, dysfunction, and possibly loss of pulses in an injured limb
   7) More than minimal blood in vomit, saliva, feces, or urine
   8) Progressive abdominal enlargement, pain, and tenderness in a woman of child-bearing age who has missed several menstrual periods

4. Suspect the bleeding early.
   Care for shock.
   Provide high-flow oxygen.
   Evacuate the patient rapidly to a hospital.

5.

Types	Causes
Hypovolemic	Decrease in circulating blood volume.
Vasogenic	Mechanisms fail that control blood vessel tone, causing the vessels to relax and enlarge. Normal blood volume becomes inadequate to fill the vessels.
Cardiogenic	Pumping function of the heart fails.

6. A
   C
   B

7. 1) Fatigue, restlessness, and anxiety, followed by confusion and mental dullness; may progress to partial or complete unresponsiveness
   2) Falling pulse pressure followed by falling blood pressure
   3) Abnormal respirations, usually rapid at first, then labored, and finally gasping
   4) Gradual increase in pulse rate; later, pulse becomes weak and thready
   5) Gradually increasing thirst; nausea followed by vomiting
   6) Severe weakness
   7) Profuse sweating
   8) Cold, clammy, and pale or cyanotic skin
   9) Dull, lusterless eyes; pupils eventually dilate
   10) Specific signs and symptoms of the underlying condition that caused the shock

8. Compensated shock: the body's response efforts keep the circulatory system functioning at a normal level
   Decompensated shock: circulatory system is starting to fail despite the body's most vigorous efforts

9. 1) First impression: Consider the mechanism of injury or nature of illness in deciding whether to anticipate shock.
   2) Perform the urgent survey, providing interventions as necessary.
   3) Control bleeding, if present.
   4) Start arrangements for rapid transport.
   5) Perform the rapid body survey.
   6) Give the patient high-flow oxygen, if available.
   7) Splint any fractures and dislocations you find.
   8) Keep the patient supine with the lower extremities elevated, unless the patient is short of breath.
   9) Maintain the patient's body temperature.
   10) Transport off the hill
   11) Perform nonurgent and ongoing surveys while awaiting transport
   12) Give the patient nothing to eat or drink.
   13) Monitor the patient frequently (ongoing survey).
   14) Give special care for specific types of shock, e.g., hypothermia.
   15) Transport the patient to a hospital as soon as possible.

10. D. On his or her back with the legs raised 12 inches

11. B. Head and shoulders raised, hips flexed, knees bent

12. Put patient in a supine position to allow cerebral blood flow to return to normal. Assess for injuries. Advise the patient to rest before resuming normal activity.

13. A release of histamine and other substances from the injured tissues causes blood vessels to leak, the blood pressure to fall, bronchial walls to swell, and smooth muscles of the bronchi and other organs to go into spasm. The patient may develop hives, acute respiratory distress, wheezing, massive swelling of the face and tongue, nausea, vomiting, cramps, diarrhea, convulsions, coma, and death.

14. Epinephrine, administered by a person properly trained or licensed. A rescuer may assist the patient in injecting the drug, if necessary.

Chapter 7 Scenarios

1. The signs and symptoms (confusion, thirst, nausea, pulse, and skin color) suggest shock. Give oxygen, arrange for immediate transport, keep warm, and elevate legs if patient allows.

CHAPTER 8 STUDY QUESTIONS

1. **Contusions** Impact with a blunt object. Underlying tissues are crushed and small blood vessels are torn, causing local bleeding and/or swelling and bluish discoloration.

   Hematoma Severe contusion resulting in larger blood vessel damage and tumor-like collage of blood in the tissues.

   Muscle Strain Injury to muscles resulting from overstretching joints or tearing of muscle.

2. 1) Apply a pressure bandage
   2) Apply a cold compress
   3) Elevate the injury
   4) Splint the injury, if appropriate
   5) Assist with evacuation as necessary

3. R: rest
   I: ice
   C: compression
   E: elevation

4. **Abrasion** A superficial injury caused by moving contact between the skin and a rough surface. Blood oozes from injured vessels.

   Laceration A tear in the skin. Bleeding may be profuse or mild depending on the size and number of injured blood vessels.

   Incision A clean laceration caused by a sharp object. Usually bleeds more because blood vessels constrict and retract less effectively.

   Avulsion A piece of skin torn loose from underlying tissues and left hanging by a flap.

   Amputation A separation of parts of the body that are torn completely free from the body.

   Puncture A wound caused by a sharp, narrow object. Rescuer should search for exit wounds.

   Impaled object An object that is protruding from a wound.

5. 1) Follow all BSI precautions
   2) Inspect the wound
   3) Control bleeding by direct pressure
   4) Prevent further contamination
   5) Cleanse the wound
   6) Apply a sterile compress and bandage
   7) Elevate and splint the injured part
   8) Arrange for tetanus prophylaxis
   9) Treat the patient for shock, if necessary

6. Placed in its normal position before applying direct pressure.

7. Initiate BSI precautions. Remove all foreign matter with sterile forceps or tweezers. Control bleeding. Wash the surrounding skin with 10 percent Betadine, soap and water, or other antiseptic solution. Generously irrigate the wound with clean, warm water or sterile physiological saline solution. Dry the wound with a sterile dressing. Apply a sterile dressing and use a suitable bandage to hold in place.

8. **Superficial (First degree)** Involves superficial layers. Skin is red, tender, painful, may be swollen.
   Partial thickness (Second degree) Involves epidermis and part of dermis. Swelling, blister formation occurs.
   Full thickness (Third degree) Penetrates three layers of tissue. Skin is "cooked" discolored. No blisters form.

9.
   1) Put out the fire and/or remove the patient from the heat source
   2) Apply cold water
   3) Perform urgent survey with attention to airway and breathing
   4) Avoid burned skin contamination and blister rupture
   5) Estimate extent and seriousness of burn
   6) Remove jewelry from a burned extremity
   7) Assess and care for additional injuries
   8) Cover the burn with sterile or clean material
   9) Watch for respiratory distress and give oxygen as necessary
   10) Immobilize a burned extremity
   11) Treat for shock, if necessary
   12) Transport patient to medical care

10.

Critical	1. Burns of any depth complicated by injury to the respiratory tract, fractures, other major injuries, or serious illnesses (pneumonia, heart failure, etc.) 2. Full- or partial-thickness burns of important areas, or burns that extend completely around a body part (circumferential burns). 3. Full-thickness burns of more than 10 percent of the body surface (more than 2 percent in young children [under age 5] and older adults [over age 55]). 4. Partial thickness burns of more than 30 percent of the body surface (20 percent in young children and older adults).
Moderate (Uncomplicated, not circumferential or involving important areas)	1. Full-thickness burns of 2 to 10 percent of the body surface (1-2 percent in young children and older adults). 2. Partial-thickness burns of 15 to 30 percent of the body in adults (10 to 20 percent in young children and older adults). 3. Superficial burns of more than 50 percent of the body surface.
Minor (Uncomplicated, not circumferential or involving important areas)	1. Full-thickness burns of less than 2 percent of the body surface. 2. Partial-thickness burns of less than 15 percent of the body surface (less than 10 percent in young children and older adults). 3. Superficial burns of less than 50 percent of the body surface.
Minimal (otherwise healthy adults only)	1. Full-thickness burns of less than 1 percent of the body surface. 2. Partial-thickness burns of less than 5 percent of the body surface. 3. Superficial burns of less than 30 percent of the body surface.

11. A. The severity, extent, and depth of the wound, and the age and condition of the patient

12. With burns caused by dry chemicals—which are activated by water—such as dry lime, sulfuric acid, and metallic sodium, or caustic soda.

13.

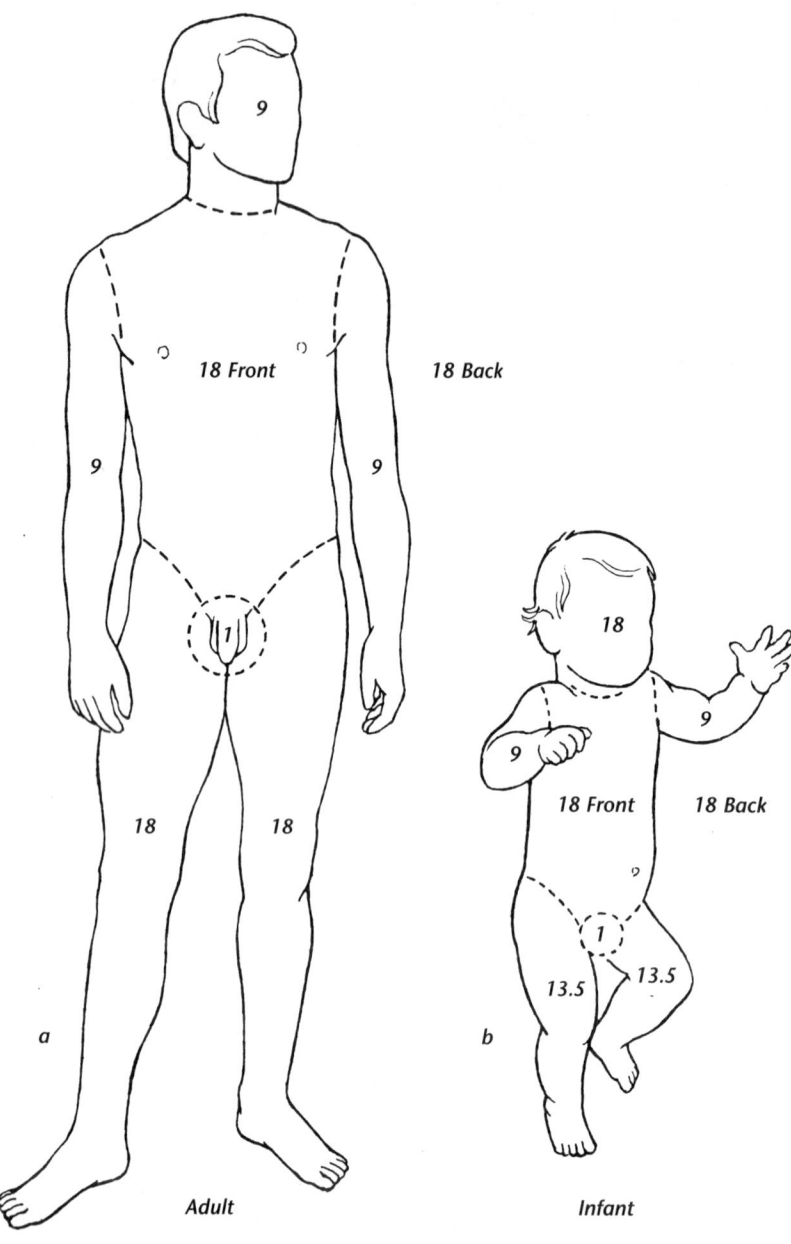

14. D. Immediate washing with large quantities of water

15. **Occlusive dressing** For sucking chest wounds and open abdominal wounds with exposed organs. Put universal dressing or layers of sterile compresses directly on wound (moistened with saline solution for abdominal wounds). Cover with sterile, airtight layer of plastic, foil, or Vaseline gauze. Seal 3 of the 4 edges tightly to skin with adhesive tape while patient holds breath after exhalation.

   Pressure Dressings To maintain direct pressure on bleeding wound. Firmly applied without interfering with circulation.

   Stabilizing Dressings To stabilize impaled object. Thick layer of sterile dressings held firmly in place with tape or roller bandages.

16. **Dressings** Clean cloth (pillowcases, sheets, towels, and sanitary napkins)

    Bandages Pack straps, belts, strips torn from clothing, cord, nylon webbing

    Cravats and Triangular Bandages Kerchiefs and bandannas

    Occlusive Dressings Rolled T-shirts, clean socks, plastic sandwich or garbage bags

17. The most comfortable

18. C. Blood vessels may become constricted as swelling occurs

19. They are less likely to restrict circulation

20. **Moving Joints** Use self-adhering roller bandage, which is elastic enough to stretch with joint motion rather than move. Make several circular turns around the limb above the joint, overlapping the upper end of the dressing. Bring bandage diagonally across the dressing and make several similar turns around the limb below the joint. Work bandage diagonally back up over the dressing. Repeat process until dressing is snug.

    Tapering Cones Use self-adhering roller bandage. Make several turns around the limb below the dressing and then continue up, over, and above the dressing, with each turn overlapping the one below by half an inch to three-fourths of an inch. Anchor the loose end to skin above dressing with vertical strips of tape.

Chapter 8 Scenarios

1. The burns are classified as partial thickness or second degree. Emergency care includes immediately removing all clothing soaked in the oil. Do not pull any clothing, rather cut it if necessary. Soak all areas in cool water or place a wet clean cloth on the affected areas for 10 minutes. Call 911 immediately and give high-flow oxygen. Perform the urgent survey assessing for other complications. Obtain a SAMPLE history. Cover the burned areas with sterile dressings.

2. Initiate body substance isolation precautions. Control the bleeding if necessary. Apply a sterile dressing and ice. Elevate the leg and complete the rapid body survey. Obtain a SAMPLE history. If the pain, bruising, and swelling is bad enough, splint and recommend the patient seek follow-up medical care for an x-ray.

3. 1) First- and second-degree flash burns to face and neck
   2) Sudden burst of flame, painful redness and blisters on face, raw feeling in throat (trachea) on inspiration
   3) BSI precautions (gloves, at a minimum)
   4) Yes, if difficulty breathing increases, give oxygen by cannula at 6 lpm (mask would be too painful)
   5) Put out fire. Move patient away from fire area. Evaluate and monitor airway. Apply cold, wet compresses initially to burn sites for about 10 minutes, then follow with dry sterile dressings. Estimate extent and depth of burns. Give oxygen by cannula. Treat for shock. Transport.
   6) Airway edema and compromise. Shock.
   7) Probably by ambulance unless airway becomes a problem, then by helicopter.

CHAPTER 9 STUDY QUESTIONS

1.

Fracture Types	General Characteristics
Closed, simple transverse fracture	One fracture line. Overlying skin is intact. Swelling and tenderness at fracture site.
Open fracture	Involves a wound of the overlying skin. Severe bleeding. Danger of contamination to fracture.
Displaced, closed, simple fracture	Bone ends are moved out of their normal alignment.
Comminuted, closed fracture	Has two or more fracture lines with three or more fragments.
Greenstick, closed fracture	Is an angulated fracture through part of the bone shaft. Occurs only in elastic bones as seen in children.
Spiral, closed fracture	Fracture line spirals around the shaft of the bone. Caused by rotational (twisting) forces.

2. A. Involves a bone broken into more than two fragments

3. Probing with the examiner's fingertip

4. Bleeding into small blood vessels

5. B. Dislocation

6. Stretching and tearing of the joint capsule and ligaments

7. The force is less severe, therefore the tearing of joint muscles is not as great. No displacement of bone ends is present.

8. **Fractures**
   1) Suitable mechanism of injury
   2) Pain
   3) Tenderness
   4) Deformity
   5) Sound
   6) Function
   7) Swelling and ecchymosis
   8) Crepitus and false motion
   9) Wounds
   Dislocations
   1) Mechanism of injury
   2) Pain
   3) Deformity
   4) Loss of normal joint motion
   5) Swelling and tenderness over the joint
   Sprains
   1) Tenderness
   2) Swelling and ecchymosis
   3) Pain at site of injury
   4) Some loss of joint function

9. Circulation, motion, sensation

10. 1) Perform urgent survey
    2) Determine mechanism of injury
    3) Expose and assess site of major injury indicated by patient
    4) Assess circulation and nerve supply below injury
    5) If pulse is rapid and/or breathing labored and these changes are not explained by the major injury, assess neck and chest (followed by abdomen and pelvis if appropriate)
    6) Assess any additional pain sites indicated by patient

11. 1) To prevent the jagged fragments of broken bones in fractures from grinding against each other or causing further damage to nerves, blood vessels, and other tissues
    2) To prevent accidental conversion of a closed fracture to an open fracture
    3) To reduce pain, swelling, and bleeding
    4) To prevent shock
    5) To allow greater ease in transport
    6) To prevent long-term disability and decrease rehabilitation time

12. Spinal fractures and fractures near or associated with the knee, wrist, elbow, and shoulder joints

13. D. Ankle, lower leg, midfemur, or midhumerus

14. They are accompanied by disruption of the joint and by damage to nerves and blood vessels.

15. Initiate BSI precautions. Washing the skin around the wound with a germicidal solution, flushing the wound with sterile saline solution, keeping exposed bone ends moist, covering with a moist sterile dressing (saturated in sterile saline if available).

16. Anything by mouth

17. 1) Expose the fracture site
    2) Grasp the limb with both hands below the fracture site
    3) Assistant supports the limb by placing one hand below and one hand above the fracture site
    4) Maintain gentle traction on the limb while straightening it
    5) If necessary, rotate limb into as anatomically normal position as possible
    6) Observe bone ends and fracture site
    7) Maintain manual traction until splint is applied
    8) If resistance or severe pain occurs, stop attempts at alignment

18. 1) Pulses distal to the injury are absent
    2) The part distal to the injury turns white or blue
    3) The part distal to the injury feels cold
    4) The patient develops worsening pain in the part distal to the fracture rather than at the fracture site
    5) Ability to move parts distal to the injury is lost or impaired

19. 1) Initiate BSI precautions
    2) Expose and inspect the injury site
    3) Care for an open wound, if present
    4) If necessary, align a deformed fracture
    5) Splint the injured part
    6) Check and document circulation and nerve supply before and after alignment and splinting
    7) If circulation and/or nerve supply are impaired, attempt cautious alignment
    8) Treat sprains with support, cold packs, and by having the patient keep weight off the injured extremity
    9) Treat for shock, if necessary

20.

Type of Splint	Additional Supplies Required	Types of Injuries Used
FIXATION		
Quick Splint	Possibly additional padding	Lower legs, some dislocations
Cardboard Splint	Padding, cravats	Lower legs, arms, some dislocations
Wire, Ladder Splint	Padding, cravats, self-adhering roller bandages	Upper arms and forearms, hands, improvised splinting for legs, ankles, and feet
Malleable Metal Splint	Padding, cravats, self-adhering roller bandages	Upper arms and forearms, hands improvised splinting for rigid collar, splinting for legs, ankles, and feet
Air Splint	No additional supplies required	Forearms, upper extremity, legs, or lower extremity
Vacuum Splint	Suction pump	Forearms, upper extremity, legs, or lower extremity
Sling and Swathe	Cravats, possibly padding	Clavicles, dislocations, upper extremity
TRACTION		
Hare	All supplies provided with commercial package	Midshaft femur fracture
Sager or Kendrick Traction Device	All supplies provided with commercial package	Midshaft femur fracture
Thomas (modified)	Cravats, ankle hitch, or smaller rope for pulley system	Midshaft femur fracture
Improvised (several variations)	Single ski, two ski poles, cravats, ski pole basket spreader, grommetted tip pocket, cord, ankle hitch	Midshaft femur fracture

21. C. A traction splint

22. 1) Position the body properly on the board
    2) Immobilize shoulder girdle
    3) Immobilize pelvis girdle
    4) Immobilize lower extremities
    5) Adjust strapping
    6) Immobilize head and neck
    7) Immobilize arms with palms against thighs

23. The rigid collar is the only available device that will resist axial loading of the cervical spine

Chapter 9 Scenarios

1. First make sure transportation to the hospital is already on its way. Loosen the splint and see if this helps. If circulation continues to become impaired you may have to provide gentle flexion until resistance is met.

CHAPTER 10 STUDY QUESTIONS

1. 1) Kinetic energy
   2) Potential energy

2. 1) Rotational
    2) Bending
    3) Penetration
    4) Compression
    5) Distraction (Stretching)

3. Penetration   The wounding object is smaller in diameter and/or the force of impact is relatively greater, so that the force per unit area is great enough to drive the object through the skin. Damage to deeper tissues may be much greater than indicated by the size of the entry wound.

    Compression   The wounding object is larger in diameter and/or the force is weaker, so that the skin is not broken. Frequently damages tissues beneath the skin, causing a closed wound such as a contusion or hematoma.

    Bending   Hyperflexion and hyperextension. Stretching and compression injuries.

    Rotational   Twisting types of falls.

    Distraction   Exerting a pulling or tugging motion on a part of the body.

4. B
    C
    D
    A

5. Kinetic

6. Penetrating

7. 1) Hyperflexion type of bending trauma
    2) Vertebra compression fracture
    3) Midshaft femur fracture
    4) Hip fracture-dislocation
    5) Patella fracture
    6) Foot fracture

8. Acceleration

9. Rotational force

10. 1) Estimated speed of travel, distance of the fall, speed of the striking object
    2) Characteristics of the ground or any other surface impacted by the patient
    3) Forces inflicted on the patient's body
    4) Types of trauma involved
    5) Visible injuries
    6) Types of internal injuries possible
    7) Signs of developing shock
    8) Likelihood of a spine injury

11. Ski strap—fall—nonrotational
    Catching an edge—fall—rotational
    Excessive speed—collision—nonrotational
    Lack of ability level—fall—rotational
    Poor binding release—fall—rotational

12. B. Trauma

13. 1) Fallen from a height that is 2Ω to 3 times the body height
    2) Involved in moderate high speed accident
    3) Hit by auto going 25 miles per hour or more
    4) While skiing, collided at high speed
    5) Gun shot wound
    6) In shock or respiratory distress
    7) Unresponsive due to head injury
    8) Buried in an avalanche
    9) Struck by a falling object

Chapter 10 Scenarios

1. 1) Rotational trauma
   2) Hyperflexion injury
   3) Compression trauma

CHAPTER 11 STUDY QUESTIONS

1. | **Fractures** | **Signs and Symptoms** |
    |---|---|
    | Clavicle | Pain in the shoulder area. Patient attempts to self-splint. Dropped shoulder, swelling and tenderness over the clavicle along with some deformity. |
    | Scapula | Tenderness, swelling, and ecchymosis over scapula, with pain on attempted use of upper extremity. |
    | Upper Arm | Swelling, tenderness, and ecchymosis in deltoid muscle area; marked angulation and instability in midshaft fractures. |
    | Above the Elbow | Swelling deformity, tenderness, pain, and ecchymosis. |
    | Forearm and Wrist | Swelling, tenderness, ecchymosis, pain on motion, and usually some deformity. |
    | Hand | Obvious deformity along with swelling, tenderness, ecchymosis, and loss of function. |
    | **Sprains** | |
    | Shoulder | Joint is tender, painful and may be slightly swollen; pain is increased by use. |
    | AC Separations | Obvious, tender, shelf-like deformity at the point of the injured shoulder. |
    | Elbow | Slightly swollen, tender, and painful; pain is increased by use. |
    | Wrist | Swollen, tender, and painful to use. |
    | Hand and Finger | Swollen, tender, and painful to use. |

Dislocations

Shoulder	Shoulder looks and feels more square than a normal smooth, round shoulder. Tenderness over shoulder; patient resists attempts to bend shoulder because of pain.
Elbow	Elbow joint usually locked in slight flexion. Marked swelling, tenderness, deformity, and pain on attempted motion.
Wrist	Swelling and deformity, with pain on attempted motion of the joint.
Finger	Grossly deformed finger joint, locked in flexion, and with pain on attempted motion. Swelling can be minimal or extensive.

2. **Fractures** — **Emergency Care**

Clavicle	Splint with a sling and swathe.
Scapula	Immobilize area with a sling and swathe.
Upper Arm	For fracture below the head of the humerus, splint with sling and swathe. Do not attempt alignment of fractures near a joint. For mid-shaft fractures, align fracture, apply a padded rigid splint to outside of upper arm, and incorporate splint into a sling and swathe.
Above the Elbow	Splint the injury in the position found.
Forearm and Wrist	Splint with all-purpose, rigid forearm splint that supports hand and holds it in position of function.
Hand	Immobilize entire hand with a bulky hand dressing and rigid all-purpose forearm splint. Support with sling as appropriate.

Sprains

Shoulder	Apply cold packs and, in severe cases, a sling.
AC Separations	Limit joint motion by supporting the arm with a sling and applying cold packs.
Elbow	Apply cold packs and splint with a sling and swathe.
Wrist	Apply cold packs and, for severe sprain, splint with a rigid splint that extends at least to elbow and holds hand in the *position of function*. A sling supports arm.
Hand and Finger	Splint with a bulky hand dressing or tape so that it is held in adduction.

Dislocations

Shoulder	Splint with sling and swathe. A rolled blanket or parka may be needed as padding between upper arm and chest if arm cannot be brought against chest. Transport sitting rather than lying down.
Elbow	Check radial pulse and motion and sensation of wrist and hand. Splint injury in the position found. Take patient to hospital as soon as possible.
Wrist	Immobilize injury in position found, using a rigid splint to protect forearm and hand.

Finger — Immobilize injury in position found, usually with a modified bulky hand dressing and a rigid forearm splint to prevent wrist movement.

Note: Air splints work well with dislocations to support the extremity in an unusual position.

3. Anterior dislocation of the shoulder—patient holds arm slightly away from the chest and supports it with the opposite hand.

    Posterior dislocation of the shoulder—patient holds arm away from the body or over the head, unable to bring it near the chest.

4. A. Sling and swathe

5. D. In a sitting position and supported from behind

6. Circulatory and neurological function of the limb. If the circulation is impaired, attempts need to be made to improve circulation by gently aligning the fracture or redoing the splint. The situation becomes an emergency and the patient must be transported to a hospital as soon as possible.

7. Stabilized and immobilized in near anatomical position

8. Adducted: sprained shoulder or fractured upper arm
   Abducted: fractured clavicle

Chapter 11 Scenarios

1. Equipment needed may be padded boards, ski pole, cravats, spineboard. Since the patient cannot move the arm, it should be splinted as it is. If the patient can be splinted in the sitting position, make sure they are supported during transport. Transport will depend on the location. You could use a toboggan, ski mobile, spineboard, or a stretcher.

2. 1) Dislocated left shoulder with possible further complications, i.e., fractures, torn ligaments, soft tissue, and neurological injuries.
   2) Splint arm in position of least discomfort using blanket splint or vacuum splint. Monitor vital signs and distal circulation and sensation. Keep warm. Transport to appropriate facility.
   3) Loss of distal circulation and sensation. Hyperventilation due to pain. Fainting. Difficult to splint in position of least discomfort. Difficult to transport in toboggan due to splinting needs.
   4) Ideally, the patient is splinted with arm in position of least discomfort sitting up in the toboggan. Consider second rescuer in the toboggan to stabilize patient. Expedient transportation is vital because patient needs doctor's attention as soon as possible.

3. 1) Possible dislocated shoulder.
   2) Severe pain and unwillingness to move arm
   3) Protect yourself during the survey with gloves
   4) Oxygen could be used, but probably not necessary.
   5) Try to splint the arm in place before moving the patient. If you can't splint the arm in place, support the arm and shoulder and move the patient to a sitting position and splint in place. The distal pulse should be checked before and after any move to make sure that good CMS is maintained
   6) The biggest problem could be impaired circulation. Another problem could be watches or jewelry getting stuck from swelling.
   7) Transport the patient in the most comfortable position possible, probably sitting up.

CHAPTER 12 STUDY QUESTIONS

1. | **Sprains** | **Signs and Symptoms** |
    |---|---|
    | Knee | Look for swelling and feel for tenderness of the medial and lateral ligaments, the patellar ligament, the posterior part of the joint capsule, and the hamstring tendons. |
    | Ankle | Tenderness, swelling, and bruising over the top of the foot and around one or both malleoli |
    | **Fractures** | |
    | Pelvic | Patient will be lying down and complaining of lower abdomen pain, which is usually increased by movement. |
    | Hip | Severe pain and inability to move. Involved lower extremity is externally rotated and usually is shortened. Upper thigh below the groin or around the greater trochanter usually is tender when palpated. |
    | Femoral Shaft | Externally rotated and shortened limb, with a large, tender bulge in the thigh. Severe pain and inability to move. Fracture may be severely angulated. |
    | Above-knee Femur | Large, tender swelling in the lower thigh above the knee, with pain and inability to move the limb. |
    | Lower Leg | Patient complains of severe pain and resists movement of the leg. Swelling, tenderness, and ecchymosis usually present at fracture site. |
    | Ankle | Swelling, tenderness, and ecchymosis of tissue around the ankle joint. Patient may or may not be able to move the joint. |
    | Foot | Tenderness, swelling, ecchymosis, and occasionally deformity at fracture site. |
    | **Dislocations** | |
    | Hip | Attempted motion produces severe pain, tenderness over the upper thigh just below the groin. Check for paralysis of foot, foot drop, and numbness in the lower leg and sole of the foot. |
    | Knee | Severe pain, swelling, gross deformity of the knee, and inability to move the knee. |
    | Patella | Knee locked in flexed position, producing a marked deformity. |
    | Ankle | Tenderness, swelling, and deformity of the ankle joint, with pain on motion. |

2. A. Slightly flexed

3.

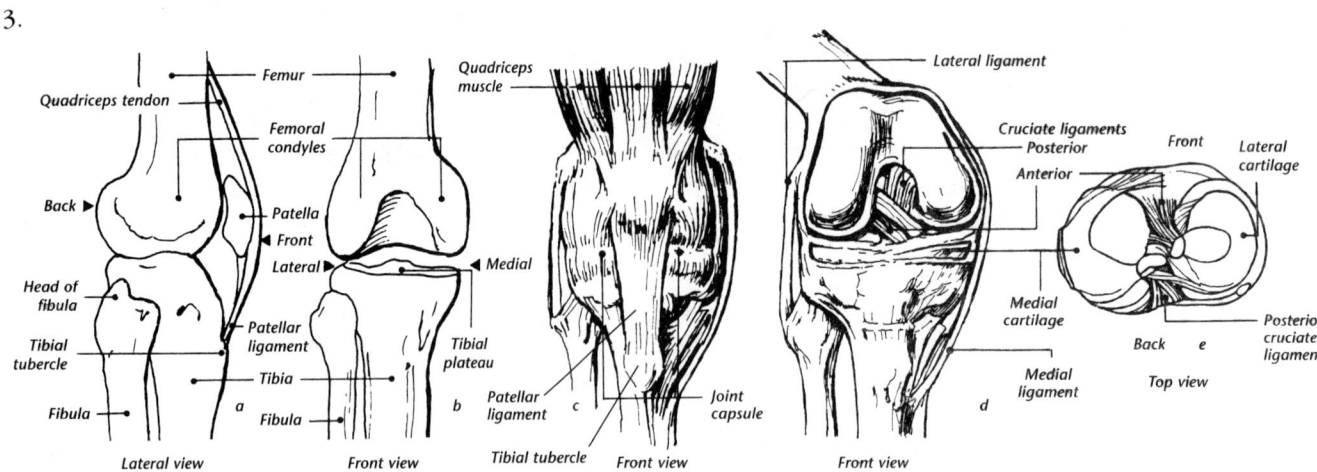

4. C. Medial collateral

5. 1) Blood in urine
   2) Severe abdominal pain
   3) Shock

6. D. Pelvis

7. C. 24 hours

8.

Sprains	**Emergency Care**
Knee	Apply cold packs and immobilize the knee with a suitable fixation splint. Advise patient to see a physician before putting weight on the extremity.
Ankle	Apply cold packs and support the ankle with a cravat ankle bandage or figure-of-eight made from elastic bandage. Severe ankle sprains should be treated with fixation splint designed for lower leg.
Fractures	
Pelvic	Immobilize on a long splint board and treat for shock, if needed.
Hip	Immobilize the patient on a long spineboard. Do not attempt to flex the hips or knees. If flexed, do not straighten. Splint against the normal lower extremity by padding between the extremities and tying the legs and thighs firmly together with cravats.
Femoral Shaft	Immobilize the extremity with a traction splint and treat for shock, if necessary.
Above-knee Femur	Check and monitor circulation and nerve supply below the injury. Immobilize the fracture with a lower-extremity fixation splint that extends to just below the groin. Do not use a traction splint.
Lower Leg	Apply fixation splint designed for the lower leg. Align fracture so foot is in its proper relationship to the leg.
Ankle	Apply a fixation splint designed for the lower leg or use a folded blanket or parka splint.
Foot	Patient should stay off his or her feet. Use boot or shoe to protect and splint the injury. Splint severe fractures with folded blanket, pillow, or folded parka.

Dislocations

Hip   Immobilize on a long spineboard. Maintain involved lower extremity in position found with pillows, wadded jackets, straps, and cravats. Transport to a hospital immediately.

Knee   Immediately check and monitor circulation and nerve supply to the extremity distal to the injury. Splint the dislocation in the position found using clamshell-type lower extremity fixation splint. Transport to a hospital immediately.

Patella   Splint in position found with clam-shell-type lower-extremity fixation splint. Check and monitor circulation and nerve supply.

Ankle   Align before splinting in lower-leg fixation splint.

9. This type of femoral fracture involves the upper part of the femur. Pulling on the iliopsoas muscle holds the upper fracture fragment in a flexed position. Attempts to straighten the hip cause severe pain.

   Place the patient on a long spineboard with the limb stabilized in position with rolled parkas or pillows. The patient may prefer to sit up during transport.

10. Immobilize in a traction splint if there are spasms of the thigh muscles
    Check distal pulse before and after applying the splint
    Check for feeling below the area of the fracture
    Monitor vitals
    Treat for shock

11. Align the fracture with axial traction to near-anatomically correct position
    Manually stabilize the extremity
    Assess the circulatory and neurological function of the limb
    Apply a splint designed for the lower leg
    Reassess the circulatory and neurological function of the limb
    Treat for shock

12. Distal pulse to verify there is no change in CMS

Chapter 12 Scenarios

1. Lower extremity injury. Call for additional patrollers, a toboggan, splinting materials, and oxygen. Perform a thorough assessment to determine if there are other injuries. Treat the open ankle injury by realigning the deformity, if not associated with the joint. Dress and bandage the open wound, splint the lower extremity, give oxygen, if necessary. Transport the patient to the aid room.

   Potential problems are the bone going back in, swelling, and infection. Equipment needed will be a soft splint such as a pillow, blanket, or air splint. A quick splint should be used with caution.

   Emergency care includes BSI, assessing the distal pulse, splinting the ankle in current position as long as there is distal circulation. Reassess distal circulation. Make sure he did not hit his head or neck. While waiting to transport, obtain a SAMPLE history and a rapid body survey.

   Perform the nonurgent survey after transporting.

2. Initiate BSI. Emergency care will be to provide the patient with oxygen and splint with a traction splint. Control any bleeding. Apply the ankle hitch while someone stabilizes the leg. Pull manual traction. Measure the traction splint against the good leg for Hare traction splint. Apply the splint, strapping the groin strap first, then apply the traction until it matches the manual traction. Close the remaining straps. Reassess circulation. Position the patient on a spineboard for transportation. Make sure he did not hit his head or neck. While waiting transport, obtain a SAMPLE history and a rapid body survey. Perform the nonurgent survey after transporting.

3. Initiate BSI. The first impression includes noting single patient and the scene is safe. Note the patient is responsive and her location. The urgent survey includes introducing yourself and asking his name and if you can help. Determine the chief complain is the injured leg. Perform the trauma history and focused body survey. This includes locating the exact injury site and assessing the distal pulse. Using a quick splint or two padded boards, splint the leg in the position found and reassess distal circulation. Make sure she did not hit her head or neck. While waiting to transport, obtain a SAMPLE history and a rapid body survey. Perform the nonurgent survey after transporting. The nonurgent survey includes reassessing distal circulation, recording vitals and performing a whole body head-to-toe survey. The ongoing survey includes monitoring the patient until advanced transportation arrives.

CHAPTER 13 STUDY QUESTIONS

1. A. Open skull fracture
   B. Brain contusion
   C. Blood clot inside the skull

2. Any loss of responsiveness

3. AVPU Scale

4. Hypoxia (insufficient oxygen)

5. True

6. An injured spine

7. Headache, nausea, vomiting, decreasing level of responsiveness, changes in the pupils, rise in systolic blood pressure or pulse pressure, slow pulse, slow and/or irregular breathing, incontinence, weakness or paralysis of one or more extremities

8. 1) Elevate the patient's head 6 inches
   2) Administer high-flow oxygen

9. 1) First impression
   a. Note presence of obstacles
   b. Note number of patients and responsiveness of each
   c. Determine the nature of the incident and MOI
   d. Evaluates the need to assess or extricate the patient
   e. Note the need for personnel or equipment
   f. Initiate BSI precautions

2) Urgent survey
   a. Determine level of responsiveness
   b. Calls for transport, equipment, assistance, and/or EMS as needed
   c. Open airway
   d. Guard cervical spine
   c. Check breathing
   d. Check circulation
   e. Control severe bleeding
      1) If labored breathing and/or fast, weak pulse, not explained by injuries, assess neck and chest, followed by abdomen, pelvis, and extremities. Care for significant injuries as discovered
   g. Obtain SAMPLE history
   h. Perform rapid body survey
   i. Determine pulse and respiration rates
   j. Stabilize and maintain body temperature
   k. Mechanically stabilize neck or place non-trauma patient in semi-prone position
   i. Transport as soon as possible
3) Nonurgent survey
   a. Assess and record LOR and vital signs
   b. Update SAMPLE history from companions
   c. Perform whole body survey
   f. Care for all problems found
   e. Arrange or provide for transportation

10. 1) Urgent survey. Treat life-threatening conditions. Give CPR and rescue breathing, and control severe bleeding as necessary. It is very important to maintain the airway.
    2) Insert an oral airway.
    3) Give oxygen in high concentration.
    4) Place the patient in a recovery (NATO) position for nontraumatic unresponsiveness or when there is no question of neck or back injury. The patient's head should be slightly higher than the feet.
    5) Dress wounds.
    6) Watch for vomiting. Use suction if necessary.
    7) Monitor vital signs and state of responsiveness.
    8) Keep the patient warm but not too warm.
    9) Keep eyelids closed to prevent eyes from drying.
    10) Watch for convulsions.

11. Putting a patient in a semi-prone position (recovery position) using a logroll. If one rescuer is available, the patient's head and neck must be stabilized as well as possible manually when the patient is turned to one side. Kneel at the patient's side, far enough away so you can roll the patient toward you. Bend the patient's far elbow and place the patient's far hand behind his or her head. Straighten the patient's near arm and place it at the patient's side with the palm against the thigh. Cross the patient's far ankle over the near ankle. With one hand behind the patient's far shoulder and the other behind the patient's far hip, roll the patient quickly onto the side toward you.

12. E
    C
    A
    B
    D

13.

Type	Signs and Symptoms	Emergency Care
Scalp Lacerations	Bleeds freely and can cause considerable blood loss	Careful, direct pressure. Be careful not to contaminate wound. Cover with sterile compress held with triangular bandage or stocking cap.
Concussions	Sees "stars," experiences confusion, loss of memory, dizziness, severe headache, weakness, and double vision or other visual changes.	Monitor and record at regular intervals the level of responsiveness, state of pupils, and other vital signs.
Brain Contusion	Small amount of swelling, prolonged loss of responsiveness, paralysis, and changes in pupils.	Take quickly to hospital and monitor airway, level of responsiveness, pupils and other vital signs. Treat unresponsiveness if it develops.
Bleeding Inside the Skull	Pressure on brain, deterioration of neurological status.	Quick transport to hospital, monitor patient closely, record findings at regular intervals, treat unresponsiveness.
Skull Fractures	Small amount of swelling, prolonged loss of responsiveness, paralysis, and changes in pupils. Possible scalp wound, cerebrospinal fluid. May produce bleeding from nose, ear, or mouth Raccoon eyes or Battle's sign	Take quickly to hospital and monitor airway, level of responsiveness, pupils and other vital signs. Treat unresponsiveness if it develops. Provide local wound care.

14. Determine and record:
   1) Level of responsiveness
   2) State of the pupils
   3) Ability to perceive touch and pain
   4) Ability to move the extremities in response to pain
   5) Observed changes
   Send recorded information with the patient to the hospital

   Signs and symptoms
   1) Decreasing level of responsiveness or difficulty in awakening the patient
   2) Nausea or vomiting that worsens or recurs
   3) Unexplained visual changes, including photophobia, double vision, blurring, blindness, or seeing "spots" or "stars"
   4) Changes in the pupils
   5) Increasingly severe headache
   6) Change in personality, memory, ability to concentrate or ability to think
   7) Weakness, paralysis, or loss of sensation, especially of one side of the body
   8) Seizure

15.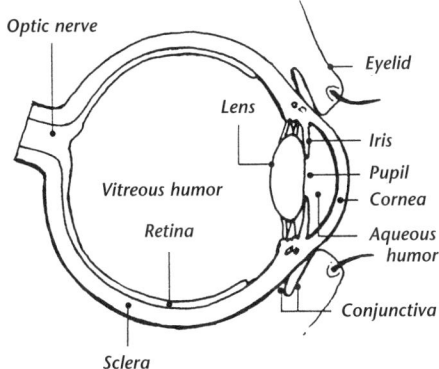

16. B. Covered

17. B. Wash the eye with a large amount of tap water

18. 1) Open and maintain the upper airway, always protecting the cervical spine
    2) Use suction if necessary
    3) Insert an oral airway if the patient is unresponsive. The patient may have to be turned onto one side so that copious secretions or bleeding can drain away
    4) Give oxygen in high concentration
    5) Stop external bleeding with direct pressure
    6) The patient may need to be immobilized on a spineboard

19. C. Maintain an open airway

20. A. On both sides

21. 1) Press the upper nostril against the septum for five minutes
    2) Place a pencil-sized roll of gauze between the upper lip and the teeth, and press inward on it for several minutes to shut off the artery to the septum
    3) Place a wad of Vaseline gauze in the bleeding nostril and press the side of the nostril against the septum
    4) Place an ice bag over the nose

22. B
    E
    C
    D
    A

23. Place the patient in the recovery position, be prepared to suction, monitor patient closely

Chapter 13 Scenarios

1. Institute BSI. The patroller's assessment should be very thorough with firm palpations with emphasis on the head, face, and neck. Calming the patient is an absolute must. The goggles and branch must be immobilized with appropriate dressings and bandages with no attempt to remove either the goggles or the branch. The patient should be secured to a spineboard and constantly monitored. Equipment: Standard toboggan rescue pack, oxygen, spineboard, blood pressure cuff and scope.

2. Ask her how she feels, has this ever happened, does she have a headache, is she in pain, can she feel her distal extremities, does her neck hurt? The problem appears to be either a concussion or a brain contusion; however, treat it as a head or neck injury with full spinal protocol.

3. Suspect a cervical spine injury especially since breathing seems to be impaired. Emergency care includes BSI, call for transportation (911), open airway with jaw-thrust, insert an oral airway, assist breathing as needed with pocket face mask until a bag-valve-mask arrives, give high glow oxygen, maintain manual cervical stabilization until the patient can have a collar and spineboard in place. Perform the body survey and transport. Perform the nonurgent survey once inside. Monitor vitals, especially the airway and breathing.

CHAPTER 14 STUDY QUESTIONS

1.

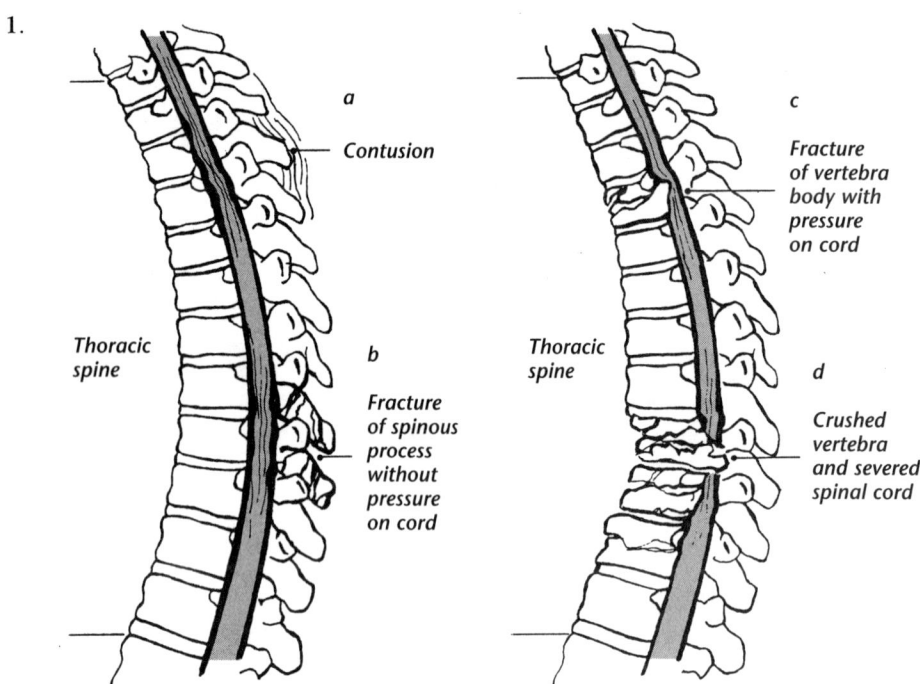

2. Prevent further injury and transport the patient without delay to a hospital

3. D. Chest muscles, or the chest muscles plus the diaphragm, may be paralyzed

4.

Spine	Spinal Cord
Pain at the injury site Localized tenderness Possible deformity or unusual position Associated soft-tissue injuries Patient self-splinting or guarding	Any or all of the Spine signs and symptoms (but not always present) Numbness Abnormal sensations Weakness or paralysis Neurogenic shock Difficulty breathing Incontinence Priapism

5. 1) Any significant injury above the clavicle, especially to the head
   2) Any injured patient with impaired responsiveness
   3) Any injury involving high kinetic energy and sudden acceleration or deceleration, especially if there is axial compression, distraction, rotation, or severe bending of the spine
   4) Persons involved in accidents while driving or riding in vehicles involved in a crash while traveling 25 mph or faster, or if another occupant of the same vehicle was killed
   5) Skiers who collide with stationary objects or other skiers
   6) Skiers who hit hard during jumps or high-speed falls
   7) Any fall from more than 2½ to 3 times the patient's height, or less if from a moving vehicle or chairlift
   8) Persons hit by falling rocks, trees, or other objects
   9) Pedestrians or bicyclists struck by motor vehicles
   10) Any surfing or shallow-water diving injury

6. 1) Perform all steps in first impression. Determine mechanisms of injury.
   2) Perform urgent survey—responsive patient—injured, while maintaining spinal precautions, including:
      a. Checking for respiratory distress.
      b. Treating for shock.
   3) Perform rapid body survey including:
      a. Ask about symptoms of injury.
      b. Ask the patient to squeeze your hands and wiggle his or her toes.
      c. Examine the injury site without moving the patient, if possible.
   4) Perform nonurgent and ongoing surveys as appropriate

7. Ask the patient to indicate the location and type of any pain and whether there is numbness, weakness, or abnormal sensations below the site of pain. Ask the patient to wiggle his or her toes and to squeeze both your hands. Check the patient's arms and legs for perceptions of pain and touch. Look for obvious injuries of the face, head, neck, and trunk, and for any obvious deformities of the spine.

8. 1) Maintain the airway and stabilization of the head and neck.
   2) Care for unresponsiveness if present.
   3) Care for urgent problems discovered during the urgent survey.
   4) Assess sensation and movement in all four extremities before and after logrolling, lifting, and placing the patient on a long spineboard.
   5) If the patient is found prone or semiprone, logroll the patient into the supine position when appropriate.
   6) Move the head and neck gently into the neutral position if not originally in that position.
   7) Monitor breathing carefully and assist it if necessary. Administer high-flow oxygen.
   8) Remove the patient's helmet, if present.
   9) Apply a rigid collar.
   10) Care for additional injuries discovered during the urgent body survey.
   11) Place the patient on a long spineboard using proper techniques (logroll, bridge lift, long-axis drag, direct ground lift and carry) or an interim short extrication device as appropriate. Immobilize the patient on the spineboard.
   12) Watch for vomiting and manage it by turning the spineboarded patient on his or her side and using suction.
   13) At regular intervals, monitor and record the patient's vital signs, ability to move, and perception of pain and touch in all four extremities.
   14) Anticipate and care for shock if it develops.
   15) Transport the patient rapidly to a hospital.

9. C. Jaw-thrust maneuver

10. The first rescuer stabilizes the patient's head and neck in the neutral, in-line position throughout the procedures and until the patient is immobilized on the long spineboard. A rigid collar should be in place. The board is placed at the patient's far side and lined up so that the patient will end up on it in the proper position.

The second and third rescuers kneel at the side of the patient to which he or she will be rolled.

The patient's legs are placed side-by-side in line with the body, the feet are tied together, and the arms are extended at the sides with the palms against the upper thighs and the elbows locked.

The second rescuer kneels at the patient's midchest, placing the hand nearest the patient's head behind the patient's far shoulder, and the other hand on the patient's far wrist.

The third rescuer kneels at the patient's knees, placing the hand nearest the patient's head on the patient's thigh just below the patient's hand. The other hand grasps both pant cuffs at the patient's ankles.

At a signal from the first rescuer, the patient's body is rolled 90 degrees onto the side, facing the two rescuers. During this, the third rescuer keeps the patient's ankles slightly off the ground enough to keep the legs in line with the body during the roll and the first rescuer watches the chest turn and rotates the head and neck in-line with the chest.

While the patient's body is on its side, an assistant pulls the board toward the patient so that its side is touching the patient's back, and tips it toward the patient at a 30-to 45-degree angle.

11. Used to put a long spineboard in place under the patient. It is a more stable lift since rescuers are in better balance.

    This method requires at least four and preferably five rescuers. The rescuer at the patient's head is the leader who maintains manual stabilization of the head and neck during the procedures and calls out the commands. A rigid collar should be in place. The patient should be supine in the neutral, anatomic position.

    1) Five is the ideal number of rescuers for this lift although it can be done with four. One rescuer is designated as the leader; preferably one who is positioned so that he or she can see the entire scene easily. An additional person is required to slide the long spineboard in place under the patient.

    2) The first rescuer is at the patient's head end, maintaining manual stabilization of the patient's head and neck. A rigid collar should be in place.

    3) Rescuers two and three are on one side of the patient, faced by rescuers four and five on the other, opposite side. The rescuers kneel close to the patient's body, with their knees 8-12 inches apart.

    4) Each rescuer butts the head against the shoulder of his or her opposite number (Fig. 14.6a). The rescuers' arms should hang freely.

    5) Rescuers two and four then place their hands at the level of the patient's shoulders and lower chest; rescuers three and five place their hands at the level of the patient's lower abdomen or upper thighs, and legs. Each hand grasps a roll of the patient's clothing directly below the rescuer's shoulders (so that lifting can be straight up).

    6) At a word from the leader, the four rescuers at the patient's sides brace their heads against their opposite partners' shoulders and prepare to lift. At a command, the patient is lifted smoothly a previously agreed upon distance (usually six to twelve inches) (Fig. 14.6b).

    7) An assistant then slides the long spineboard beneath the patient (Fig. 14.6c).

    8) In some cases, the spineboard cannot be brought close enough to the patient, and the patient must be moved a short distance. This can be done by means of a long axis drag or by the direct ground lift and carry.

12. 1) The first rescuer stabilizes the patient's head and neck by placing one hand on each side of the helmet, with the fingers holding the patient's mandible.
    2) The second rescuer prepares to take over stabilization by placing one hand behind the patient's occiput and cupping the other hand under the patient's chin
    3) The first rescuer transfers stabilization to the second rescuer, then removes the helmet strap by unfastening or cutting it, removes eyeglasses if necessary, spreads the sides of the helmet, and eases it off the patient's head
    4) The first rescuer then takes over stabilization from the second rescuer, with one hand on each side of the patient's head in the standard manner.

13. 1) Lay the board on the ground next to the patient. Undo the straps and lay them out of the way.
    2) Apply a rigid collar.
    3) Continue to stabilize the patient's head and neck in the neutral position until the patient is immobilized on the spineboard.
    4) In the case of a child with a large head, pad the board with a folded blanket under the torso area.
    5) Tie or tape the patient's ankles together.
    6) Assess and record motion and sensation below the injury immediately before—and after—transferring the patient to the spineboard.
    7) Transfer the patient to the board using one of the techniques described previously.
    8) To prevent lateral shifting of the legs, place a rolled towel against the outside of each leg (to be included in the strap that immobilizes the legs).
    9) In the case of a child, to prevent lateral shifting of the trunk, place a rolled towel or blanket on each side of the trunk (to be included in the straps that immobilize the trunk).
    10) Pad between the knees, under the backs of the knees, and under the small of the back. While doing this, avoid any unnecessary movement of the patient.
    11) Secure the patient to the board with a suitable strapping technique (see chapter 9). Secure the body before the head.
    12) Using an additional strap, immobilize the patient's upper extremities with the palms against the thighs.
    13) Add additional straps or cravats as necessary to provide adequate immobilization. To prevent axial shifting when going up or down a steep hill, include over-the-shoulder straps and groin straps.
    14) Pad between the back of the head and the board to maintain the head and neck in the neutral position.
    15) Immobilize the head and collared neck with a commercial head immobilizer, or with a rolled towel on each side and straps across the brows and across the rigid collar.

14. Short spineboard: when a patient if found sitting or in a difficult-to-extricate position.
    Standing spineboard: when a patient with a neck or back injury is standing or walking around.

Chapter 14 Scenarios

1. Stabilize the head and neck manually. This is done to maintain spinal integrity and prevent further injury.

2. 1) Probable cervical spine injury, minor head injury (concussion).
    2) Head plant is a significant mechanism of injury. Initial appearance, patient reports positive sign of pain in neck immediately following injury, the tingling when trying to sit up. Assessment confirms tingling.
    3) Protective ski gear will suffice as there is no presence of anticipation of body fluids.
    4) Yes, administer high flow (15 lpm), high concentration oxygen (partial rebreather)
    5) Assessment, spinal precautions, treat for shock, oxygen, cervical collar, spineboard with full immobilization, transportation.
    6) Problems to be anticipated stem from not immobilizing and further damage. If pressure is not relieved, possible respiratory compromise.
    7) Full body immobilization, quick (not scoop and run) transportation to base facility, ambulance transportation to hospital.

3. 1) Indications of a head injury, minor concussion, and injury to the upper back and neck. The patient may have "cleaned his clock," but more serious injury must be considered.
    2) Factors include the event, skier in the air, and a hard landing on his upper back and or the back of his head. The evidence that the patient was initially unresponsive is important and needs to be elicited from bystanders if not observed. The history and interview adds to your conclusions. Body survey will confirm complaints of pain on palpation in the upper back area.
    3) Gloves for assessment process.
    4) Oxygen is appropriate, flow rate 15 lpm, high concentration via nonrebreather mask.
    5) Manually guard cervical spine upon arrival. Urgent survey. Simultaneously interview bystanders, have partner do it if possible. Rigid collar. Mechanical immobilization on a spineboard. Reevaluate neurological condition in extremities. Oxygen administration upon equipment arrival. Load into a toboggan. Transportation to an aid facility.
    6) Patient may lapse into full unresponsiveness with corresponding airway management issues, patient's breathing may become less consistent. Shock.
    7) Transport patient head uphill in toboggan to aid facility. EMS transport to hospital
    8) Area incident/accident report with witness statements noted to confirm history.

CHAPTER 15 STUDY QUESTIONS

1. D. Inhalation

2. Open Chest Wounds — Any penetration of the chest wall—by an object, e.g. ice axes, ski pole tips, tree branches, knives, or because of high velocity, e.g., bullets

    Closed Chest Wounds — Compression ("blunt") trauma—When a skier collides with a fixed object such as a tree or other object

3. The underlying injuries to lungs, heart, and/or blood vessels and the resulting interference with respiratory and circulatory system function

4. 1) Pain at the injury site
    2) Respiratory distress
    3) Cough
    4) Failure of normal chest wall motion
    5) Shock
    6) Coughing up blood
    7) Cyanosis
    8) Open wound
    9) Deviation of trachea to one side
    10) Subcutaneous emphysema
    11) Myocardial contusion

5. Flail chest

6. 1) First Impression: What happened? Determine mechanism of injury. Initiate BSI.
    2) Urgent survey:
       - airway, breathing, circulation, bleeding. Basic life support techniques as required. Rescue breathing, CPR, control of bleeding.
       - If chest injury is suspected or pulse or breathing abnormal, assess neck and chest.
       - Obtain trauma history and confirm MOI. Conducts focused body survey, provides care for chief complain.
       - Performs rapid body survey, SAMPLE history, interventions and rapid transport
    3) Nonurgent survey: vital signs, history, and whole body survey.
    4) Ongoing survey: Record and monitor vital signs and patient's condition at regular intervals.

7. **Rib Fractures**   Caused by falls and collisions. Very painful; pain typically increases when breathing and coughing. Patient usually prefers to sit up.

   Penetrating Injuries   Caused by penetrating object generally injuring heart, lungs, and blood vessels. Can cause air and/or blood to leak into the pleural cavity. Patient complains of pain, is always short of breath, usually prefers to sit up, and may be cyanotic. May cough up blood.

   Compression   Caused by sudden, massive, crushing injury. Swelling and cyanosis of the upper body; distension of neck veins and bulging of eyes; shock; severe respiratory distress; and cyanosis.

   Injuries to Back of Chest   Trauma effecting lungs and kidneys. Pain in back of chest.

   Pneumothorax   Caused by internal spontaneous rupture, penetrating wound or laceration by sharp ends of broken rib. Condition includes pain, respiratory distress, and decreased motion of the affected side of the chest during breathing.

   Tension Pneumothorax   Serious complication of pneumothorax. Severe, rapidly progressive respiratory distress; a weak, rapid pulse; falling blood pressure; bulging of the chest wall tissues between the ribs and above the clavicles on the involved side; engorgement of the neck veins; deviation of the trachea to the opposite side; and cyanosis.

   Hemothorax   Caused by bleeding from vessels in the lung or chest wall that have been damaged by a closed or open chest injury. Similar to pneumothorax except that significant blood loss into the pleural space may cause shock.

   Subcutaneous Emphysema   Injury to air-containing parts of respiratory tract in chest and neck allowing air to escape into tissues. Crackling sensation under the skin. Other signs are those of the underlying injury.

   Myocardial Contusion   Blunt injury to chest involving heart and lungs. Fast or irregular heartbeat. May cause heart failure or shock.

   Pericardial Tamponade   Accumulation of fluid around the heart interfering with heart's ability to relax between contractions. Weak, fast pulse, falling blood pressure, and progressive decrease in the difference between systolic and diastolic pressure. Neck veins engorge and the face swells.

   Injury to the Great Vessels   Crushing or penetrating chest injuries lacerating vessel walls or fracturing entire vessels. Usually rapidly fatal due to massive bleeding.

8. 1) Open and maintain the upper airway
   2) Give rescue breathing, if needed
   3) Give oxygen in high concentration
   4) Allow patient to sit up if he or she prefers to do so
   5) Cover a sucking chest wound with an airtight dressing.
   6) Stabilize a flail chest
   7) Control external bleeding
   8) Stabilize an impaled object in place
   9) Monitor vital signs
   10) Splint simple rib fractures for comfort
   11) Transport immediately

9. Out

10. Lift a corner of the dressing and pull the sides of the wound apart to see if air whistles out

11. C. Stabilizing the impaled object in place

12. B. Pneumothorax

13. D. Pericardium

Chapter 15 Scenarios

1. Tension pneumothorax. Emergency care includes calling for transportation immediately, opening and maintaining the airway, and giving high flow oxygen. Be prepared to assist in breathing. Perform a rapid body survey and care for any other injuries. Obtain a SAMPLE history. Perform the nonurgent survey once inside and monitor vitals, especially airway and breathing.

2. 1) Initial assessment suggests an open chest injury with poor vital signs, urgent transportation needs and a difficult extrication scene.
   2) Patient apparently hit something in the brush causing the chest injury. Patient's speed suggests continued movement after injury. Although no physical evidence indicates spine injury, mechanism of injury prevents it from being ruled out. Bystanders may provide additional clues and can be of assistance when initially stabilizing patient. The patient's worsening condition is most probably due to a tension pneumothorax building up. Unless ALS intervention is available on scene, the patient must be rapidly transported to a physician or hospital.
   3) Gloves during assessment process.
   4) Oxygen at high concentration is an essential part of treatment. The earlier the better. High liter flow (15 lpm) with a nonrebreather mask is indicated.
   5) Rapid transportation is the first priority. Following assessment, the patient needs spinal packaging and oxygen immediately upon arrival of equipment. Use bystanders to assist you in stabilizing patient and possibly begin extrication until other patrollers arrive. Manual stabilization, rigid collar and spineboard. High concentration oxygen. Transportation head uphill to physician or hospital. Physician intervention is appropriate if available.
   6) Patient condition worsens, breathing becomes more labored, slow, and may need to be manually assisted.
   7) Rapid but stable transportation is essential, patient transported head uphill with a patroller monitoring constantly.
   8) Area accident report and an area incident report if required by policy for the race event, accident investigation by area policy.

3. 1) Assume head and neck injuries, closed flail chest.
   2) Cyanosis, unresponsiveness, chest compromise, and respiratory distress.
   3) Give high flow (15 lpm) oxygen, rescue breathing may be necessary.
   4) Oral airway, oxygen, stabilize head and neck. Immobilize on a spineboard, stabilize flail chest segment, rapid evacuation off the mountain, immediate transport to hospital facility.
   5) Vascular shock; respiratory distress; hypothermia; deficient airway if not maintained; vomiting.
   6) Supine on a spineboard, head uphill in toboggan, rapid transport to hospital.

CHAPTER 16 STUDY QUESTIONS

1. 1) Sharp or high-velocity objects that create an opening
   2) Punctures
   3) Lacerations

2. 1) Compression trauma
   2) Contusions
   3) Lacerations
   4) Ruptures
   5) Shear injuries

3. 1) Stomach
   2) Intestines
   3) Gallbladder

4. Contents of liquid or semisolid material is highly irritating and infectious. It spills into the peritoneal cavity, producing a painful, inflammatory reaction called peritonitis.

5. 1) Liver
   2) Spleen
   3) Kidneys

6. Damage causes severe bleeding. Blood irritates the peritoneum.

7. 1) Abdomen usually becomes rigid and distended
   2) Pulse faster and weaker
   3) Normal bowel sounds disappear as inflammation and infection paralyze intestines
   4) Intestines enlarge and fill with fluid
   5) Hypovolemic shock due to bleeding
   6) Abdominal pain (increased by moving)
   7) Inability to locate pain precisely

8. Fractures of the overlying ribs or adjacent vertebrae

9. 1) Tenderness
   2) Swelling
   3) Ecchymosis
   4) Hypovolemic shock
   5) Usually blood in the urine

10. Lacerated bladder or tear in the urethra

11. Application of a cold pack and temporary stabilization of the groin area with clothing or an athletic-supporter-like garment made of triangular bandages

12. Control bleeding by local pressure. Anchor dressings with a diaper-like arrangement made from triangular bandages or use tight-fitting underpants.

13. 1) First impression: Ask the patient to describe the circumstances of the accident. Note the mechanism of injury: will it produce a significant abdominal or pelvic injury? Initiate BSI.
    2) Urgent survey
       - Give basic life support, as needed. Follow up a rapid and/or weak pulse and/or labored breathing by assessing the neck and chest.
       - Determine the characteristics of the pain. Assess abdomen and pelvis while patient lies supine with knees bent.
       - Inspect and palpate for open wounds, bleeding, bruises, swelling, tenderness, muscle rigidity, and abdominal distention.
       - Obtain trauma history and confirm MOI
       - Conduct focused body survey. Treat any wounds found.
       - Anticipate nausea and vomiting.
       - Transport off hill
    3) Nonurgent survey
       - Perform whole body survey. Assess remainder of body.
       - Collect any voided urine and inspect for blood.
       - Reassess and record the vital signs at regular intervals.
    4) Ongoing survey: Record and monitor vital signs and patient's condition at regular intervals.

14. Universal dressing or several layers of sterile compresses moistened with sterile physiological saline or with the cleanest water available to which one-half teaspoonful of salt has been added per quart. Cover this with a layer of clean (preferably sterile) airtight materials (such as Vaseline gauze, foil, plastic wrap, or a plastic bag) to keep the organs from drying out.

15. 1) Keep the patient warm and recumbent in the position of greatest comfort.
    2) Control external bleeding by direct pressure.
    3) Give nothing by mouth.
    4) Maintain the airway. Manage vomiting, using suction if necessary. Assist ventilation as needed.
    5) Bandage wounds.
    6) Protect eviscerated organs with a sterile, moist occlusive dressing.
    7) Stabilize an impaled object in place.
    8) Monitor and record vital signs, change in location or character of pain, amount of distention, vomiting, description of vomitus, amount and description of urine, and any other changes.
    9) Anticipate and treat shock.
    10) Use the PASG if possible to treat intra-abdominal or pelvic bleeding and stabilize a fractured pelvis.
    11) Immobilize patient with fractured pelvis on a long spineboard
    12) Transport to a hospital.

16. A. Treat the patient for shock and rapidly transport to medical care

Chapter 16 Scenarios

1. Suspect an acute abdomen problem, possibly an appendicitis. Emergency care includes: initiate BSI precautions, determine what happened, perform the urgent survey. Perform a SAMPLE history, anticipate vomiting. Transport in a position of comfort (semiprone with knee bent up). Request an ambulance if she does not have anyone she is with to take her to the hospital immediately.

2. 1) Blunt trauma to abdomen, possible ruptured spleen as area of impact is immediate to spleen.
   2) The point of impact on the snow gun is the principle evidence along with assessment findings and elevated pulse, a detailed examination of abdomen including palpation.
   3) Glove during assessment; be aware of possible vomiting.
   4) Yes. Major internal bleeding indicates need for high flow (15 lpm) and high concentration delivery of oxygen as soon as possible.
   5) This is a "load and go" incident. Transportation is the highest priority—get loaded and move to base facility. Call for oxygen, but do not wait.
   6) Major complication is shock and additional blood loss.
   7) High priority is transport. Get to base, use oxygen if available, but not wait at scene.
   8) This is a case needing full incident investigation including any witness statements and photographs as the situation involves a snow gun.

CHAPTER 17 STUDY QUESTIONS

1. During the urgent survey, obtain a medical (OPQRST) history and conduct a focused body survey of the area of chief complaint. Pursue symptoms of fever, pain, weakness, respiration, distress, and variations of normal function.

2. **Complaints**   **Signs and Symptoms**

   Respiratory infections   Shortness of breath which is due to nasal stuffiness caused by swelling of nasal passages, sneezing, scratchy throat, flu symptoms, earache. Also pneumonia, pleurisy, and bronchitis—lower respiratory tract infections.

Pulmonary edema	Bubbly sounds, wheezes, and rattle heard by unaided ear, shortness of breath, coughs frequently, easier to breathe in a sitting position, produces frothy pink sputum.
Emphysema	Enlarged chest, prolonged exhalations, shortness of breath, coughing and wheezing. Inability to walk very far without supplemental oxygen.
Asthma	Periodic attacks of coughing, wheezing, and dyspnea. Shortness of breath.
Pulmonary embolism	Respiratory distress, cough, spitting up blood, chest pain that worsens with breathing and coughing.
Airway obstruction	Crowing type of stridor. Related to trauma, unresponsiveness, or accidental inhalation of small foreign bodies or food.
Malignant disease	Chronic cough, blood in sputum, progressive shortness of breath, weight loss, chronic hoarseness.
Hyperventilation	Increase in rate and depth of breathing caused by altitude, nausea, or emotional reaction. Interference with normal function of muscles and nerves, causing coldness, numbness, tingling of hands, feet and mouth, feeling of lightheadedness and increased shortness of breath.

3. C
   A
   D
   B

4. **General Measures**
   1) Allow the patient to assume the most comfortable position if there is no chance of a spine injury.
   2) Give high-flow oxygen, if available, to any patient with moderate to severe respiratory distress.
   3) Perform the Heimlich maneuver for an adult or a modification of it for an infant or child if there is acute upper-airway obstruction due to a foreign body.
   4) If ventilations appear to be ineffective, i.e., too fast, slow, or shallow, assist ventilation using a pocket mask or bag-valve-mask with supplemental high-flow oxygen (see chapter 6).

5. A. Lung

6. C. Respiratory distress

7. B. Pulmonary edema

8. A. Emphysema

9. 1) First impression: Person appears to have an illness (not an injury). Initiate BSI.
   2) Urgent survey:
      - Introduce self. Ask, "Can I help you? What's the trouble?"
      - Give BLS and otherwise care for any urgent problems discovered. Note signs and symptoms, vital signs.
      - Obtain medical history. Ask patient to describe problem and elaborate. Assess vital signs.
      - Perform a focused body survey, head and neck. Assess the chest.
      - Provide care for chief complaint. Interventions as needed
      - Perform rapid body survey, SAMPLE history, interventions, and rapid transport as needed

3) Nonurgent survey:
- Assess and record LOR and vital signs
- Update SAMPLE history
- Perform whole body survey
- Care for all problems

4) Ongoing survey: Record and monitor vital signs and patient's condition at regular intervals.

10. 1) Position of comfort
    2) Keep warm
    3) Give oxygen
    4) Transport

11. 1) Chest pain with fever and associated with deep breathing
    2) Chest pain with fever, shortness of breath, weakness and/or cold sweating
    3) Sub-sternal chest pain, crushing, squeezing, heavy
    4) Chest pain that radiates to neck, jaw, left shoulder, left arm, or both shoulders

12.

Complaint of Pain	Signs and Symptoms
Chest wall	Pain on breathing, pain on use of upper extremity, point tenderness
Due to heart disease	Angina pectoris, or myocardial infarction [identify specific signs]
Due to respiratory disease	Sore throat, sub-sternal irritation, lateral chest pain, coughing, deep breathing
Due to gastrointestinal distress	Indigestion, burning in nature, sub-sternal location, occasionally radiates to neck or one shoulder, frequently relieved by antacids
Associated with stress and anxiety	Sustained contraction of chest wall, chronic ache, may be accompanied by indigestion

13.

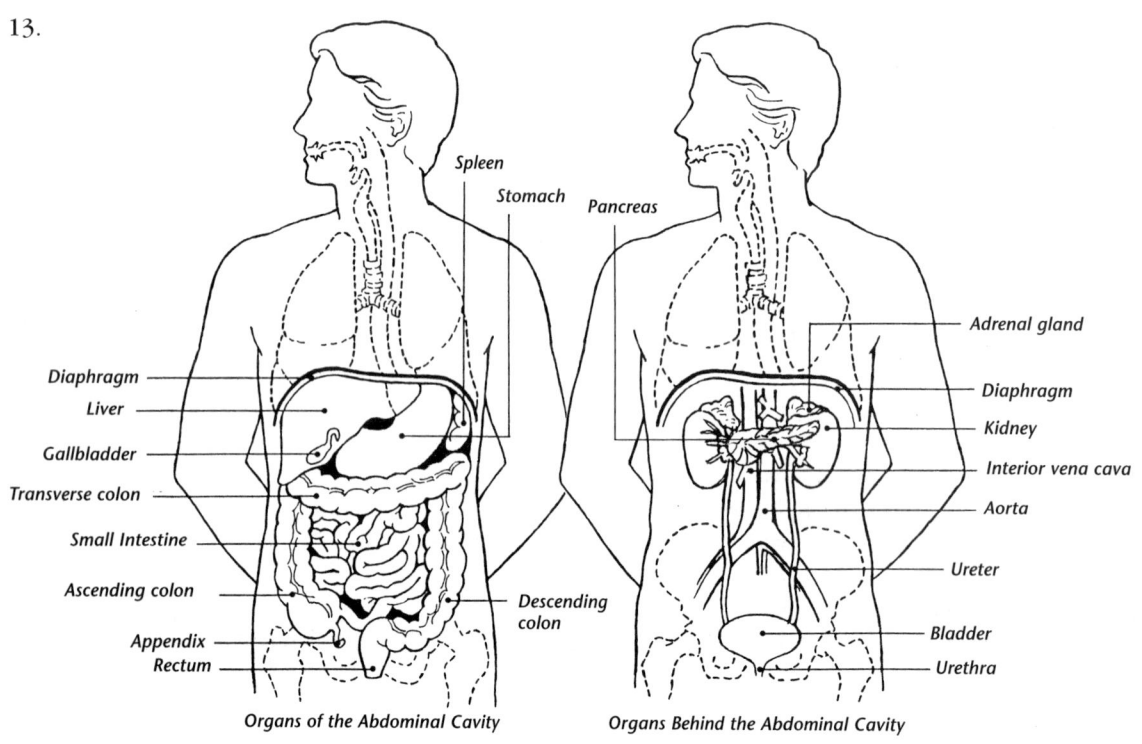

Organs of the Abdominal Cavity   Organs Behind the Abdominal Cavity

14.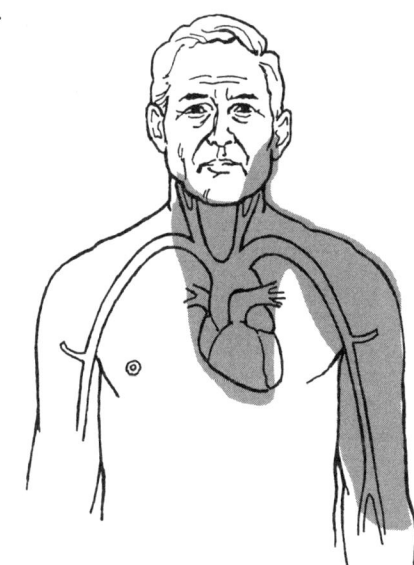

15. | Gastrointestinal Complaint | Signs and Symptoms | Emergency Care |
| --- | --- | --- |
| Indigestion | Heartburn, pain, nausea, vomiting | Antacids |
| Nausea and vomiting | Reaction to stimuli or other effects | Mild: wait a few hours and give water, sweet tea, 7-up
Serious: prevent dehydration, give liquids |
| Diarrhea | Passage of soft or liquid stool, dehydration | Control by diet or non-prescription preparations.
Severe: medical care |
| Blood in stools | Bright red - lower GI tracts
Dark red/brown: serious condition | Evacuate to hospital |
| Colic | Intermittent, severe abdominal pain | Apply heat to abdomen |
| Constipation | Passage of hard, dry stools at less than normal intervals | Eat quantities of cooked fruit and vegetables; increase water intake |
| Difficulty in swallowing | Problem swallowing | See physician |
| Jaundice | Yellow discoloration of skin | See physician promptly |
| Acute abdomen | Pain without diarrhea; fever, tenderness, rigidity of abdominal muscles, nausea, vomiting | Keep patient lying down. Don't give anything by mouth. Monitor vital signs, treat for shock, evacuate to hospital without delay |

Genitourinary Complaints	Signs and Symptoms	Emergency Care
Painful urination	Urination at frequent intervals, occasional blood in urine	Adequate fluid intake, encourage to seek medical attention
Blood in urine	Blood in urine, pain	Seek medical attention
Incontinence	Uncontrolled passage of urine or feces, moderate to severe diarrhea, epileptic seizure, senility, overuse of drugs or alcohol, spinal cord injury, severe illness or injury	Seek medical attention
Inability to urinate	Severe pain, inability to urinate	Allow privacy, position of choice, warm water, running water
Abnormal menstrual flow	Spotting, excessive flow/length	Seek medical attention
Urethral/vaginal discharge	Discomfort, irritation, discoloration/foul smelling discharge	Seek medical attention

Miscellaneous Complaints	Signs and Symptoms	Emergency Care
Vertigo, lightheadedness	Unsteady, whirling sensation, severe nausea/vomiting, lying flat relieves symptoms, sitting up brings dizziness, ringing in ears, lightheadedness	Seek medical attention
Headache	Throbbing, possible nausea, possible abnormal vision	Previous successful remedies (aspirin, etc.) Chronic problems: seek medical attention
Pain in lower back	Pain between fourth and fifth lumber vertebra or fifth lumber vertebra and sacrum, may radiate into one or both buttocks, may involve sciatic nerve, increased by bending, stooping, lifting, and twisting; tenderness/tightening of muscles on either side of lumbo-sacral region	Lying in a knee bent position, non-prescription analgesics, local heat to back, exercises

16. F
 D
 C
 A
 B
 E

17. 1) Keep the patient lying down in the most comfortable position
 2) Do not give the patient anything by mouth. Watch for vomiting. Monitor upper airway.
 3) Monitor vital signs and record any new developments in signs and symptoms
 4) Give high-flow oxygen if available.
 5) If shock occurs, elevate the patient's legs 12 inches
 6) Transport rapidly to a hospital

18. 1) Serial vital signs
    2) Any major events or changes

19. 1) Duration of illness
    2) Time
    3) Manner and circumstances of onset
    4) Getting better or worse
    5) Association with body position
    6) Change in time and location
    7) Constant or intermittent symptoms (weakness, light-headedness, or excessive fatigue, any bleeding)
    8) Has injury or illness happened previously

20. A. Colic

Chapter 17 Scenarios

1. 1) Hyperventilation
   2) Reassuring him and having him breathe into a sack to increase oxygen intake
   3) He may faint

CHAPTER 18 STUDY QUESTIONS

1. A characteristic type of pain that occurs when the heart muscle is temporarily starved for oxygen. It usually appears during physical exertion or emotional stress, when the heart requires more oxygenated blood than the narrowed coronary arteries can deliver.

2. Any sudden episode of a malfunction of the heart

3. Death of a portion of the heart muscle

4. Angina pectoris

5. Patient's head and chest should be raised to counteract shortness of breath. Patient's feet should be elevated about 12 inches from ground to facilitate treatment of shock.

6. 1) Cardiac arrest
   2) Cardiogenic shock
   3) Pulmonary edema

7. Cerebrovascular accidents (strokes)

8. B. On his or her side, with the head and shoulders raised

9. **Signs and Symptoms**
   Heart attack 1) Pain described as squeezing or crushing, or a sensation of pressure
   2) Pain beneath the sternum, typically radiating to the throat, jaw, left shoulder, and left arm
   The pain occasionally radiates to both shoulders, both arms, and the epigastrium
   3) Anxiety and fear of death
   4) Respiratory distress
   5) Pale, cold clammy skin
   6) The pulse can be normal or subnormal
   7) Blood pressure can be normal or abnormal
   8) The patient usually prefers to sit up
   9) Complications: cardiac arrest, cardiogenic shock, and pulmonary edema

Stroke (CVA)
1) Impairment of responsiveness
2) Weakness or paralysis, usually on one side of the body
3) Drooling, difficulty in swallowing, slurred speech
4) Upper airway obstruction may occur
5) The patient's head and eyes may be turned to one side
6) Occasionally, convulsions may occur
7) Headache and dizziness may occur
8) Blood pressure can be normal or high
9) Aphasia

Emergency Care

Heart attack
1) Keep the patient in the most comfortable position
2) Give oxygen in high concentration
3) Calm and reassure the patient
4) Shield the patient from bystanders
5) Watch for complications
6) Monitor and record vital signs
7) Give CPR, if necessary
8) Provide rapid access to an EMS or ACLS team

Stroke (CVA)
1) Give general care for unresponsiveness, as appropriate
2) Maintain the upper airway
3) Use suction, if necessary
4) Give oxygen in high concentration
5) Monitor and record vital signs, particularly the level of responsiveness
6) Keep the patient lying down with the head and upper body slightly elevated Do not use a pillow
7) Avoid casual conversation within the patient's hearing
8) Give nothing by mouth
9) Evacuate the patient to a hospital

10. An AED is a battery-operated device equipped to immediately identify shockable rhythms using two electrodes attached to the patient's chest. This device requires special training, certification, and licensing (in some states) and is an operational decision made by area management.

11. Using a standard toboggan, the "leap frog" technique is recommended. It entails alternating between periods of CPR and periods of transport. Stop CPR only long enough to lift the patient into the toboggan, continuing it until actual transport begins. Stop CPR and run the toboggan for about 30 seconds. Then stop the toboggan, park it across the fall line, and administer one minute of CPR. Repeat this sequence until you reach the bottom of the hill or terrain flat enough that CPR can be administered while the toboggan is moving.

12.

Category	Hypoglycemia	Ketoacidosis
Onset	Rapid	Gradual
Mental Status	Personality changes, confusion, sleepiness, altered responsiveness, or unresponsiveness	Same
Respirations	Usually normal	Rapid, deep
Pulse	Rapid	Rapid, weak

Blood pressure	Normal	Low
Skin	Pale, moist	Flushed, dry, warm
Breath	Normal	Fruity odor
Weakness, fatigue	Weakness	Both
Headache	Frequent	Occasional
Hunger	Yes	No, except by history.
Thirst	No	Severe
Seizures	Not rare	Rare
Shock	Rare	May occur
Abdominal pain	Rare	May occur
Blood glucose (by test strip or glucose meter)	Low (less than 50 mg/dl*)	High (greater than 300 mg/dl)
Treatment:		
General care for unresponsiveness	As needed	As needed
Sugar	Yes—urgent	If in doubt about diagnosis
Response to treatment	Rapid, to sugar	Slow (Observable in hospital)

13. A disease in which a young person is unable to produce any insulin

14. A disease in which a person can produce insulin but not enough for his or her needs

15. A sudden transient alteration of normal brain function

16. 1) Protect the patient from self-injury
    2) Do not restrain the patient
    3) After the seizure is over, open and maintain the airway and give additional care for unresponsiveness, as needed
    4) Assess the patient for injuries
    5) Allow the patient to rest until he or she is fully responsive and functional
    6) Ask about seizure medication
    7) Advise the patient to see a physician if there is no history of seizure
    8) Manage aberrant behavior
    9) Encourage a medical follow-up

17. D. Protect the patient from injury

18. A condition in which, when inhaled, the carbon monoxide combines with the hemoglobin of the red blood cell and makes the cell unable to carry oxygen

19. A. Carbon monoxide

20. When a drug changes a body's physiology so that lack of the substance causes physical illness, and the drug is needed to feel normal

21. **Substance Abuse**

    Signs and Symptoms

    1) Central nervous system depression
    2) Central nervous system stimulation
    3) Changes in the appearance of the eyes
    4) Changes in the nose
    5) Changes in the skin
    6) Psychiatric changes

    Emergency Care

    1) Open and maintain the airway
    2) Give general care for unresponsiveness
    3) Monitor and record vital signs
    4) If breathing is depressed, stimulate the patient and give rescue breathing as necessary
    5) Treat shock if it develops
    6) Calm an agitated patient
    7) Do not leave the patient alone until he or she is turned over to the EMS system
    8) Treat convulsions, if present
    9) Preserve vomitus, bottles, pills, and other drug paraphernalia and send the material to the hospital with the patient

22. A, B
    C
    E
    D

23. C. Narcotics

24. D
    I
    A
    F
    G
    E
    H
    B
    C

Chapter 18 Scenarios

1. Heart attack. Emergency care includes call for transportation (911) immediately. Perform the urgent survey. Obtain a SAMPLE history and assist the patient in taking medication if he takes any such as nitroglycerin. Provide high flow oxygen. Keep the patient calm and in a comfortable position until the ambulance arrives. Monitor vitals closely.

2. Diabetic coma. Emergency care includes call for transportation (911). Perform the urgent survey, looking for a medic alert tag. Obtain a SAMPLE history. Place the patient in a semi-prone position and monitor airway, being prepared to suction. Measure blood sugar if able. Continue to monitor the patient until the ambulance arrives.

3. Stroke. Emergency care includes call for transportation (911), then perform the urgent survey. Perform the ABCs and insert an oral airway. Obtain a SAMPLE history and make sure there are no other injuries. Provide high-flow oxygen and transport to the aid room, keeping the head elevated slightly. Perform a nonurgent survey and obtain vitals. Monitor the patient's ABCs closely until the ambulance arrives.

4. Place the patient in a semi-prone position, call for transport (911), and monitor closely.

5. 1) An acute asthma attack.
   2) The patient's reported activity immediately preceding the event, pertinent past medical history, and assessment result is consistent with an acute asthma attack.
   3) The presence of respiratory secretions suggest that at least gloves are required. Your ski clothing will protect all other areas.
   4) Oxygen should be administered using a low flow (4 lpm) initially. If there is cyanosis or severe respiratory distress, provide high flow oxygen and be prepared to assist ventilation in the event of respiratory arrest.
   5) Get the patient to the most comfortable position for respiratory ease, usually in a sitting position. Transport and maintain in this position, assist the patient using his prescribed inhaler.
   6) Heightened anxiety on the patient's part who cannot breathe, possible respiratory failure from carbon dioxide, narcosis with the use of high flow oxygen.
   7) Maintain the patient in a sitting position and transport to the base facility.

CHAPTER 19 STUDY QUESTIONS

1.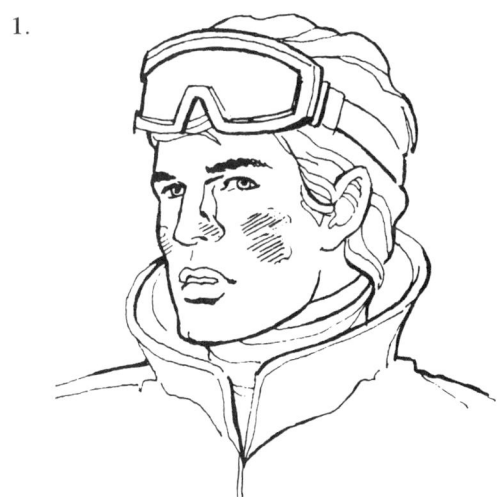

2. 1) Second degree—Blisters form within minutes and enlarge, filled with pink or reddish fluid.
   2) Third degree—Small blisters with reddish blue or purplish fluid. Surrounding skin is red or blue; frostbitten part is cool and numb, stiff.
   3) Fourth degree—Numb, cold, bloodless, white to dark purple in color, quickly develops gangrene.

3. Superficial—only the skin is frozen
   Deep—both skin and underlying tissues are frozen

4. Rapid rewarming in a water bath of 102 to 108 F

5. It may lead to gangrene.

6. B
   A
   C

7. Mild—90°F and above
   Severe—below 90°F

8. Immersion — In cold water. From exposure to cold rain and high wind.

   Field — In healthy individuals in the outdoors—skiers, climbers, hikers, lost hunters. May accompany injuries occurring outdoors in cold weather.

   Urban — In individuals with a physical predisposition, disability, or illness. Has a high mortality rate.

   Submersion — Near drowning in cold water (below 70 degrees F or 21 degrees C), combined with hypoxia.

9. **General Measures:** Stabilize the body temperature by preventing further heat loss
   Mild Hypothermia: Rewarm the patient as safely as possible. Rewarm the body core in advance of the shell if possible
   Severe Hypothermia: Treat the patient gently to avoid precipitating ventricular fibrillation. Stabilize patient, avoid fast rewarming, and treat dehydration

10.

	Signs and Symptoms	**Emergency Care**
Heat Stroke	Hot, flushed skin. Patient may or may not sweat. Rapid pulse that later becomes thready. Variable blood pressure. Confusion, weakness, dizziness, headache. Patient complains of feeling very hot. Later complications—Nervous system: agitation, delirium, stupor, seizures, and coma. Digestive system: nausea, vomiting, diarrhea, and blood in stool. Shock. Abnormal bleeding.	Move the patient to a cool environment. Immediately cool the patient by any available means. Give care for unresponsiveness as needed. Monitor and record vital signs. Give care for shock, as needed. Give care for convulsions, if needed. Give oxygen in high concentration. Transport the patient to a hospital as fast as possible, continuing cooling en route.
Heat Exhaustion	Confusion, restlessness, anxiety. Weakness. Thirst, Cold and clammy skin. Fast and/or thready pulse. Blood pressure may be normal or low. It may drop when the patient sit up. Profuse sweating. Temperature may be normal or slightly elevated.	Move the patient to a cool environment. Keep the patient lying down. If the patient is able to swallow, give him or her mildly salted liquids. If improvement is not rapid, evacuate the patient to a hospital.

11. Fatigue, weakness, headache, and loss of appetite, nausea, vomiting, and shortness of breath on exertion. Patient appears pale and ill, may feel lightheaded, and has edema in ankles and poor urine output.

12.

	HACE	**HAPE**
Early Symptoms	Symptoms of AMS, but worse (headache, nausea and vomiting, insomnia) Ataxia Altered mental status	Cough. Increasing respiratory distress. Mild chest pain. Weakness.
Late Symptoms		Cyanosis. Severe cough with abundant frothy, pink sputum. Rapid pulse, severe respiratory distress. Audible gurgling sounds in the chest.

13. Rapid descent to a lower altitude

14. A. Sitting

15. 1) Recognize the problem and stop further ascent.
    2) Descend rapidly.
    3) Give oxygen in high concentration, if available.
    4) Keep the patient in the most comfortable position. Sitting is preferable.
    5) Treat headache with mild analgesics.
    6) Give care for unresponsiveness, if necessary.

16. Physical sunscreens block sunlight mechanically with opaque greases. They are particularly suitable for small areas such as the nose and lips.
    Chemical sunscreens rely on chemical agents to selectively filter out harmful rays.

17. Apply sunscreen 1 to 2 hours before sun exposure and reapply it several times during the day.

18. C. Sunburn of the conjunctiva

19. An irritation of the skin that resembles a first-degree sunburn. Treat windburn by applying soothing, greasy ointments or lotions.

20. 1) Be aware of possible dangers, especially live wires
    2) Perform a rapid and thorough first impression and urgent survey
    3) Start basic life support rapidly, if indicated. Do not give up on CPR or rescue breathing too soon.
    4) Consider the possibility of a neck and other injuries from a fall.
    5) Give high-flow oxygen
    6) Care for altered responsiveness as needed
    7) Perform the rapid body survey and take care of additional injuries, if present
    8) Transport the patient rapidly to a hospital
    9) Perform the ongoing survey en route.

21. Hypoxia, hypothermia, injuries, and shock

22. Open airway, start rescue breathing. Add insulating materials over and around the patient. Give oxygen in high concentration and flow rate. After ABCs completed, perform focused body survey, manage hypothermia, and treat any fractures or other injuries.

Chapter 19 Scenarios

1. Mechanism of injury: Have to assume a fall into an object that fractures the arm; cold exposure, two plus hours. Objective: Assess and maintain the airway; immobilize and splint the fractured humerus; eliminate or reduce heat loss and stabilize hypothermia. The local rescue objectives should be brought in as much as appropriate. Equipment: items available that are described in the pack and request an additional sleeping bag; oxygen and passive rewarming equipment. Emergency Care: Assess and identify all physical injuries; verify and maintain the airway; reposition the patient to minimize surface contact; immobilize arm; insulate the patient with equipment available; prepare for rapid evacuation; do not try to rewarm externally.

2. 1) Hypothermia; diabetes with mild hypoglycemia
   2) 34 degrees, windy, misty rain, no hat, skiing four hours, hypoglycemic, shivering, tired, poor memory, difficulty with motor skills
   3) Yes, mask at 12 lpm
   4) Administer oral glucose, provide a hat, zip jacket, and blanket. Administer oxygen, then transport and rewarm. Possibly administer warmed IV fluids.
   5) Further disorientation, confusion, unresponsiveness
   6) Prompt transport off hill by toboggan. If stabilization proceeds without difficulty in aid room, no hospital transport necessary.

3. 1) Hypothermia. Could possibly be hypoglycemia.
   2) No hat, rain, wet, fatigued, confusion, shivering, core temp, no breakfast
   3) Oxygen not indicated
   4) Give sugar on hill. Get skier out of cold, provide insulation over and under; remove wet clothing. Gradual rewarming.
   5) None expected if treated.
   6) Emergency transport not necessary.

4. 1) Has acute mountain sickness
   2) Ascent to high altitude, headache, shortness of breath, and nausea
   3) Oxygen if necessary, 1 to 2 lpm
   4) Treat either with descent to a lower altitude or rest and light diet before resumption of skiing.
   5) HACE or HAPE may develop
   6) Transport to lower altitude. No hospital care necessary if symptoms subside.

CHAPTER 20 STUDY QUESTIONS

1. Neonate: birth to 4 weeks
   Infant: 1 to 12 months
   Toddler: 1 to 3 years
   Preschooler: 3 to 5 years

2. - smaller body mass
   - thinner skin
   - a larger ratio of body surface area to mass
   - a larger, heavier head in relation to body size, supported by a relatively weaker neck
   - a relatively larger tongue
   - smaller airway passages
   - a more elastic but weaker skeleton (because ligaments may be stronger than their associated bones)
   - faster heart and breathing rates
   - higher metabolic rates and oxygen requirements
   - less effective control of body temperature
   - the ability to compensate for developing shock to the extent that a drop in blood pressure occurs later than in adults.
   - (in the young infant) a preference for breathing through the nose rather than the mouth

3. Brachial

4. Respiratory arrest or shock

5. Have the parent hold the mask for the child
   Insert oxygen tube in the bottom of a paper cup
   Use blow-by oxygen by holding the end of the tube two inches from the face

6. They have smaller air passages and a larger tongue

7. Anything greater than 2 seconds is considered abnormal, more than 5 seconds is a sign of shock

8. Response to verbal stimuli consists of such things as turning in response to the parent's voice, eye opening, crying, nonverbal noises or calming Grade behavior compared to normal children of the same stage of development

9. They have large heads, increased body surface area in comparison to the body mass, and more labile body temperature control.

10. Obtain as complete a SAMPLE history as possible from patient, parent, or companions; perform a rapid body survey or whole body survey on both responsive and unresponsive patients starting with uninjured areas first and assess painful areas and head last.

11. Strong respiratory efforts tend to retract the sternum and muscles between the ribs rather than expand the chest.

12. High-flow oxygen and rapid transport

13. True

14. Immediately control any external bleeding, administer high-flow oxygen, care for special injuries such as fractures, and rapidly transport the patient to medical care.

15. Fractures (especially greenstick) more common than sprains; internal chest injuries without overlying rib fractures; breathing impeded; injuries to internal organs; head and neck injuries

16. The spineboard must be designed so that the number and location of the strap holes will accommodate the body size of the patient. Padding of 2 to 3 inches must be placed beneath the trunk of the patient to maintain the neutral anatomical position of the head and neck.

17.

SPECIFIC INJURY/ILLNESS	EMERGENCY CARE
Burns	See a physician for all burns. For moderate or critical burns administer high-flow oxygen, assist with breathing, rapidly transport to hospital
Poisoning	Pay attention to LOR, ABCs, obtain detailed history, call poison control center or hospital ER
Drowning	Remove from water, give basic life support, add high-flow oxygen as soon as possible, remove wet clothing, take temperature
Seizures	Help patient lie down in open area away from obstacles. After seizure open and maintain airway as necessary and perform urgent survey
Hyperthermia	Rapidly cool the patient by whatever means are available and immediately transport to medical care
Hypothermia	Stabilize the body temperature by preventing further heat loss. Rewarm the patient as safely as possible. Rewarm the body core in advance of the shell, if possible. Treat patient gently, give fluids
Severe Infection (Sepsis)	Give high-flow oxygen and rapidly transport to medical care. Do not cool, but remove excess layers of clothing.
Dehydration	Immediately transport to medical care. Administer high-flow oxygen and offer fluids
Child Abuse	Convey suspicions to EMS or other medical personnel who will then contact the proper authorities

Chapter 20 Scenarios

1. Suspect a femur injury, shock, and a possible head injury. Emergency care includes call for transportation (911), then begin the urgent survey. Explain to the father that in order for you to provide the best care for his son, you need his help in remaining calm and accepting what you do. Obtain SAMPLE history from the father. Have the father use his jacket to help keep his son warm and calm. Have the father help stabilize his head and neck until more help arrives since full neck and back precautions will be used. Call for oxygen, toboggan, spineboard, and pediatric traction splint. Apply oxygen, traction splint, and spineboard/collar. Maintain body temperature. Transport and perform a nonurgent survey once inside. Have the father gather equipment and have his vehicle ready to go on to the hospital while you are waiting for the ambulance. Continue to monitor vitals.

2. Younger child: Injuries may include rib fractures or soft tissue injuries to underlying organs. Pain could just be related to emotional state of patient. Emergency care should include splinting if necessary, transport patient in most comfortable position, monitor breathing closely and treat any other injuries.

Older child: Injuries may include sprain or dislocation of shoulder but of greater concern is a possible cervical spine injury. Patroller should check CMS of extremities. Emergency care should include placing patient on a spineboard with a cervical collar, monitor CMS and level of responsiveness closely and transport to a medical facility.

CHAPTER 21 STUDY QUESTIONS

1.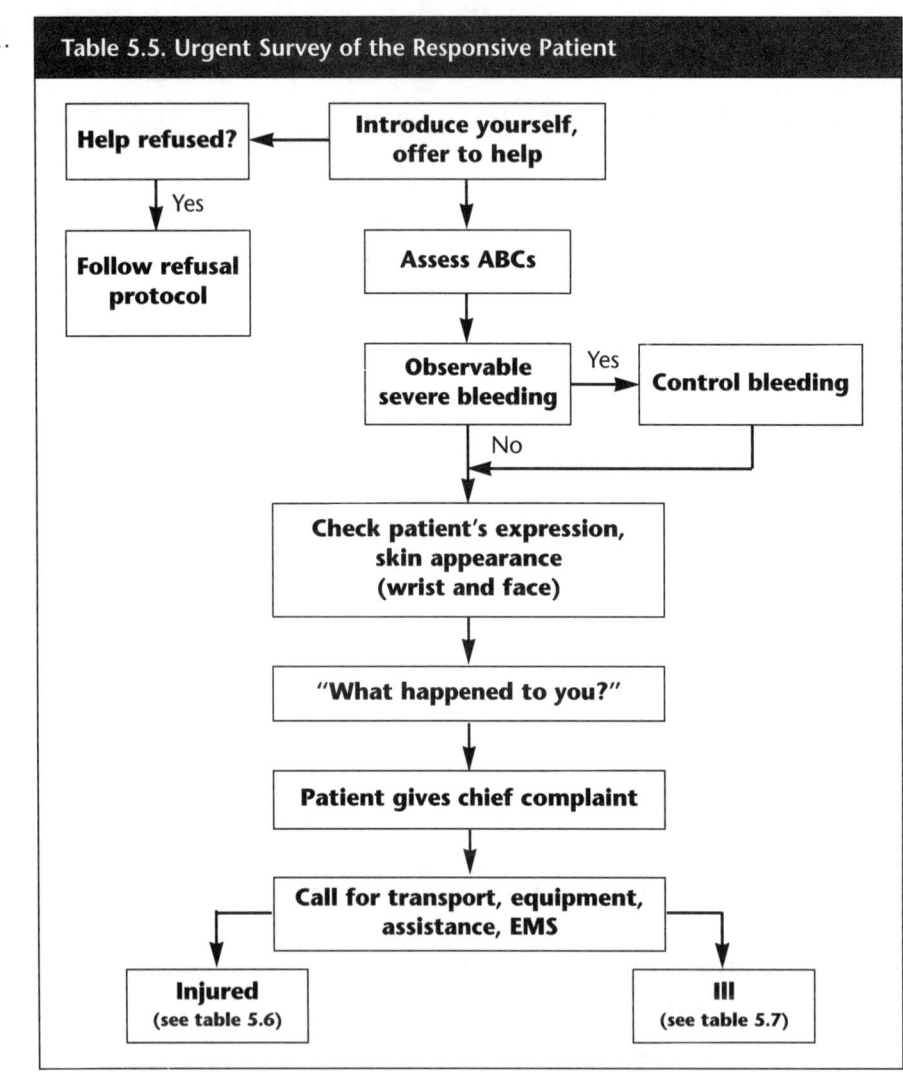

2. Determining whether the patient is injured or has a medical complaint

3.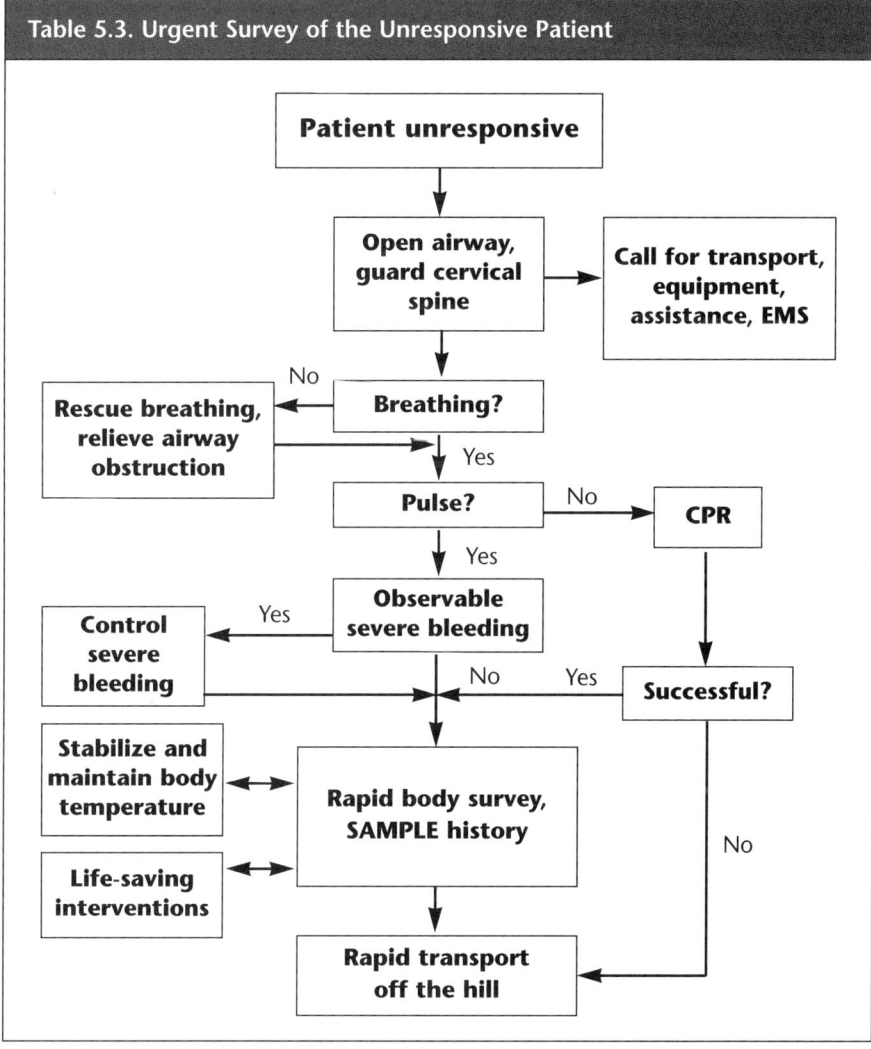

Table 5.3. Urgent Survey of the Unresponsive Patient

4. Determining whether the unresponsiveness is due to injury (trauma) or to an illness (medical)

5.
   1) Head injury, especially with alteration of responsiveness of five minutes or more or an open skull fracture
   2) Unresponsiveness due to any cause
   3) Shock due to any cause
   4) Fracture of the femur, pelvis, or of two or more long bones
   5) Flail chest, sucking chest wound, tension pneumothorax, or any other chest injury with respiratory distress
   6) Any illness with respiratory distress
   7) Cervical spine injury, especially with paralysis, loss of sensation, shock, or labored breathing
   8) Open wound of abdomen
   9) Traumatic amputation of the arm, forearm, thigh, or leg
   10) Crushing injury of abdomen or pelvis, i.e., spleen
   11) Heart attack, especially cardiac arrest
   12) Stroke
   13) Anaphylactic shock
   14) Internal bleeding

6. 1) Major eye injuries
   2) Injury to the blood or nerve supply to an extremity
   3) Crushing injury to an extremity
   4) Hip, knee, or ankle dislocation
   5) Fractures or fracture-dislocations near the elbow or knee
   6) Open fractures
   7) Back injury, especially with weakness, paralysis, or loss of sensation

7. A patient who is unresponsive or has an altered mental status. A potential neurological emergency may exist.

8.

Location of Pulse	Advantages/Disadvantages	Single Blood Pressure Value
Carotid	Always reliable. / Not the first choice for a responsive patient.	Greater than 60mm Hg
Radial	Convenient. / Not reliable in shock or cold environment.	Greater than 80mm Hg
Femoral	Usually measurable. / Difficult to obtain.	Greater than 70mm Hg

9. A measure of skin perfusion, the rate of blood flow through the small skin vessels. Helpful in suspecting early shock.

10. Contusion with swelling, fracture of the nose, facial bones, or jaw.

11. Compare the two sides of the body. Ask, "Can you feel your legs and feet? Do they feel normal, numb, or tingly?" Scrape the skin of the patient's thighs, legs, and feet with a fingernail. Ask separately, "Can you flex and extend your hip, knee, and ankle, and wiggle your toes?"

12. 1) Evidence of lethal injury such as decapitation, severe head injury, massive open wounds of the head, chest, or abdomen; consumption of the body by fire, or a severing injury of the trunk
    2) Careful assessment shows no respirations, pulse, or detectable heartbeat over a period of several minutes
    3) No response to painful stimuli
    4) Widely dilated pupils that do not respond to light
    5) Pale, cool skin, blue lips and nails
    6) Rapidly glassing eyes
    7) Relaxed body sphincters, evacuation of body wastes

13. **...an ill patient complaining of pain**
    Find where it hurts, then get patient to elaborate. Note whether pain changes in response to breathing, coughing, motion, or change in position. Indications may include: common medical emergencies such as chest pain, heart attack, or acute abdomen

    ...an ill patient with a fever or an acute infection
    Find out what part of the body is involved. Indications for upper or lower respiratory infection.

    ...an unresponsive patient with strong pulse at normal rate
    May be due to uncomplicated head trauma or a medical condition such as stroke, drug overdose, or seizure

    ...an unresponsive patient with weak, fast pulse
    Quickly check capillary refill, examine skin, and blood pressure. Probably in shock if the blood pressure is normal or low, the skin perfusion abnormal as shown by delayed capillary refill; the breathing rate increased, and/or the skin cold, pale or blue, and moist. A rising pulse also suggests shock, possible multiple injuries from trauma

    ...a patient with slow pulse
    Environmental (cold) problem, serious head injuries, high spinal cord injuries, and some types of heart disease.

    ...a responsive patient with rapid pulse with normal skin color, moisture, temperature
    Suspect heart problem

    ...a patient with rapid pulse with red, hot skin, elevated temperature
    Significant infection, heat stroke

    ...a patient with high blood pressure
    Chronic hypertension, stress (painful injuries), strenuous exercise, head injury

    ...a patient with normal blood pressure
    Evaluate mechanism of injury, gain other information, think about early stages of shock and possibility of other serious conditions

    ...a patient with low blood pressure
    Heart attack or shock: if accompanies fast and/or weak pulse and rapid respirations

    ...a patient with increased respiratory rate
    Low blood oxygen, disturbance in lung integrity, or respiratory dynamics from fever, hypoxia, lung disease

    ...a patient with decreased respiratory rate
    Hypothermia, severe hypoxia, brain damage due to stroke, increased intra-cranial pressure, head injury, drug overdose, cyanosis, altered mental status

14.

Look	Feel	Listen	Smell
Facial expression	Skin temperature and moisture	Abnormal sounds during breathing or talking such as wheezes, stridor, rhonchi, frequent coughing, hoarseness, weak voice	Alcohol
Skin color and moisture	Tenderness		Fruity order of diabetic ketoacidosis
Open wounds, bleeding, impaled objects, exposed external organs	Enlarged lymph nodes		Urinous odor of kidney failure
Scars	Swellings	Audible bowel sounds	Odor of urine or feces in incontinence
Abnormal discharges	Indentations		
Bruises	Deformities		
Swellings	Crepitus (grinding of bone ends)		
Deformity, asymmetry, abnormal position, abnormal shortening	Subcutaneous emphysema		
	Abdominal masses		
Missing or displaced body parts	Deviated trachea		
	Peripheral pulses		
Abnormality of superficial veins			
Capillary refill time			
Symmetrical chest expansion			
Effort required to breathe			
Abdominal distension			
Movement of extremities			
Medic alert tags/bracelets			
Jewelry on injured extremities			

15. At a minimum, use rubber (latex) gloves, and pocket mask or mouth shield. Local protocols should also be listed.

Chapter 21 Scenarios

1. First impression indicates there is a low level of responsiveness, so call for transportation (911). Perform the urgent survey and determine all the injuries. Because of the LOR, be prepared for the patient to become unresponsive. Prepare for vomiting and monitor the airway. Immobilize the jaw with a cravat while waiting for help/toboggan to arrive. Provide high-flow oxygen and package using full spinal immobilization. Transport to the aid room and perform the nonurgent survey. Monitor vitals until the ambulance arrives.

2. First impression indicates the location may soon be unsafe, so protect yourself and move both patients to a safer location. Problems may include more fire and possibly an explosion. Call for transportation (911), and additional help. Triage the patients starting with the burn patient to make sure clothing is still not burning. Quickly cut away any burning material. Survey the other patient to determine the extent of his injuries. Provide high-flow oxygen for the burn patient and transport him first. As soon as possible get a burn sheet or cool water on his burns. Protect the burns. Monitor both patients until EMS arrives.

3. The mechanism of injury indicates the following possible problems: head injury, neck injury, back injury, leg injury and possibly internal bleeding. Since the area is out of bounds, an investigation with pictures should probably begin. Start BSI precautions and call for transportation (911). Begin the rapid survey to determine the extent of injuries. Control any bleeding. Obtain a SAMPLE history. Stabilize the head and neck. The patient should be extricated with full spinal immobilization. Maintain body heat, provide high-flow oxygen as soon as it arrives. Perform the nonurgent survey once transported to the aid room. Monitor vitals until EMS arrives.

CHAPTER 22 STUDY QUESTIONS

1. Techniques designed to move the patient (without causing further injury to the patient or endangering the rescuers) from the original location to a place where it is more conducive to continue emergency and package the patient for transport.

2. 1) By knocking a rock (or other debris) down onto the patient
   2) Dislodging the patient from a stable position

3. Rescuers with training and experience in this environment

4. 1) Position 1: Supine, with back straight, eyes front, and extremities straight with palms against the sides of the thighs
   2) Position 1a: Supine, but head, neck, back, and extremities can be rotated, bent, or in any position other than in Position 1
   3) Position 2: On the side, but with back straight, eyes front, and extremities straight
   4) Position 2a: On the side, but with head, neck, back, and extremities in any position other than anatomical position
   5) Position 3: Prone, except that the head is usually turned to the side
   6) Position 3a: Prone, with head, neck, back, and extremities in any other than the neutral anatomical position

5. One

6. 1) Head
   2) Shoulders
   3) Hips

7. The leader usually is located at the patient's head or at the site of the most severe injury, maintaining manual stabilization and giving the appropriate signals to the other rescuers.

8. Sideways

9. C. Hips and legs rather than the back

10. Emergency moves are used when there is an immediate need to move the patient whether or not enough help is available. The main danger is aggravating a spine injury.

    Non-emergency moves suggest that the patient should be stabilized before being moved, i.e., urgent survey, urgent care given, fractures splinted, neck and back stabilized, body temperature maintained. Enough help and all equipment is on hand.

11. 1) Immediate danger to the patient or rescuers
    2) Approaching bad weather
    3) Inability to access the patient for care
    4) The need to gain access to other patients with life-threatening injuries
    5) The need to move a patient to a flat, level surface to perform CPR

12. Fireman's Drag—Removing a responsive patient from a low, confined space where there is room for only one rescuer and for removing a patient from a smoke-filled room, since the freshest air is near the floor.

    Fireman's Carry—Removing a patient quickly from a hazardous area when patient is unresponsive or unable to support him or herself by walking or leaning on the rescuer.

    Human Crutch—A person who is responsive and not seriously ill can be assisted in walking to safety.

    Front Cradle—A person who is small and light when spine injury is unlikely.

    Back Carry—One-person carry for a responsive patient without serious injury. Making a sling seat aids the process.

13. 1) Requires 4 to 6 rescuers
    2) First rescuer at the head, rescuers 2, 3, (4, 5) along either side of patient kneeling close to patient
    3) Rescuers 2-5 butt their head against the shoulder (or shoulder-to-shoulder) of the rescuer opposite them
    4) Rescuers place hands under patient alternating with the rescuer across from them
    5) Leader (usually at the head) verifies that all rescuers are ready and then gives the word to lift patient (rescuers use arms only) only high enough to allow sixth rescuer to slide a spineboard under the patient

14. Use if the rescuers must first carry the patient some distance. The rescuers simultaneously stand on command and walk in unison while carrying the patient. The procedure is reversed to lower the patient to the ground or into a litter.

Chapter 22 Scenarios

1. Start BSI precautions and call for transportation (911). Begin the urgent survey to determine the extent of injuries. Call his supervisor to make him aware of what has happened. Also call for additional help to help with the equipment pinning him down. Suspect possible internal bleeding or even a back injury. The patient should be extricated with full spinal immobilization. Maintain body heat, provide high flow oxygen as soon as it arrives. Perform the nonurgent survey once transported to the aid room. Monitor vitals until EMS arrives.

CHAPTER 23 STUDY QUESTIONS

1.

Alpine Skiing	Nordic Skiing	Snowboarding	Monoskiing	Tubing
Soft-tissue injuries	Knee	Ankle	Lacerations	Soft-tissue injuries
Lower leg and knee fractures, sprains	Thumb	Wrist	Ankle injuries	Head and spine injuries
Head, spine, chest, abdominal trauma injuries	Acromioclavicular separations	Knee		Multiple fractures
	Clavicle fractures	Shoulder		
Shoulder injuries	Wrist fractures	Face		
Skier's thumb	Ankle injuries	Head		
ACL	Severe eye injuries	Fracture of lateral projection of talus bone		
	Upper extremity stress fractures	Fractures of vertebrae, sacrum, and femur		
	Skier's toe			

2. Skier's thumb that occurs when a skier tries to break a fall with an outstretched hand while holding onto a ski pole. The thumb is bent back on impact, spraining or fracturing the medial structures of the first thumb joint.

3. Falls and collisions

4. **Rotational**—foot rotates outward and forces the leg outward at the knee (twisting)
   Nonrotational—fall forward tending to bend leg over the front edge of the ski boot (nontwisting)

5. 1) Sprained or ruptured ligaments of the knee or ankle
   2) Sprained or fractured ankle
   3) Fracture of one or both bones of the leg

6. 1) Sprained ankle or knee
   2) Ruptured Achilles tendon
   3) Fractured ankle
   4) Boot-top lower-leg fracture
   5) Sprained hand, wrist, or shoulder
   6) Dislocated shoulder
   7) Fractured clavicle, arm, forearm, or hand

7. Ability, experience, equipment, slope conditions, natural obstacles, speed, physical condition.

8. a) If you fall, stay down
   b) Do not attempt to sit down if you lose control
   c) If in danger of losing balance, bend knees slightly, get hips above knees, and keep your skis together and arms forward
   d) Do not straighten legs completely or move hand backward
   e) Take the Vermont Safety Research ACL Awareness training program

9. a) Ski under control
   b) Avoid the skier below you
   c) Do not obstruct the trail
   d) Yield to others when entering a trail
   e) Use devices to prevent runaway skis
   f) Keep off closed trails

10. To keep the patient's weight from jamming the injured extremity against the end of the toboggan during a downhill ride.

11. **Head downhill**—patients with shock, hypothermia, lower-extremity injuries, and abdominal injuries (unless short of breath)
    Head uphill—patients with injuries to the head, face, neck, chest, and upper extremity, as well as for patients who are short of breath, unresponsive, heart attack suspects, and when the terrain is very steep
    On injured side—patient with unilateral chest injury
    Semiprone or recovery position—patients with nausea and vomiting, and unresponsive patients for nontraumatic reasons

12. Most life-threatening condition

13. Extremities (especially lower), spinal injuries (compression trauma); head and neck trauma; avalanche burial and drowning; overuse injuries

14. Abrasions, contusions, lacerations, fractures, concussions

15.
Commercial Backcountry Toboggans	**Improvised Backcountry Toboggans**
Lighter (than alpine toboggans)	Weaker (than commercial backcountry types)
Smaller (than alpine toboggans)	More difficult to handle in snow
Long front handles	More difficult to pull long distances
	One or more pair of skis held together by a frame or aluminum flashing and plastic
	Handles for ski poles or ropes

Chapter 23 Scenarios

1. A possible ACL injury because the foot rotated in, the weight was on the downhill ski, and she heard her knee pop. Transport head downhill and injury uphill.

2. Assessment:
   First impression: location of patient, bike, or log, level of responsiveness
   Urgent survey: Introduce yourself, obtain permission to treat, ask: "What happened? Where do you have pain? Did you hit your head? Do you have any pain in your neck or back?" Perform the rapid body survey. Survey shoulder, palpate shoulder, neck, back, and possibly head), check CMS distally
   Injuries: Possible shoulder dislocation or fractured clavicle, may have head and neck injuries
   Transportation decision: if head and neck injuries are not indicated, patient may require a ride or may be able to walk out
   Emergency care: Mobilize arm and shoulder, a sling and swathe may splint it in position found, check CMS distally after splinting, transport

CHAPTER 24 STUDY QUESTIONS

1. When there are more patients than rescuers

2. Those for whom what is done will make a difference

3. 3
   2
   4
   1
   3
   2
   1
   3

4. Priority, Handling, Color Code, Description, Examples

Table 24.1. Summary of Triage Categories

Priority	Handling	Color Code	Description	Examples
1	Immediate	Red	1. Hypoxia or shock is present or pending. 2. Survival is likely with rapid care and transport. 3. Care is not time-consuming.	Upper airway obstruction, chest injury, burns with respiratory distress, major bleeding, pericardial tamponade, shock, deteriorating head injuries, altered mental status, medical emergencies
2	Delayed	Yellow	1. Serious injuries are present without hypoxia or shock. 2. Patient is able to wait more than 45 minutes before transport. 3. Patient requires more care than red-priority patients and has less of a chance of survival.	Severe burns without respiratory distress, back or spinal cord injuries, multiple or major fractures, stable abdominal injuries, eye injuries, severe head or chest injuries
3	Hold	Green	1. Injuries are not life-threatening. 2. Patient may be ambulatory. 3. A minimum of emergency care is needed. 4. Patient is able to wait several hours before transport.	Closed fractures, minor burns, psychological problems, localized soft-tissue injuries, uninjured to be accounted for
4	Dead	Black	1. Vital signs are absent or soon to be absent.	Cardiac arrest, respiratory arrest, obvious lethal injuries, obvious death

5. START (Simple Triage and Rapid Treatment) is designed to be used by the first rescuer(s) responding to the incident and rapidly identify salvageable, high-risk patients
   1) Register a first impression and report to your base station so that help can be obtained and resources mobilized
   2) Identify patients with minor injuries who are not at risk
   3) Assess each patient's respiration and provide appropriate salvaging maneuvers
   4) Assess each patient's circulation and provide appropriate salvaging maneuvers
   5) Assess each patient's mental status
   6) Identify those who, for practical purposes, are dead

6. Comparison Between Standard and Triage Assessment

Standard Assessment	Triage Assessment (Survival Scan)
1. A—Open the airway and guard the cervical spine. Ask, "Are you okay?"	1. Open the airway with the jaw-thrust maneuver. Tell the patient not to move his or her head and neck.
2. B—Assess breathing. Give rescue breathing if required.	2. Assess breathing. Do not give rescue breathing. Have a green-priority patient keep the airway open if needed.
3. C—Assess circulation and bleeding. Assess the carotid or radial pulse. Control bleeding if required. Give CPR if necessary.	3. Assess the radial pulse. If it is weak or absent, check for bleeding and elevate the patient's legs 12 inches. Do not give CPR. Have a green-priority patient put direct pressure on a bleeding site if necessary.
4. Conduct an urgent body survey if the patient is unresponsive or critical, otherwise do a focused trauma or illness survey.	4. Assess the patient's mental status. Can he or she follow simple commands?
5. Conduct a nonurgent survey.	5. Conduct further assessment and provide care when time and additional help permit.

7. The average amount of time that elapses before a patient with serious or multiple injuries starts to deteriorate rapidly

8. A. Circulatory
   B. Respiratory
   C. Nervous

Chapter 24 Scenarios

1. #1 in first toboggan on a spineboard; #3 in second toboggan on a spineboard; until toboggans return, remaining patroller should treat #2 and #4 and reassure #5

2. 1) BSI precautions include gloves at a minimum. Consider different gloves for each patient.
   2) This will be a patient-by-patient decision based on assessment and availability. Highest identified need gets oxygen soonest upon its availability.
   3) First impression, resource requests for personnel and equipment, triage assessment of patients, patient care as time permits after triage. Maintain command and assign personnel to most serious injuries as they arrive on the scene. You provide initial care to the three with life-threatening conditions after completing triage. Conduct initial airway maintenance immediately.
   4) Confusion, chaos, public reaction, media, local public safety agencies arriving, lack of immediate resources, you are by yourself for five minutes, stress.
   5) As personnel arrive, assign one individual to coordinate the movement of patients to an intermediate location or directly transfer to EMS as available. Consider staging of ambulances and any helicopters.
   6) Initially use triage tags. Later complete detailed documentation. Obtain same from EMS. Detailed incident report, witness, statements, and other as directed by management.

CHAPTERS 25, 26, 27, AND 28 STUDY QUESTIONS

1. 1) Ingestion
   2) Inhalation
   3) Injection
   4) Absorption through the skin or mucous membranes

2. 1) Inappropriate behavior or disturbances of responsiveness
   2) Suspicious materials
   3) Unusual odors
   4) Convulsions
   5) Shock
   6) Gastrointestinal symptoms
   7) Excessive salivation or perspiration
   8) Abnormal pulse and/or respirations
   9) Dilation or constriction of pupils
   10) Redness, blistering, stains, or burns on the skin
   11) Patient (or witness) reporting having ingested, inhaled, or injected a substance

3. **Summary of Assessment and General Care for Poisoning**
   1) Survey the scene.
   2) Conduct the urgent survey and care for urgent problems. Monitor airway and breathing.
   3) Obtain the SAMPLE history from the patient or witnesses. If you decide that poisoning is possible or likely, try to identify what was taken, in what amount, how, when, and why.
   4) Call EMS for an emergency ambulance.
   5) Call the regional poison control center or hospital emergency department for instructions and provide any recommended additional emergency care.
   6) Save containers, poisonous substances, vomit, etc., and send this material along with the patient to the hospital.
   7) Conduct an ongoing survey, frequently monitoring the patient's airway, breathing, and level of responsiveness.
   8) Provide suction, rescue or assisted breathing, CPR, and treatment for shock and convulsions as needed.
   9) Rapidly transport the patient to a hospital.

4. 1) Remove all watches, rings, and bracelets from an involved extremity before swelling starts
   2) Place a cold pack on the injection site to slow absorption, except in the case of snakebite
   3) Treat subcutaneous and intermuscular (not intravenous) injections with commercial negative pressure device.
   4) Transport to the hospital

5. Circulatory disturbances: heart abnormalities or shock
   Gastrointestinal disturbances: nausea, vomiting, diarrhea, and cramps
   Central nervous system symptoms: convulsions, excitement and hyperactivity or depression, mental confusion, altered mental status and unresponsiveness
   Skin irritation: itching, redness, burning, swelling, blisters, and rash
   Swollen mucus membranes

6. Colorado tick fever, Rocky Mountain spotted fever, Lyme disease, and ehrlichiosis

7. 1) Do not run or walk
    2) Get out of snake's striking distance
    3) Remove jewelry from bitten extremities
    4) Use a commercial negative pressure suction device
    5) Splint the bitten extremity. Assess circulation periodically for problems encountered with swelling
    6) Mark the boundary of swelling with a pen and write the time the mark was made on the skin. Repeat procedure every 15 minutes
    7) Transport patient to emergency department
    8) Treat for shock
    9) Do not make incisions, use tourniquets or constricting bands, apply ice or cold water, or give electric shocks.

8. 1) Stop bleeding by direct pressure
    2) Irrigate the wound thoroughly with clean water or sterile saline solution
    3) Wash the wound thoroughly with soap and water
    4) Soak wound with antiseptic solution
    5) Leave wound open and cover with sterile dressing
    6) Splint large extremity wounds
    7) Transport to emergency department as soon as possible

9. 1) Do not attempt to capture animal. Contact animal control personnel
    2) Avoid being bitten or allowing the animal's saliva to come in contact with non-intact skin
    3) If animal is killed, save the head and ship it on ice to the state health lab for testing
    4) Patients bitten by a confirmed rabid or uncaptured animal should receive rabies vaccination

10. 1) The patient's initial rectal temperature and any subsequent readings
    2) The water temperature
    3) The patient's age
    4) The probable length of submersion
    5) The emergency care that has been given
    6) Any other important factors, e.g., other injuries discovered

11. 1) Turn patient to supine position, guarding neck if indicated
    2) Open and maintain airway
    3) BSI as possible
    4) Give rescue breathing
    5) Remove patient from water on long spineboard or use multiple-rescuer direct lift
    6) Start CPR, if appropriate, as soon as on dry land or suitable firm surface
    7) Give high-flow oxygen
    8) Anticipate vomiting
    9) Take rectal temperature
    10) Transport to hospital as soon as possible

12. First stage   From the onset of regular contractions until the lower end of the uterus—the cervix—is completely stretched open.

    Second stage   From the time the baby starts to leave the uterus until it is completely outside the mother's body.

    Third stage   From the delivery of the baby to the delivery of the placenta.

13. 1) The onset of regular uterine contractions that are 5 minutes or less apart in a woman at or near term.
    2) A sudden gush of fluid from the vagina.
    3) Passage of more than a small amount of bloody mucous.

14. 1) The woman has had one or more previous children and the head is visible during a contraction
    2) The woman is having her first child and the visible part of the head is larger than a fifty-cent piece
    3) Contractions are less than 3 minutes apart and lasting more than 60 seconds, the woman is bearing down hard with each contraction and feels like she needs to move her bowels

15. **Complications of Childbirth**

    Nonbreathing baby
    - Give CPR (Note: do not attempt to resuscitate a baby with strong odor, large blisters, very soft head, or obvious deformities)
    - Take mother and baby to hospital as soon as possible

    Abnormal presentation or prolapsed cord
    - Support the baby's body in the position it is delivered
    - Create an airway for the head if its delivery is delayed
    - Cover a prolapsed umbilical cord with a clean towel moistened with saline. Take mother to hospital without delay in knee-chest position.
    - Keep head away from the prolapsed cord if possible
    - Transport to the hospital.

    Abnormal bleeding
    Before or during the first stage of labor:
    - Immediate transport to the hospital
    - Patient on left side
    - Treat for shock, if necessary

    During the third stage:
    - Treat for shock
    - Give oxygen at high concentration and flow rate
    - Tie and cut the umbilical cord and encourage the mother to breast feed to stimulate the uterus to contract
    - Take soaked pads to the hospital

    Prolonged delivery
    - If there is no progress in delivery signs after 20 minutes, stop what you are doing and take the woman to the hospital

16. B. Cervical vertebrae

17. C. Be performed so that weight is widely distributed over the ice surface

STUDY NOTES

FOUND AN ERROR?

We've done everything to ensure that the
information in this study book is totally correct.
But sometimes errors do occur.
If you find that any of the information
contained in this study book
is inaccurate or out of date,
please let us know about it
so we can correct our files and
ensure that the next edition
is even more accurate.

Take a minute to fill out the
infomation and return to us at:

Education Department
National Ski Patrol
133 South Van Gordon Street, Suite 100
Lakewood, CO 80228-1706

FAX 1-800-222-I SKI

STUDY NOTES

STUDY NOTES